CASE STUDIES

Stahl's Essential Psychopharmacology

Volume 2

CASE STUDIES Stahl's Essential Psychopharmacology

Volume 2

Stephen M. Stahl

University of California at San Diego, CA, USA
University of Cambridge, Cambridge, UK

and

Thomas L. Schwartz

SUNY Upstate Medical University, Syracuse, NY, USA

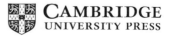

CAMBRIDGE
UNIVERSITY PRESS

CAMBRIDGE
UNIVERSITY PRESS

University Printing House, Cambridge CB2 8BS, United Kingdom

Cambridge University Press is part of the University of Cambridge.

It furthers the University's mission by disseminating knowledge in the pursuit of education, learning and research at the highest international levels of excellence.

www.cambridge.org
Information on this title: www.cambridge.org/9781107607330

© Stephen M. Stahl and Thomas L. Schwartz 2016

First published 2016
6th printing 2021

Printed in Singapore by Markono Print Media Pte Ltd

A catalogue record for this publication is available from the British Library

Library of Congress Cataloguing in Publication data
Stahl, Stephen M., 1951– author. | Schwartz, Thomas L., author.
Case studies : Stahl's essential psychopharmacology / Stephen M. Stahl and Thomas L. Schwartz.
Cambridge, United States : Cambridge University Press, 2016.
LCCN 2015041120 | ISBN 9781107607330 (paperback : volume 2)
LCSH: Mental illness – Chemotherapy – Case studies. | Mental illness – Chemotherapy – Examinations, questions, etc. |
Psychopharmacology – Case studies. | Psychopharmacology – Examinations, questions, etc. | BISAC : MEDICAL / Mental Health.
LCC RC483.S66 2016 | DDC 616.89/18–dc23
LC record available at http://lccn.loc.gov/2015041120

ISBN 978-1-107-60733-0 Paperback

Contents

Introduction

Following on from the success of the launch volume of *Case Studies* in 2011, we are very pleased to present a second collection of new clinical cases. *Stahl's Essential Psychopharmacology* started in 1996 as a textbook (currently in its fourth edition) on how psychotropic drugs work. It expanded to a companion *Prescriber's Guide* in 2005 (currently in its fifth edition) on how to prescribe psychotropic drugs. In 2008, a website was added (**stahlonline.org**) with both of these books available online in combination with several more, including an *Illustrated* series of books covering specialty topics in psychopharmacology. The *Case Studies* shows how to apply the concepts presented in these previous books to real patients in a clinical practice setting.

Why a case book? For practitioners, it is necessary to know the science and application of psychopharmacology – namely, both the mechanism of action of psychotropic drugs and the evidence-based data on how to prescribe them – but this is not sufficient to become a master clinician. Many patients are beyond the data and are excluded from randomized controlled trials. Thus, a true clinical expert also needs to develop the art of psychopharmacology: namely, how to listen, educate, destigmatize, mix psychotherapy with medications, and use intuition to select and combine medications. The art of psychopharmacology is especially important when confronting the frequent situations where there is no evidence on which to base a clinical decision.

What do you do when there is no evidence? The short answer is to combine the science with the art of psychopharmacology. The best way to learn this is probably by seeing individual patients. Here we hope you will join us and peer over our shoulders to observe 30 complex cases from our own clinical practice. Each case is anonymized in identifying details, but incorporates real case outcomes that are not fictionalized. Sometimes more than one case is combined into a single case. Hopefully, you will recognize many of these patients as similar to those you have seen in your own practice (although they will not be exactly the same patient, as the identifying historical details are changed here to comply with disclosure standards, and many patients can look very much like many other patients you know, which is why you may find this teaching approach effective for your clinical practice).

We have presented cases from our clinical practice for many years online (e.g., in the master psychopharmacology program of the Neuroscience Education Institute (NEI) at neiglobal.com) and in live courses (especially at the annual NEI Psychopharmacology Congress). Over the years, we have been fortunate to have many young psychiatrists from our universities, and indeed from all over the world, sit in on our practices to observe these cases, and now we attempt to bring this information to you in the form of a second case book.

The cases are presented in a novel written format in order to follow consultations over time, with different categories of information designated by different background colors and explanatory icons. For those of you familiar with *The Prescriber's Guide*, this layout will be recognizable. Included in the case book, however, are many unique sections as well; for example, presenting what was on the author's mind at various points during the management of the case, and also questions along the way for you to ask yourself in order to develop an action plan. There is a pretest, asked again at the end as a posttest, for those who wish to gain CME credits (go to **neiglobal.com** to answer these questions and obtain credits). Additionally, these cases incorporate ideas from the recent changes in maintenance of certification standards by the American Board of Psychiatry and Neurology for those of you interested in recertification in psychiatry. Thus, there is a section on Performance in Practice (called here "Confessions of a psychopharmacologist"). This is a short section at the end of every case, looking back and seeing what could have been done better in retrospect. Another section of most cases is a short psychopharmacology lesson or tutorial, called the "Two-minute tutorial," with background information, tables, and figures from literature relevant to the case in hand. Shorter cases of only a few pages do not contain the tutes, but get directly to the point, and are called "Lightning rounds." Drugs are listed by their generic and brand names for ease of learning. Indexes are included at the back of the book for your convenience. Lists of icons and abbreviations are provided in the front of the book. Finally, this second collection updates the reader on the newest psychotropic drugs and their uses, and adopts the language of *DSM-V.*

The case-based approach is how this book attempts to complement "evidence-based prescribing" from other books in the *Essential Psychopharmacology* series, plus the literature, with "prescribing-based evidence" derived from empiric experience. It is certainly important to know the data from randomized controlled trials, but after knowing all this information, case-based clinical experience supplements that data. The old saying that applies here is that wisdom is what you learn *after* you know it all; and so, too, for studying cases after seeing the data.

A note of caution: we are not so naïve as to think that there are not potential pitfalls to the centuries-old tradition of case-based teaching. Thus, we think it is a good idea to point some of them out here in order to try to avoid these traps. Do not ignore the "law of small numbers" by basing broad predictions on narrow samples or even a single case.

Do not ignore the fact that if something is easy to recall, particularly when associated with a significant emotional event, we tend to think it happens more often than it does.

Do not forget the recency effect, namely, the tendency to think that something that has just been observed happens more often than it does.

According to editorialists,[1] when moving away from evidence-based medicine to case-based medicine, it is also important to avoid:
– Eloquence or elegance-based medicine
– Vehemence-based medicine
– Providence-based medicine
– Diffidence-based medicine
– Nervousness-based medicine
– Confidence-based medicine

We have been counseled by colleagues and trainees that perhaps the most important pitfall for us to try to avoid in this book is "eminence-based medicine," and to remember specifically that:
– Radiance of gray hair is not proportional to an understanding of the facts
– Eloquence, smoothness of the tongue, and sartorial elegance cannot change reality
– Qualifications and past accomplishments do not signify a privileged access to the truth
– Experts almost always have conflicts of interest
– Clinical acumen is not measured in frequent flier miles

Thus, it is with all humility as practicing psychiatrists that we invite you to walk a mile in our shoes; experience the fascination, the disappointments, the thrills, and the learnings that result from observing cases in the real world.

Dr. Schwartz would like to sincerely thank Stephen Stahl, Rich Davis, Steve Smith, Lou Achille, Richard Marley, and the Neuroscience Education Institute team for training, teaching, mentoring, and emphasizing that learning can be difficult and fun simultaneously.

Stephen M. Stahl, MD, PhD

Thomas L. Schwartz, MD

[1] Isaccs D and Fitzgerald D. Seven alternatives to evidence based medicine. *British Medical Journal 1999; 319:7225.*

CME information

Release/expiration dates

Print monograph released: April, 2016
Electronic books released: May, 2016
CME credit expires: September, 2018

Overview

This book is a series of case studies in psychiatric disorders, all adapted from real practice, that provide a glimpse into what cases look like after the first consultation and over time, living through the treatments that work, the treatments that do not work, the mistakes, and the lessons to be learned.

Target audience

This activity has been developed for prescribers specializing in psychiatry. All other healthcare providers interested in psychopharmacology are welcome for advanced study, especially primary care physicians, nurse practitioners, psychologists, and pharmacists.

Need for this content

Mental disorders are highly prevalent and carry substantial burden that can be alleviated through treatment; unfortunately, many patients with mental disorders do not receive treatment or receive suboptimal treatment. There is a documented gap between evidence-based practice guidelines and actual care in clinical practice for patients with mental illnesses. This gap is due, at least in part, to lack of clinician confidence and knowledge in terms of appropriate usage of the diagnostic and treatment tools available to them. To help address clinician performance deficits with respect to diagnosis and treatment of mental disorders, this book provides education regarding: (1) diagnostic strategies that can aid in the identification and differential diagnosis of patients with psychiatric illness; (2) effective clinical strategies for monitoring and treating psychiatric patients; and (3) new scientific evidence that is most likely to affect clinical practice.

Learning objectives

After completing this book, you should be better able to:
- Diagnose patients presenting with psychiatric symptoms according to best practice standards
- Implement evidence-based psychiatric treatment strategies designed to maximize adherence and patient outcomes
- Integrate novel treatment approaches into clinical practice according to best practice guidelines

- Assess treatment effectiveness and make adjustments as needed to improve patient outcomes

Accreditation and credit designation statements

The Neuroscience Education Institute (NEI) is accredited by the Accreditation Council for Continuing Medical Education (ACCME) to provide continuing medical education for physicians.
The Neuroscience Education Institute designates this enduring material for a maximum of 55.0 *AMA PRA Category 1 Credits™*. Physicians should claim only the credit commensurate with the extent of their participation in the activity.

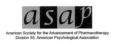

The American Society for the Advancement of Pharmacotherapy (ASAP), Division 55 of the American Psychological Association (APA), is approved by the American Psychological Association to sponsor continuing education for psychologists. The ASAP maintains responsibility for this program and its content.
The American Society for the Advancement of Pharmacotherapy designates this program for 55.0 CE credits for psychologists.
Nurses: for all of your continuing nursing education (CNE) requirements for recertification, the American Nurses Credentialing Center (ANCC) will accept *AMA PRA Category 1 Credits™* from organizations accredited by the ACCME. The content of this activity pertains to pharmacology and is worth 55.0 continuing education hours of pharmacotherapeutics.
Physician assistants: the National Commission on Certification of Physician Assistants (NCCPA) accepts *AMA PRA Category 1 Credits™* from organizations accredited by the American Medical Association (AMA) (providers accredited by the ACCME).
A certificate of participation for completing this activity is available.
Note: the content of this print monograph activity also exists as an electronic book under the same title. If you received CME credit for the electronic book version, you will not be able to receive credit again for completing this print monograph version.

Optional posttest and CME credit instructions (see p. 441)

Peer review

This material has been peer-reviewed by an MD to ensure the scientific accuracy and medical relevance of information presented and its independence from commercial bias. NEI takes responsibility for the content, quality, and scientific integrity of this CME activity.

Disclosures

It is the policy of NEI to ensure balance, independence, objectivity, and scientific rigor in all its educational activities. Therefore, all individuals in a position to influence or control content are required to disclose any financial relationships. Although potential conflicts of interest are identified and resolved prior to the activity being presented, it remains for the participant to determine whether outside interests reflect a possible bias in either the exposition or the conclusions presented.

Disclosed financial relationships with conflicts of interest have been reviewed by the NEI CME Advisory Board Chair and resolved.

Authors/developers

Thomas L. Schwartz, MD

Professor and Vice Chair, Department of Psychiatry, SUNY Upstate Medical University, Syracuse, NY

No financial relationships to disclose.

Stephen M. Stahl, MD, PhD

Adjunct Professor, Department of Psychiatry, University of California, San Diego School of Medicine, San Diego, CA

Honorary Visiting Senior Fellow, University of Cambridge, Cambridge, UK

Director of Pharmacotherapy, California Department of State Hospitals, Sacramento, CA

Grant/research: Alkermes, Clintara, Forest, Forum, Genomind, JayMac, Jazz, Lilly, Merck, Novartis, Otsuka America, Pamlab, Pfizer, Servier, Shire, Sprout, Sunovion, Sunovion UK, Takeda, Teva, Tonix

Consultant/advisor: Acadia, BioMarin, Forum/EnVivo, Jazz, Orexigen, Otsuka America, Pamlab, Servier, Shire, Sprout, Taisho, Takeda, Trius

Speakers Bureau: Forum, Servier, Sunovion UK, Takeda

Board Members: BioMarin, Forum/EnVivo, Genomind, Lundbeck, Otsuka America, RCT Logic, Shire

Meghan Grady (posttest questions author)

Director, Content Development, Neuroscience Education Institute, Carlsbad, CA

No financial relationships to disclose.

The **peer reviewer** has no financial relationships to disclose.

Disclosure of off-label use

This educational activity may include discussion of unlabeled and/or investigational uses of agents that are currently not labeled for such use by the Food and Drug Administration (FDA). Please consult the product prescribing information for full disclosure of labeled uses.

Disclaimer

Participants have an implied responsibility to use the newly acquired information from this activity to enhance patient outcomes and their own professional development. The information presented in this educational activity is not meant to serve as a guideline for patient management. Any procedures, medications, or other courses of diagnosis or treatment discussed or suggested in this educational activity should not be used by clinicians without evaluation of their patients' conditions and possible contraindications or dangers in use, review of any applicable manufacturer's product information, and comparison with recommendations of other authorities. Primary references and full prescribing information should be consulted.

Cultural and linguistic competency

A variety of resources addressing cultural and linguistic competency can be found at this link: **nei.global/CMEregs**

Provider

Provided by the Neuroscience Education Institute.
Additionally provided by the American Society for the Advancement of Pharmacotherapy.

Support

This activity is supported solely by the provider, Neuroscience Education Institute.

List of icons

Icon	Description
	Pre- and posttest self-assessment question; question
	Patient evaluation on intake; Patient evaluation on initial visit
	Psychiatric history
	Social and personal history
	Medical history
	Family history
	Medication history
	Current medications

	Psychotherapy history; psychotherapy moment
	Mechanism of action moment
	Attending physician's mental notes
	Further investigation
	Case outcome; use of outcome measures
	Case debrief
	Take-home points
	Performance in practice: confessions of a psychopharmacologist
	Tips and pearls
	Two-minute tutorial

Abbreviations

5-HT	serotonin	CACNA1C	calcium channel, voltage-dependent, L-type, alpha 1c subunit
5-HT1A, -2A, -2C, -7, etc.	serotonin (receptors)		
AA	Alcoholics Anonymous	CAD	coronary artery disease
AAPA	American Academy of Physician Assistants	CAM	complementary alternative medicine
AAWG	antipsychotic-associated weight gain	CBT	cognitive behavioral therapy
ACC	anterior cingulate cortex	CIDP	chronic inflammatory demyelinating polyneuropathy
ADHD	attention deficit hyperactivity disorder		
AIMS	Abnormal Involuntary Movement Scale	CIT	combination-initiation-treatment
AMA	American Medical Association	CME	continuing medical education
AN	anorexia nervosa	CNE	continuing nursing education
ANCC	American Nurses Credentialing Center	CNS	central nervous system
		COMT	catechol-O-methyltransferase
APA	American Psychological/ Psychiatric Association	COPD	chronic obstructive pulmonary disease
ASAP	American Society for the Advancement of Pharmacotherapy	CPAP	central positive airway pressure
ASD	autism spectrum disorder	CRSD	circadian rhythm sleep disorder
AUD	alcohol use disorder		
BMI	body mass index	CSF	cerebrospinal fluid
BN	bulimia nervosa	CT	computerized tomography
BPDO	borderline personality disorder	D2	dopamine-2 receptor
		D3	dopamine-3 receptor
BZ	benzodiazepine	DA	dopamine
BZRA	benzodiazepine receptor agonist	DAT	dopamine transporter
		DBS	deep brain stimulation

DBT	dialectical behavior therapy	HTN	hypertension
		IBS	irritable bowel syndrome
DDP	dynamic deconstructive psychotherapy	IDS	Inventory of Depressive Symptomatology
DED	depression–executive dysfunction syndrome	IOR	ideas of reference
		IPT	interpersonal psychotherapy
DID	dissociative identity disorder	LAT	lateral hypothalamus
DLPFC	dorsolateral prefrontal cortex	LC	locus coeruleus
DM2	diabetes type II	MAOI	monoamine oxidase inhibitor
DR	dorsal raphe	MDD	major depressive disorder
DRD2	D2 receptor gene	MDE	major depressive episode
DRI	dopamine reuptake inhibitor	MDQ	Mood Disorder Questionnaire
ECT	electroconvulsive therapy	M-PPPT	Manualized psychopharm-acopsychotherapy
EEG	electroencephalogram		
EKG	electrocardiogram	MRI	magnetic resonance imaging
EMR	electronic medical record		
EpCS	epidural prefrontal cortical stimulation	MST	magnetic seizure therapy
		MT1	melatonin-1 receptor
EPS	extrapyramidal syndrome	MT2	melatonin-2 receptor
ERP	exposure and response prevention therapy	MT3	melatonin-3 receptor
		MTHFR	methylene tetrahydrafolate reductase
FDA	Food and Drug Administration	NA	Narcotics Anonymous
FM	fibromyalgia	NAC	N-acetyl cysteine
fMRI	functional magnetic resonance imaging	NaSSA	noradrenergic and specific serotonergic antidepressant
GABA	gamma-aminobutyric acid		
GAD	generalized anxiety disorder	NCCPA	National Commission on Certification of Physician Assistants
GERD	gastroesophogeal reflux disease		
		NDRI	norepinephrine–dopamine reuptake inhibitor
GI	gastrointestinal		
GIT	gastrointestinal tract	NE	norepinephrine
HA	histamine	NEI	Neuroscience Education Institute
H1	histamine-1 receptor		

NET	norepinephrine transporter	RAS	reticular activating syndrome
NMS	neuroleptic malignant syndrome	RLS	restless legs syndrome
		SAD	social anxiety disorder
NRI	norepinephrine reuptake inhibitor	SAMe	S-adenosyl methionine
OCD	obsessive compulsive disorder	SARI	serotonin antagonist reuptake inhibitor
		SCN	suprachiasmatic nucleus
ODD	oppositional defiant disorder	SDA	serotonin–dopamamine antagonist
OFC	orbitofrontal cortex	SERT	serotonin transporter
OROS	osmotically controlled-release oral delivery system	SGRI	selective GABA reuptake inhibitor
OSA	obstructive sleep apnea	SJS	Stevens–Johnson syndrome
PAM	positive allosteric modulators	SNRI	serotonin–norepinephrine reuptake inhibitor
PCP	primary care physician	SODAS	spheroidal oral drug absorption system
PD	panic disorder	SPARI	serotonin partial agonist reuptake inhibitor
PDP	psychodynamic psychotherapy	SPMI	severe and persistent mental illness
PDSQ	Psychiatric Diagnostic Screening Questionnaire	SRI	serotonin reuptake inhibitor
PET	positron emission tomography	SSRI	selective serotonin reuptake inhibitor
PHQ-9	Patient Health Questionnaire	SUD	substance use disorder
PMDD	premenstrual dysphoric disorder	TBI	traumatic brain injury
		TCA	tricyclic antidepressant
PME	premenstrual exacerbation	TD	tardive dyskinesia
PMS	premenstrual syndrome	TEN	toxic epidermal necrolysis
PPPT	psychopharmaco-psychotherapy	TMJ	temperomandibular joint
PTSD	post-traumatic stress disorder	TMN	tuberomammillary nucleus
QIDS	quick inventory of depressive symptomatology	TMS	transcranial magnetic stimulation
		TRA	treatment-resistant anxiety

TRD	treatment-resistant depression	VMPFC	ventromedial prefrontal cortex
URI	upper respiratory tract infection	VNS	vagus nerve stimulation
VLPO	ventrolateral preoptic area	VTA	ventral tegmental area

The Case: Achieving remission with medication management augmented with pet therapy

The Question: Do avoidant symptoms respond to medication management?

The Dilemma: Psychotherapy may not alleviate personality traits

Pretest self-assessment question (answer at the end of the case)

Which antidepressant monotherapy most mimics the classic two-drug augmentation strategy where a partial selective serotonin reuptake inhibitor (SSRI) responder has the anxiolytic buspirone (BuSpar) added in an adjunctive manner?

A. Vilazodone (Viibryd)
B. Mirtazapine (Remeron)
C. Aripiprazole (Abilify)
D. Nefazodone (Serzone)
E. Vortioxetine (Brintellix)

Patient evaluation on intake

- 51-year-old woman states that she "doesn't care anymore"
- She has "fought her way off alcohol and out of the housing shelter and people are still not very nice"
- "Alcoholism took away my things" and she "is struggling to get them back"

Psychiatric history

- Patient had been without major psychiatric symptoms until she was in her 30s
- Was gainfully employed as an office manager but began to drink alcohol as stress at work and home mounted
  - Became a daily drinker with clear tolerance to increasing amounts of alcohol, and a failure to fulfill social roles and obligations as a result
  - Lost her job and her family, then became homeless and lived in a shelter
  - Attended Alcoholics Anonymous (AA) and became sober
    - Now, has been sober for at least 10 years
- However, she has not been able to return to gainful employment due to depression and anxiety
  - Works intermittently and volunteers at some local events
  - Prefers to meet and befriend people who will automatically accept her and not reject her
  - Often is very sensitive to criticism

1

- These efforts are often thwarted as the patient frequently becomes dysphoric and isolative, but then blames others for not checking on her, helping her, or caring about her
- This dynamic sets up more depression and anxiety as a result
- She admits to full major depressive disorder (MDD) symptoms
  - She has passive suicidal thoughts only in that she "doesn't care if she were to die in her sleep as she wouldn't mind"
  - Denies guilt/worthlessness symptoms but is often agitated
  - Poor concentration, low energy, and amotivation are evident
  - Mood is constricted and often dysphoric
- Additionally, she "worries about everything" all the time, cannot focus, and is tense
  - Feels she was like this before the alcohol use disorder (AUD) and MDD started
  - These worry symptoms get worse when the MDD escalates
  - Admits that her drinking lowered this type of anxiety effectively
- There is no evidence of psychosis, mania, other anxiety, or other substance use disorder (SUD)
- She has relatively few friends but has strong but tenuous family ties in the region
  - Feels overly criticized, judged, or put down, which causes her to isolate herself more and become depressed

Social and personal history

- Graduated high school and worked successfully as an office manager for many years
- Married and is divorced and single now
- Now is estranged from her grown daughter
- Does not use drugs or alcohol and has been sober for more than 10 years

Medical history

- Osteoporosis with falls and fractures
- Chronic inflammatory demyelinating polyneuropathy (CIDP)
- Essential familial tremor

Family history

- The patient admits a family history of
  - MDD in sister
  - GAD in sister and an aunt
  - AUD throughout extended family

Medication history

- Very few treatments were given with the previous provider, who utilized mostly low-dose selective serotonin reuptake inhibitor (SSRI) antidepressants, and focused more on weekly psychodynamic psychotherapy (PDP) as the treatment of choice with an area therapist
- Currently, perhaps 20% global improvement in intensity and duration of depressive symptoms at most is noted, but still has issues with generalized anxiety disorder (GAD) and avoidant traits after two years of weekly PDP

Psychotherapy history

- Two years of weekly PDP
- Several years of supportive psychotherapy prior
- Regular use of 12-step AA groups
- Small, unsustained responses to these psychotherapeutic interventions outside maintenance of full sobriety are noticed

Patient evaluation on initial visit

- Gradual onset of MDD symptoms after sobriety achieved
- Mounting social stressors regarding finances, housing, and family issues were the likely triggering set of events
- This is associated with a premorbid GAD and avoidant personality traits
  - Patient admits difficulty making and maintaining friendships
  - She will often only approach others if guaranteed of being liked or accepted
  - When stressed or depressed, she will often isolate herself and become interpersonally detached
  - This makes it hard for her to re-engage her friendships, leaving her feeling more alone, abandoned, and angry
    ○ Two years of psychotherapy have only minimally lessened this maladaptive set of traits
- MDD is moderate; she is not suicidal
- She has been compliant with medication management and psychotherapy sessions
  - Reports no current side effects
- She has good insight into her anxious-depressive symptoms but not her avoidant patterns

Current medications

- Sertraline (Zoloft) 100 mg/d (SSRI)

Question

In your clinical experience, do patients with avoidant personality traits or disorder respond to antidepressants?

- Yes
- No
- Sometimes

Attending physician's mental notes: initial evaluation

- This patient has chronic MDD
- When MDD is in remission, she seems to be left with anxiety and avoidant traits
  - These residual symptoms predispose her to more stress and resultant major depressive episodes (MDEs)
- She has not seen full remission of *all* psychiatric symptoms in last 10 years
- She does function relatively well with regard to activities of daily living and has reasonable social support
- Her initial failure currently to a moderate-dose of SSRI is not alarming as only about one-third of patients remit on initial treatment
  - However, she likely has failed with two to three SSRIs now, at varying doses at a multitude of previous providers
- She seems to be failing to respond to a reasonable course of psychotherapy
- She is solidly sober, compliant, verbal, and engaging, which helps her prognosis

Question

Which of the following would be your next step?

- Increase the sertraline (Zoloft) to the full approved dose of 200 mg
- Switch to a non-SSRI as she has failed this antidepressant mechanism of action repeatedly
- Augment the current SSRI with another agent to increase response
- Combine the current SSRI with a second antidepressant to increase response
- Do nothing additionally outside continuing PDP
- Change from a PDP approach to either interpersonal psychotherapy (IPT) or cognitive behavioral psychotherapy (CBT)

Attending physician's mental notes: initial evaluation (continued)

- This patient seems to be on the gold standard approach to treating MDD but being on a few SSRIs in a row makes little sense and likely offers little hope for remission

- Her prognosis seems fair in that she is relatively undertreated with regard to antidepressant trials
  - However, there is concern that her avoidant traits have been addressed for two years with minimal insight and reduction of these behaviors
- She does meet criteria for MDD, GAD, AUD in full sustained remission, and likely, a Cluster C personality disorder

Further investigation

Is there anything else you would especially like to know about this patient?

- What is CIDP and are there any implications in treating her psychiatric symptoms?
  - CIDP is chronic inflammatory demyelinating polyneuropathy, and leads to a common type of damage to nerves outside the brain and spinal cord (peripheral neuropathy)
  - It usually affects both sides of the body equally
  - The cause is an abnormal immune response against peripheral nerves
  - The specific onset triggers vary, but an initial bout of Guillane–Barré syndrome often proceeds CIDP. In many cases, the cause cannot be identified
  - CIDP is often associated with chronic hepatitis, diabetes, HIV, inflammatory bowel disease, systemic lupus erythematosus, lymphoma, and thyrotoxicosis
  - Patients often present with difficulty walking due to weakness, difficulty using arms and hands or legs and feet due to weakness, facial weakness, sensation changes (usually affects feet first, then the arms and hands), numbness or decreased sensation, pain, burning, tingling, or other abnormal sensations
  - As this is not a central nervous system (CNS) disease, depression and anxiety are not often presenting symptoms but may result secondarily due to disability and social dysfunction
  - CIDP outcomes vary
    - The disorder may continue, progressing over the long term, or may have repeated episodes of symptoms
    - Complete recovery is possible, but permanent loss of nerve function is not uncommon

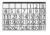

Case outcome: first interim follow-up visit four weeks later

- Insists on continuing psychotherapy as a treatment of choice as she is worried about further medication use and exhibits some hypochondriacal thought processes

- Motivational and educational techniques are utilized to work with the patient regarding accepting medication changes that might better improve her psychiatric symptoms
- Specifically, the serotonin-only SSRI agents are described in layman's terms, and other available antidepressants with different mechanisms of action are also described
- Patient responds well to the analogy that some antibiotics do not clear infections so that another antibiotic with a new mechanism is tried to relieve this type of suffering
- Refuses polypharmacy but does eventually agree to switch from the SSRI monotherapy to a norepinephrine–dopamine reuptake inhibitor (NDRI) monotherapy approach with bupropion-SR (Wellbutrin-SR)
  - This new monotherapy is titrated up to 400 mg/d (200 mg twice a day) ultimately
- Calls prior to her appointment and states that she has no side effects except initial insomnia
  - For this, trazodone (Desyrel) 50 mg at bedtime is started to compensate
    - It is explained to her that it is also an antidepressant that has sedating properties that often improves sleep for patients
    - She feels comfortable with this polypharmacy as the trazodone is not being dosed fully as an antidepressant
- Overall, she has more energy and feels brighter, but still admits to social isolation, some increase in general worries, and feels more tense overall

Question

Would you increase her current medications or change strategies?

- No, the bupropion-SR is already at its highest approved dose. Waiting for clinical effectiveness is warranted
- Perhaps increase the trazodone, despite its risk of sedation, toward 400 mg /d in divided doses to obtain its maximal antidepressant effect instead of its current hypnotic-only effect
- Perhaps add a new SSRI or other serotonergic agent to treat her remaining symptoms
- Perhaps add a benzodiazepine (BZ) anxiolytic agent to treat her remaining symptoms

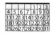

Case outcome: second interim follow-up visit at two months

- Given better rapport and trust, the patient agrees to start an SSRI in addition to her bupropion-SR and trazodone combination
  - Now titrated up to escitalopram (Lexapro) 10 mg/d

- This approach allows the patient to maintain the bupropion-SR NDRI improvements (drive, motivation, energy) and wait for further effectiveness and residual symptom reduction (anxiety, agitation, avoidance)
- Adds serotonin facilitation (in addition to the existing norepineprhine/dopamine facilitation), hopefully to lower remaining anxiety and avoidant traits
- Remembering that SSRIs alone have failed to accomplish this in the past
- Patient now appreciates the need for combining antidepressants in a rational polypharmacy approach as single agents have not garnered her a remission of symptoms in many months
- Sleep improves remarkably and she is tolerating all three agents well
- She is felt to be 30% better

Attending physician's mental notes: interim follow-up visit at three months

- Despite being a little better, the patient is treatment resistant to the SSRI plus NDRI trial
- She is maximized on a combination of antidepressants that produce robust activity via serotonin reuptake inhibitor (SRI), norepinephrine reuptake inhibitor (NRI), and dopamine reuptake inhibitor (DRI) mechanisms. These transporters are all effectively inhibited now
- She has a clinically meaningful partial response but she is not a 50% responder
- As the MDD seems to be lifting, the anxiety and avoidance appear to be more problematic now to the patient
- She is side effect free, which is positive

Question

What would you do next?

- As she is a partial responder, maximizing her SSRI further makes sense
- As she is a partial responder, maximizing her serotonin antagonist reuptake inhibitor (SARI, trazodone) makes sense
- As she is a partial responder, has now failed three to four SSRIs, one NDRI and PDP, and would combine with an evidence-based augmentation agent, i.e., atypical antipsychotic, in addition to the current medications
- Consider adding a BZ anxiolytic to better treat her anxiety symptoms

Attending physician's mental notes: second interim follow-up visit at three months

- As this patient is now more legitimately treatment resistant, continues with comorbid anxiety, personality traits, and has a history of AUD, will want to avoid controlled, or addiction-prone, medications *if possible*
- The SSRI mechanism has been maximized a fair amount over the years, yielding only partial improvements
  - Further attempts with these agents is likely futile
- Utilizing another serotonin-enhancing agent with a different mechanism of action may be helpful

Case outcome: interim follow-up visits through six months

- The patient continues the SSRI, NDRI, and SARI combination strategy as discussed previously, but agreed to be treated further with buspirone (BuSpar), which is approved for GAD and has considerable evidence for adjunctive MDD treatment
  - This drug facilitates serotonin neurotransmission further by providing 5-HT1A receptor partial agonism
  - She is titrated to 30 mg/d
- Each added medication seems to have reduced particular symptoms
  - Bupropion-SR (Wellbutrin-SR) improved energy and motivation with NDRI properties
  - Trazodone (Desyrel) improved sleep with SARI properties
  - Escitalopram (Lexapro) improved some of her generalized anxiety, worry, and restlessness with SSRI properties
  - Buspirone (BuSpar) improved her remaining GAD symptoms and depressive sadness and despondency with 5-HT1A agonism properties
- Continues to engage in avoidant, maladaptive, isolating behaviors when stressed
  - She has clear symptom reduction for many of her psychiatric disorders, but she still has psychosocial disability from her personality traits
  - From a wellness point of view, she is not in remission

Question

What would you do next?

- Escalate her current polypharmacy regimen as most agents here have some room to reach the maximum approved daily dose
- Augment with an antiepileptic such as gabapentin (Neurontin) or pregabalin (Lyrica) to treat her avoidance further
- Augment with an atypical antipsychotic to treat her avoidance further
- Augment with a BZ anxiolytic to treat her avoidance further

- Return to psychotherapy as the treatment of choice for treating personality traits now that her other psychiatric symptoms are greatly reduced

Attending physician's mental notes: interim follow-up visits through 12 months

- Patient is doing very well and perhaps is in remission from GAD and MDD
- Still experiences depressive symptom worsening or experiences increases due to adjustment disorders that nearly tip her back into full MDEs
- Each of these situations are evaluated and processed using IPT techniques such as encouraging affect, clarification, communication analysis, and decision analysis
  - The novelty of this approach seems reasonable and salient to the patient and she makes attempts to use these techniques in her social circles
  - The patient develops some ability to monitor herself and her reactions to others, isolates herself less but still continues with her personality traits to a moderate degree, especially when stress levels are high

Case outcome: interim follow-up visits through 24 months

- The patient is side effect free
- Despite initial misgivings about polypharmacy, there has been gradual improvement and this regimen has not hurt her with any excessive side-effect burden issues, and she is accepting that each additional medication has brought further benefit
- A different psychotherapeutic approach has been helpful to a certain degree, but there is not a remission of her avoidant traits and when activated, these predispose her to depressive relapse
- Weekly IPT sessions are converted to monthly therapy booster sessions to maintain gains
- Neurologist states that the CIDP has lessened but her essential tremor is worsening perhaps due to the CIDP, secondary to her antidepressants, or due to her familial tremor history
- The patient is now alcohol sober for 12 years, and she is started on chlordiazepoxide (Librium) with reasonable reductions in her tremors

Case debrief

- Two-thirds of depressed patients have some degree of treatment-resistant depression (TRD)
- Treatment resistance in this case appeared to be low initially but was complicated by her anxiety, personality, and substance dependence comorbidities

- This is a good example for the use of rational polypharmacy where drugs of different chemical classes and pharmacodynamic mechanisms are added sequentially to combat specific psychiatric symptoms
- This is a good example of how to use rational sequential psychotherapy
  - Each new medication added sequentially appeared to specifically improve certain subsets of MDD and GAD symptomatology and were well documented for every step in the medical record
- In this case, she was maximized on supportive-eclectic psychotherapy, then PDP, then IPT, with modest results. This may be akin to switching aggressively among antidepressant monotherapies
- This is also a good, albeit unfortunate, example of a patient who obtains very good symptom reduction, but does not achieve wellness with regards to gainful employment and interpersonal interactions
- Interestingly, another provider added a BZ anxiolytic to be used as an anti-tremor agent
  - After many years of alcohol sobriety, adding a gamma-aminobutyric acid (GABA)ergic BZ might be considered risky for addiction as alcohol utilizes the same mechanism of action
  - A 10 mg daily dose of escitalopram (Lexapro) and 30 mg of buspirone (BuSpar) daily actually lowered this patient's avoidant traits and helped allow her to move apartments to a better place, reconnect with estranged family members, and seek out people when stressed instead of avoiding them
- Shortly after this, the patient took in a stray one-eyed dog that required a prescription and a letter written to her housing board regarding its therapeutic value
  - Pet therapy might be considered yet another rational sequential psychotherapy endeavor
  - With this intervention, the patient achieved full sustained remission of her symptoms and has not had a recurrence of her psychiatric symptoms in many years
- She did not relapse into drinking or ever misuse the BZ over the next several years

Take-home points

- Many patients do not remit with SSRI treatment
- Switching monotherapies is a reasonable option, but as treatment resistance increases, then rational polypharmacy may be warranted to treat individual residual symptoms
  - CBT is likely the most extensively studied psychotherapy in the treatment of MDD and GAD, but other techniques such as PDP and IPT may also be effective

- Using an adequate dose for an adequate duration of these therapy techniques is important and similar to those utilized for antidepressant dose and duration strategies
- Using too little for too short a time likely will not be effective in treating depression
• Sometimes, personality disorder traits respond to medications

Performance in practice: confessions of a psychopharmacologist

What could have been done better here?
• After two to three years of PDP, should a move to a different psychotherapy have occurred sooner?
• Should one of her initial monotherapy treatments have been maximized instead of going from one drug to several drugs so quickly?
Possible action items for improvement in practice
• Research data for specific manualized psychotherapy approaches for depressive and anxiety disorders
  - Many of these trials use similar approaches methodologically and statistically as do trials studying antidepressant agents
    ○ Seek out providers who can perform these as outcomes validated in the evidence base; may be passed on to the patient
• Many short textbooks are available that review these specific psychotherapy approaches and can offer some techniques that can be utilized in psychopharmacology sessions
• Be aware of your abilities so as to always be providing psychopharmacopsychotherapy (PPPT), as discussed later

Tips and pearls

• When patients have true psychiatric comorbidities, consider a rational polypharmacy approach where additional medications are added that have at least regulatory approval for one of the psychiatric disorders at hand
• In this case, the addition of buspirone and ultimately chlordiazepoxide, two agents approved for GAD but not for MDD is suggestive of this point
• Both of these agents also have lesser supportive evidence in the treatment of MDD and even less for the treatment of personality disorder, but often are helpful in these clinical situations
• Atypical antipsychotics have the pharmacodynamic underpinnings to be reasonable anxiolytics as well
  - But currently have no approvals for GAD or personality disorder, although the evidence base is progressing, especially for quetiapine-XR (senoquel XR) in GAD

– Choosing an atypical antipsychotic in this case may have been effective and warranted, but the evidence base for the utilized treatments may be more medicolegally protective given the anxiety approvals that exist for buspirone and chlordiazepoxide, and likely the patient's pre-existing familial tremor and CIDP may have made her more prone to tardive dyskinesia (TD), extrapyramidal syndrome (EPS), and greater movement disorder burden

Psychotherapy moment

Assume that when you are providing pharmacotherapy that you are also providing psychotherapy. (You can take that pharmaco out of the therapist, but you cannot take the therapist out of the psychopharmacologist.)

Ideally, all psychopharmacologists should be aware of and grounded in solid supportive therapeutic techniques. PPPT may be considered a bare bones way to always stay grounded in the psychotherapeutic aspect of a medication management session.

In an era of psychopharmacolgists being asked to see more patients per hour, it is easy to feel a loss of empathy and to identify patients as numbers, statistics, similar to a busy medical or surgical office approach, where volume of patient care is needed to maximize the business aspect of practice. Alternatively, there may be a shortage of psychiatric care providers; therefore, there is an urgency to see as many patients as possible in a short amount of time. A model of providing manualized PPPT (M-PPPT) might be theorized, modeled, learned, and incorporated into clinical psychopharmacological practice in the same amount of time that it takes to read this psychotherapy section of a psychopharmacology book.

The goal of M-PPPT is to develop a basic psychotherapy treatment for use by busy psychopharmacologists when providing a medication management-only model of care. The psychopharmacologist must be aware and want to maintain the psychotherapeutic stance while in the daily practice of providing psychopharmacology to patients. To be realistic, some psychopharmacologists are burned out, never liked training or providing psychotherapy, or find psychotherapy draining when compared to medication management sessions. Burned-out psychopharmacologists may blame their employer or the insurance companies for creating the mill-like atmosphere of some practices, but some psychopharmacologists use this as a rationalization, because they may not want to admit; (1) they do not want to embrace psychotherapy as a technique, either (a) due to philosophical stance, (b) the sometimes draining nature of psychotherapy, (c) the learning curve of psychotherapy; or (2) the fact that it is often more lucrative to provide a higher volume of shorter medication management visits per day. Given these suppositions or limits, M-PPPT is time limited and concise, enabling psychiatric symptom reduction to be achieved within the course of usual medication management-only sessions. Interventions have an easy learning curve so that these applications may immediately be implemented into the most stoic medications-only approach model of practice.

M-PPPT increases awareness toward the use of "common factors" felt to be universal to most psychotherapies. This simplistic approach is often taught initially in nurse practitioner or psychiatric residency training, or may be used later as a "vocational rehabilitation tool" for the veteran prescriber. Using a checklist approach, a psychopharmacology session may be broken down into sections, and both psychopharmacology and psychotherapy may be employed in unison. It is recommended that at the time of outpatient admission and diagnosis, a few weekly medication *plus* psychotherapy sessions be used with gradual transitioning toward psychopharmacology-only sessions as treatment and response progress. A typical M-PPPT checklist might involve the following:

Psychopharmacology components

- Review previous note prior to session
- Check rating scales prior to session
- Ask about current positive or negative stressors
- Lethality risk assessment
- Review current pivotal target symptoms
- Review medication list
- Review side effects
- Review medical problems
- Check vitals
- Provide informed consent
  - Positive and negative medication effects
  - Rationale for psychotherapy as adjunctive treatment

Psychotherapy

- Provide psychoeducation about diagnosis and medication options
- Provide >3 core psychotherapy skills from the following list:
  - motivation
  - empathy
  - openness
  - collaboration
  - warmth
  - positive regard
  - sincerity
  - corrective experience
  - catharsis
  - establish goals

     – establish time limit
     – establish patient effort needed

Documentation

- Compile note
- Contact collaterals

This basic checklist is a manual. It covers the basic processes of a gold standard medication management visit, but at the same time, it works to orient the psychopharmacologist to stay equally focused upon providing core psychotherapy techniques in session. This type of approach was utilized in every case in the book. Outcomes, both good and bad, discussed in this book are presupposed to be due to psychopharmacologic manipulation, but the reader should be cautioned that psychopharmacology requires a fair amount of psychotherapy to optimize adherence, compliance, response, remission, wellness, and quality of life.

Two-minute tutorial

SSRI ± 5-HT1A partial agonism for treating depression: introduction to vilazodone's mechanism of action and clinical therapeutics

- In this case, one of the rational polypharmacy approaches was to augment the SSRI escitalopram (Lexapro) with the serotonergic anxiolytic buspirone (BuSpar)
- This two-drug approach allows for inhibition of the serotonin transporter (SERT) plus partial agonism of the 5-HT1A receptor
- In this case, these two mechanisms were employed sequentially, not as a combination-initiation-treatment (CIT)
- Vilazodone (Viibryd) and vortioxetine (Brintellix) are some of the most recently approved antidepressants, and combine these two mechanisms in one pill and are effectively CIT
- Vilazodone is in a new class of antidepressants, delineated as a serotonin partial agonist reuptake inhibitor (SPARI) as it is a dual-acting serotonin reuptake inhibitor plus 5-HT1A partial receptor agonist
  - This mechanism of action presumably increases serotonergic neurotransmission
    - Partial agonism properties at *presynaptic* somatodendritic 5-HT1A autoreceptors may theoretically enhance serotonergic activity and contribute to antidepressant actions
    - Partial agonism properties at *postsynaptic* 5-HT1A receptors may theoretically diminish sexual dysfunction caused by serotonin reuptake inhibition
    - Notice for vilazodone, it is active pre- and postsynaptically, which is fairly unique as far as antidepressant treatments are concerned

- ○ Its notable side effects, given its robust serotonergic activity, include:
  - ▪ Nausea, diarrhea, vomiting, insomnia, dizziness
- Dosing therefore has to be titrated to minimize gastrointestinal (GI) side effects
- The usual dose is 40 mg/d
- The drug is available in 10 mg, 20 mg, and 40 mg tablets
- The drug is titrated initially at 10 mg/d; increased to 20 mg/d after one week; increased to 40 mg/d after one more week, and should be taken with food
- Drug–drug interactions are possible as this drug is a substrate for the CYP450 3A4 enzyme system
- Inhibitors of CYP450 3A4, such as nefazodone, fluoxetine, fluvoxamine, and even grapefruit juice, may decrease the clearance of vilazodone and thereby raise its plasma levels
- Dose should be reduced to 20 mg when co-adminstered with these strong CYP3A4 inhibitors
- Inducers of CYP450 3A4, such as carbamazepine, may increase clearance of vilazodone, and thus lower its plasma levels and possibly reduce therapeutic effects
- Alternatively, vortioxetine (Brintellix) could be started. It has fewer GI side effects during titration, and its sexual dysfunction and weight-gain propensity profiles may not be as favorable as vilazodone but are likely safer than SSRI and serotonin–norepinephrine reuptake inhibitor (SNRI) drugs.
- The usual dose is 20 mg/d and need not be taken with food
- The drug is available in 5 mg, 10 mg, and 20 mg tablets
- The drug is titrated initially at 10 mg/d; increased to 20 mg/d after a few weeks if not effective
- The 5 mg dose is used in those who cannot tolerate the 10 mg tablet
- This drug is a CYP450 2D6 substrate and should be used at 10 mg/d maximum in those who are poor metabolizers or who take a 2D6 inhibitor (fluoxetine, paroxetine, bupropion, etc.)
- This drug additionally antagonizes 5-HT3, 5-HT7, 5-HT1B/D receptors whereas buspirone or vilazodone do not

Posttest self-assessment question and answer

Which antidepressant monotherapy most mimics the classic two-drug augmentation strategy where a partial SSRI responder has the anxiolytic buspirone (BuSpar) added in an adjunctive manner?

A. Vilazodone (Viibryd)
B. Mirtazapine (Remeron)
C. Aripiprazole (Abilify)
D. Nefazodone (Serzone)
E. Vortioxetine (Brintellix)

Answer: A
As noted earlier, vilazodone is a SPARI medication that utilizes the two mechanisms in one pill. Vortioxetine does utilize SSRI and 5-HT1A partial agonism but also antagonizes 5-HT1B/D, 5-HT3, and 5-HT7 receptors, making it an incorrect answer as it appears to manipulate more than a buspirone plus SSRI combination would. Mirtazapine is a norepinephrine agonist selective serotonin antagonist and does not use either an SSRI or a 5-HT1A receptor mechanism. Aripiprazole does have a significant 5-HT1A receptor agonism but has no SSRI component. Nefazodone has a weak SSRI component, blocks 5-HT2A receptors, but does not have a 5-HT1A agonist action.

References

1. Shy ME. Peripheral neuropathies. In: Goldman L, Ausiello D, eds. *Cecil Medicine*, 23rd edn. Philadelphia, PA: Saunders Elsevier, 2007; Ch. 446.
2. Fava GA, Ruini C, Rafanelli C. Sequential treatment of mood and anxiety disorders. *J Clin Psychiatry* 2005; 66:1392–400.
3. Hooker SD, Freeman LH, Stewart P. PET therapy research: a historical review. *Holist Nurs Pract* 2002; 16:17–23.
4. Stahl SM. *Stahl's Essential Psychopharmacology: The Prescriber's Guide*, 5th edn. New York, NY: Cambridge University Press, 2014.
5. Schwartz TL, Stormon L, Thase M. Treatment outcomes with acute pharmacotherapy/psychotherapy. In: Schwartz TL, Petersen T, eds. *Depression: Treatment Strategies and Management*. New York, NY: Informa, 2006; Ch. 4.
6. Stahl SM. The 7 habits of highly effective psychopharmacologists: overview. *J Clin Psychiatry* 2000; 61:242–3.
7. Gabbard GO. *Psychodynamic Psychiatry in Clinical Practice: The DSM-IV Edition*. Washington, DC: American Psychiatric Press Inc, 1994.
8. The scientific status of psychotherapies: a new evaluative framework for evidence-based psychosocial interventions. In: David D, Montgomery GH, eds. *New Evaluative Framework for Evidence-Based Psychotherapies*. Hoboken, NJ: American Psychological Association, Wiley Periodicals Inc., 2011; pp. 89–99.
9. Deranja E. When medications fail: using psychotherapy in the psychopharmacology setting. *Clin Neuropsychiatry* 2011; 8:81–94.
10. Bandelow B, Chouinard G, Bobes J, et al. Extended-release quetiapine fumarate (quetiapine XR): a once-daily monotherapy effective in generalized anxiety disorder. Data from a randomized, double-blind, placebo- and active-controlled study. *Int J Neuropsychopharmacol* 2010; 13:305–20.

11. Bogenschutz MP, Nurnberg GH. Olanzapine versus placebo in the treatment of borderline personality disorder. *J Clin Psychiatry* 2004; 65:104–9.

12. Schwartz TL. Integrating psychotherapy and psychopharmacology: outcomes, endophenotypes, and theoretical underpinnings regarding effectiveness. In: Reis de Oliveira I, Schwartz TL, Stahl SM, eds. *Integrating Psychotherapy and Psychopharmacology*. New York, NY: Routledge Press, 2014; Ch. 2.

13. Stahl SM, Moore BA, eds. *Anxiety Disorders: A Concise Guide and Casebook for Psychopharmacology and Psychotherapy Integration*. New York, NY: Routledge Press, 2013.

14. Reis de Oliveira I, Schwartz T, Stahl SM, eds. *Integrating Psychotherapy and Psychopharmacology*. New York, NY: Routledge Press, 2014.

The Case: The luteal, jaw-moving woman with paranoid paneling

The Question: Can premenstrual hormone fluctuations affect established psychiatric symptoms?

The Psychopharmacological dilemma: Finding an effective regimen for recurrent TRD while juggling complex clinical variants and side effects

Pretest self-assessment question (answer at the end of the case)

Which of the following are approved treatments for premenstrual exacerbation (PME) of existing depressive disorders?

A. Fluoxetine
B. Sertraline
C. Desvenlafaxine
D. Bupropion
E. A and B
F. None of the above

Patient evaluation on intake

- 42-year-old woman with a chief complaint of depression

Psychiatric history

- The patient had onset of depression in late teens. These episodes were often limited and likely adjustment disorder episodes
- Depression became more prominent and pervasive and she developed a chronic low-level depression consistent with dysthymia
- Since her late 20s, she has also had full MDD episodes lasting two to 24 weeks in duration, which were at times incapacitating
- Appears at times to have full inter-episode recovery from her depressive symptoms
- Many of the stress-induced depression exacerbations suggest a paranoid personality style noted in her interpersonal interactions
- She also mentions having PMS (premenstrual syndrome) and feels that her symptoms often are worse during her menstrual cycle
- History includes no previous psychiatric hospitalizations, nor any suicide attempts
- A review of psychiatric systems revealed no anxiety disorder, schizophrenia, mania, or substance misuse history
- However, she admitted to experiencing hallucinations (predominantly when depressed) where the wood grain paneling in her house (that resembles eyes and faces) would talk to her

- Her only previous treatment was with fluoxetine (Prozac) up to 40 mg/d, which she reports was intermittently and only partially effective and was discontinued the previous year
- Engagement in sporadic eclectic and supportive psychotherapy is noted

Social and personal history

- Grew up with separated parents
- Had difficulties with grades throughout school
- Ultimately achieved an associate's degree
- Works as an artist and seamstress periodically
- Is married but is estranged at times

Medical history

- Stress urinary incontinence
- Migraines
- Trigeminal neuralgia
- She currently takes trospium, hydrocodone as needed, carbamazepine for these conditions

Family history

- Anxiety disorder in mother
- AUD in father

Current psychiatric medications

- An SNRI, duloxetine (Cymbalta) 120 mg/d, was started and titrated in lieu of fluoxetine (Prozac) by her primary care provider and she states it is for incontinence

Question

Based on what you know about this patient's history and current symptoms, would you consider her to fall within the TRD spectrum?

- Yes
- No

Would you continue the SNRI duloxetine monotherapy?

- Yes, but increase the dose above the approved 120 mg/d
- Yes, but add an augmentation or combination therapy
- No, taper off and try a new monotherapy
- No, taper off and try a new CIT where two antidepressants are started simultaneously

PATIENT FILE

Attending physician's mental notes: initial evaluation

- Nothing unexpected on mental status examination
- Because she has had numerous recurrences, this makes her illness appear to be somewhat unstable; she has not shown any overt signs of bipolarity but does have clear mood lability due to hormonal changes with menses, and also due to social stressors, which are suggestive of mild-moderate personality disorder, as well as somatic illness. She also has unique quasi-psychotic features of auditory and visual illusions verses hallucinations, which may be suggestive of dissociative features or schizotypal traits, not just psychotic depression
- The best diagnosis for this patient may be MDD, recurrent unipolar disorder at this time
- During ongoing care, will need to better assess for personality disorder, premenstrual dysphoric disorder (PMDD), and psychotic disorder
- Continuing duloxetine (Cymbalta) above the 120 mg/d Food and Drug Administration (FDA) limit seems ill-advised as she has had little response to the full dose and has failed a therapeutic selective serotonin reuptake inhibitor (SSRI), fluoxetine (Prozac), in the past. The SSRI and SNRI mechanisms have failed to treat her to remission
- Given her lability and treatment-resistant status, the patient was offered a choice of an atypical antipsychotic to augment her current SNRI

Further investigation

Is there anything else you would especially like to know about this patient?

- What about details concerning the diagnosis of PMDD and of her hallucinations, and about the treatments given and the responses to those treatments for her depression?
- During the past year on her SNRI, she states she is about 30% better and has a less labile affect, but still has most of her MDD symptoms, but to a "lesser degree"
- She has had PMS for many years. Screening for PMDD is positive, but confounded by the fact that she is depressed often, if not routinely, outside of her luteal phase. It appears she is regularly depressed, but during the luteal phase, she becomes more depressed. This is a premenstrual exacerbation (PME) of an existing unipolar MDD. PMEs occur when depressed patients suffer an exacerbation of MDD symptoms during the luteal phase. She has failed to respond to one of the FDA-approved medications for PMDD (fluoxetine [Sarafem]). The other FDA approval is for sertraline (Zoloft)
- During the past year she has also complained of continuing migraines and urinary problems, which are bona fide medical conditions but may also be considered psychosomatic in that her depression likely makes them worse and more complicated to treat

Question

Based on what you know about this patient's history, current symptoms, and treatment responses, are you convinced she has TRD with PMEs?

- Yes
- No

Would you combine her SNRI with an atypical antipsychotic as suggested?

- Yes, but keep the atypical antipsychotic at a low dose for depression treatment
- Yes, increase the atypical antipsychotic to a moderate to high dose to treat her affective lability and psychosis
- No, I'd use a different medication approach altogether

Attending physician's mental notes: initial evaluation (continued)

- The patient is clearly depressed and obviously is worse in her luteal phase. Adding another agent with more serotonergic potential (serotonin [5-HT] receptor modulating agents with 5-HT2A, 5-HT2C, 5-HT1A mechanisms) seems reasonable, as long as informed consent about side effects is given
- Ways to treat her PMEs could be to add buspirone (BuSpar) for its 5-HT1A receptor partial agonism activity. Augment with trazodone (Desyrel, Oleptro) for its 5-HT2A receptor antagonism activity. Change to vilazodone (Viibryd) as it is an SSRI with pre- and postsynaptic 5-HT1A partial agonist properties. Some of the atypical antipsychotics possess some of these serotonergic mechanisms and could be utilized as well
- The mood lability never consists of sustained hypomania, thus bipolarity is ruled out. She clearly has mood lability whether due to PMEs or social stressors. Alternatively, the *DSM-V* now allows the specifier of having *mixed features* even when MDD is the principal diagnosis. In this case, the patient meets full MDD criteria and if she were to have an additional three classic symptoms of (hypo)mania simultaneously, then she would meet this specifier
- The paranoid personality traits become more evident over time and predispose her to stressful interactions
- She does have frank hallucinations when she looks at the grain of her wood paneling in her house. She interacts verbally with them. This occurs predominantly when she is stressed and depressed. They can be mood congruent or incongruent. Culturally she feels it is acceptable as she is interacting with relatives who have passed away

Case outcome: interim follow-ups through six months

- Because of her resistant depression, SSRI and SNRI failure, she was placed on off-label ziprasidone (Geodon) 20 mg twice a day with food (required for adequate absorption and bioavailablity) while continuing her SNRI duloxetine (Cymbalta). She wanted to avoid weight gain, and at the time, no atypical antipsychotic was FDA approved for depression augmentation. Ziprasidone is fairly benign for metabolically induced weight gain (antipsychotic-associated weight gain [AAWG]). It also has theoretical antidepressant potential as it antagonizes 5-HT2A receptors, partially agonizes 5-HT1A receptors, and acts as a weak SNRI pharmacodynamically

- Unfortunately, she experienced akathisia and it was discontinued
- Next, as she was educated about the rationale of the atypical antipsychotic family of medications, she agreed to start aripiprazole (Abilify) as it has similar serotonergic properties. As it also causes akathisia, it was started at 2.5 mg/d and gradually increased over several weeks for effect up to 15 mg/d
- Six months later she was "80%–90% better" and doing well clinically on the SNRI plus atypical antipsychotic combination. She had 10 lbs of AAWG as her only side effect. Blood pressure and metabolic parameters were normal
- As she was doing well, she was advised to continue her medication regimen as it is

Question

Considering her current regimen and its risk/benefit profile, what would you do next?

- Keep the regimen as it is
- Lower the aripiprazole (Abilify) gradually, as she is in remission for a few months and the risk for movement disorders is higher in affective disorder patients, and continue her duloxetine (Cymbalta) alone
- Keep regimen as it is, but add a weight-losing medication such as orlistat (Xenical), topiramate–phentermine combination (Q-Symia), naltrexone–bupropion combination (Contrave), lorcaserin (Belviq), or off-label metformin (Glucophage) to mitigate the AAWG and avoid future metabolic disorder

Attending physician's mental notes: nine months

- The patient, after two decades, is in remission. This SNRI plus atypical antipsychotic combination appears to have treated her recurrent MDD and affective lability
- She still experiences some PMEs but these are less severe and better tolerated than baseline, and she is less labile with regard to social stressors
- The atypical antipsychotics do carry TD and metabolic risks with long-term use

- MDD guidelines would suggest that as she has had three or more MDEs, effective medicines should be continued to prevent future recurrence. She is less than one year in remission
- There is risk for TD and metabolic syndrome and these should be monitored routinely, and informed consent should be given throughout ongoing treatment
- For example, annual AIMS (Abnormal Involuntary Movement Scale) and blood work to detect elevated lipids and blood sugars should be considered
• She experiences rare to absent illusions/hallucinations

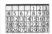

Case outcome: interim follow-ups through nine months

The chief complaint is now PMS that has been mitigated partially so far
• After discussion of these options, the patient wishes to continue her current regimen
• A few months later, her primary care physician (PCP) calls and states the patient has lateral jaw movements and feels she should be seen for this
• Patient arrives and has involuntary, intermittent lateral jaw movements. AIMS examination is positive for new-onset TD

Question

Would you continue her aripiprazole (Abilify) for her TRD?

• Yes
• No

Attending physician's mental notes: nine-month follow-ups

• TD can become permanent, thus discontinuing the atypical antipsychotic makes sense to the clinician and the patient
• The patient is aware that her MDD may recur and that increased visits and monitoring are needed as recurrence rate could be as high as 90% within a year
• To avoid MDD recurrence and withdrawal dyskinesia, the atypical antipsychotic is discontinued over two to three weeks. The jaw movements subside over a few months. She is now diagnosed with temperomandibular joint (TMJ) syndrome as a result of her previously excessive jaw movements
• The PMEs exacerbate, her stress-induced interpersonal issues escalate, but her depression is relatively stable while she is off the atypical antipsychotic and only on the SNRI

Question

If she gradually relapses into MDD, what would you consider?

- Add a formal psychotherapy such as PDP or dialectical behavioral psychotherapy (DBT)
- Add another atypical antipsychotic at risk of recurrent TD
- Try another monotherapy (non-SSRI, non-SNRI) antidepressant approach
- Try another augmentation approach (lithium, buspirone [BuSpar]), mood stabilizer such as gabapentin (Neurontin) or divalproex (Depakote)
- None of these

Attending physician's mental notes: interim follow-up through nine months (continued)

- Lithium
  - Could help to boost her mood and mitigate risk of future relapse
  - If added, may still need to watch for weight gain and lithium toxicity
  - Will need laboratory follow-ups (cell blood count, creatinine, thyroid panel, drug levels, etc.)
- Buspirone (BuSpar)
  - May help boost mood, as this has been an effective augmentation strategy for patients with MDD in some off-label trials and in clinical practice. The aripiprazole (Abilify) utilized a similar 5-HT1A partial receptor agonism so that buspirone may be the closest, non-TD-inducing mechanistic relative to aripiprazole
  - However, it does not have 5-HT2A or dopamine-2 (D2) receptor antagonism
  - Therefore, it may not be as calming, sleep promoting, or mood lability dampening
- Other atypical antipsychotics (quetiapine [Seroquel-XR], lurasidone [Latuda])
  - Another trial is too risky given her recent TD remission, unless other non-TD-inducing treatments fail first
  - Clozapine (Clozaril) could be an option if an antipsychotic is clinically warranted
- Mood stabilizers
  - The epilepsy drugs may be used as mood stabilizers and some can help mood lability in bipolar patients (per the FDA). Off-label data suggests this may help in personality disorders as well. Consider bipolar-approved sodium channel blocking lamotrigine (Lamictal) or carbamazepine (Equetro) or GABAergic divalproex (Depakote) as such. The calcium channel blocking medications gabapentin (Neurontin) and pregabalin (Lyrica) have off-label data suggesting more anxiolytic properties instead of mood stabilization properties

Case outcome and multiple interim follow-ups to 24 months

- The patient was encouraged to add the 5-HT1A receptor partial agonist, buspirone (BuSpar), to her duloxetine (Cymbalta) and it was titrated to 45 mg/d
- This failed and her MDD re-emerged at moderate levels with clear PMEs
- Instead of combining other medications or augmenting her duloxetine (Cymbalta) again, the patient chose to taper off all medications and "start from scratch" as she had lost faith in the duloxetine, which was only marginally effective before the atypical antipsychotic augmentation
- TD has fully resolved
- Other monotherapies are offered, such as an NDRI, bupropion (Wellbutrin-XL), a noradrenergic and specific serotonergic antidepressant (NaSSA), mirtazapine (Remeron), or another SNRI (venlafaxine [Effexor-XR], desvenlafaxine [Pristiq], levomilnacipran [Fetzima])
- The patient was switched from her SNRI plus Buspirone combination onto initial monotherapy with desvenlafaxine (Pristiq), another SNRI
  - This SNRI is utilized as it may have greater norepinephrine transporter (NET) inhibition properties. In other words, it may be a more effective norepineprhine reuptake inhibitor (NRI)
- Titrated initially to 100 mg/d with minimal effect
- Simultaneously, the patient's obstetrician/gynecologist placed her on low-dose diazepam (Valium) 5–10 mg/d as needed as a muscle relaxant given her complaints of PMS to that clinician
- Desvenlafaxine (Pristiq) was raised to 200 mg/d with a solid clinical response and no side effects. Unfortunately, mood lability with PMEs continued despite depression symptoms being remarkably lowered
- It was suggested to take 200 mg/d desvenlafaxine routinely but to raise it to 300 mg/d during her luteal phase PMEs
- This alternating dosing approach plus low-dose BZ was effective and she was maintained on this combination of SNRI plus BZ with very good symptom control (depression, PMEs, personality disorder-related lability, hallucinations)

Case debrief

- The patient has a lengthy history of recurrent MDD, ranging from low levels to full MDEs. They appear unipolar in nature and have been responsive to antidepressant plus augmentation approaches
- This case was difficult in that she did achieve remission for the first time in many years with the addition of an atypical antipsychotic Unfortunately, this class of agents are often effective in the treatment of MDD but carry the risk for TD, which she did develop
- This case was also complicated in that she had PMEs, personality disorder traits, and some somatic symptoms that were difficult to

navigate. However, once the MDD symptoms lessened, these complicating factors also improved

- The clinician tried to pharmacodynamically re-create her aripiprazole (Abilify) by using buspirone (BuSpar), to no avail. Next, working with the patient's desires to keep medication at a minimum, staying within a trusted class of medication (SNRI), she was able to be titrated to a significantly higher than usual but approved dose (desvenlafaxine [Pristiq] 300 mg/d), where she began a gradual and sustained response
- The low-dose diazepam (Valium) also likely improved her stress-induced lability issues as well, and was a serendipitous addition by an outside provider

Take-home points

- It can be difficult to determine whether certain symptoms are from depression, stress, personality, medical, or cultural variables
- Working with a few medications and maximizing their doses for therapeutic effects makes clinical sense until side effects occur and change the risk/benefit analysis
- Side effects ultimately make clinicians change treatments, sometimes in the face of remission, which is clinically difficult in that the next set of medications may work better, worse, or the same – or may have different or worse side effects
- Often during these medication switches, patients are undertreated initially with low doses or due to new side effects and the risk of depressive relapse is high
- In this case, the patient was titrated rapidly to a moderate-high SNRI dose in order to achieve a better therapeutic effect more quickly to avoid relapse. This was successful. Side effects were alleviated and depressive remission was restored on a minimum of medications

Performance in practice: confessions of a psychopharmacologist

- *What could have been done better here?*
  - Should more pressure for psychotherapy (dynamic, dialectical, or otherwise) have been given, noting her personality traits?
  - This might have alleviated the need for an atypical antipsychotic trial and the emergence of TD
- *Can one really "re-create" a complex medicine like the atypical Abilify (aripiprazole)?*
  - 5-HT1A partial agonism could come from buspirone (BuSpar) as in this case
  - 5-HT2A antagonism could come from nefazodone (Serzone) or trazodone ER (Oleptro)

- Cannot easily obtain dopamine-3 (D3) partial receptor agonism from another agent (e.g., ropinirole, pramipexole)
- Do not want to get D2 receptor antagonism from another typical or atypical antipsychotic agent, or more TD could occur
- Perhaps it was over zealous, too theoretical, and a waste of time attempting the buspirone (BuSpar) augmentation

Tips and pearls

- Treatment for PMDD (in the absence of true MDD and other anxiety disorders) exists through FDA approvals for Sarafem (fluoxetine) and Zoloft (sertraline) in the US
- PMEs of existing MDD can be clinically treated by facilitating luteal phase serotonin, perhaps by increasing SSRI or SNRI monotherapy doses during the luteal phase and then reducing it again

Two-minute tutorial

Tardive dyskinesia

- Long-term blockade of D2 receptors in the nigrostriatal dopamine (DA) pathway can cause upregulation of those receptors, which may lead to the hyperkinetic motor condition known as TD
- Often characterized by facial and tongue movements (e.g., tongue protrusions, facial grimaces, chewing) as well as quick, jerky limb movements
- This upregulation may be the consequence of the futile attempt of the neuron to overcome drug-induced blockade of its D2 receptors. Notice the increase in receptors in the image to the right in the following figure:

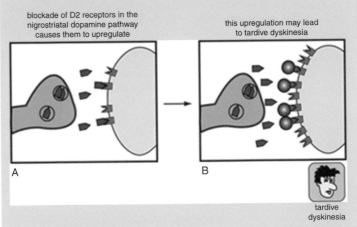

Figure 2.1. Upregulation of receptors in TD.

Tardive dyskinesia facts

- 17%–28% untreated, drug-naïve schizophrenics or in their normal unaffected twins, may show idiopathic, non-drug-related dyskinesia
- TD occurs more often with typical antipsychotics but is clearly possible with atypical antipsychotics
- As an example, risperidone's annual incidence for TD is 0.4% compared to that of 5% for typical antipsychotics
- D2 receptor antagonism in the striatum is the principal etiology suspected in TD
- Damage to striatal GABA interneurons, and cholinergic interneurons, is a likely cause of TD in some cases
- Outside D2 receptor antagonism, the atypical antipsychotics affect other receptors (5-HT2A antagonism), which may mitigate and lessen TD risk. They are associated with less risk of causing structural damage and provoking persistent, dynamic alterations in neurotransmitter systems involved in motor control
- Brain morphometric changes also differ, where typical antipsychotics may lead to increased caudate, putamen, and thalamus volumes, and atypical antipsychotics may only lead to increased thalamus volumes suggesting less risk of neurodegenerative brain changes in the basal ganglia with these agents

Tardive dyskinesia treatments

- If the patient is on a typical antipsychotic, a switch to an atypical antipsychotic may be warranted
    - Discontinue anticholinergic therapy as this may lower TD movements
    - Switch to clozapine (Clozaril/Fazaclo/Versacloz) as it has the lowest TD risk in this class
- Initiate a suppressive therapy with a conventional typical antipsychotic as increasing muscle rigidity (parkinsonism) may lower TD symptoms by "masking" TD movements
- Experimentally use tetrabenazine, donepezil, melatonin, branched-chain amino acids, dextromethorphan, vitamin E, or vitamin B6
- Risk relapse and consider staying on the antipsychotic but with a dose reduction
- Some patients with localized TD may respond to botulinum toxin (Botox) injections

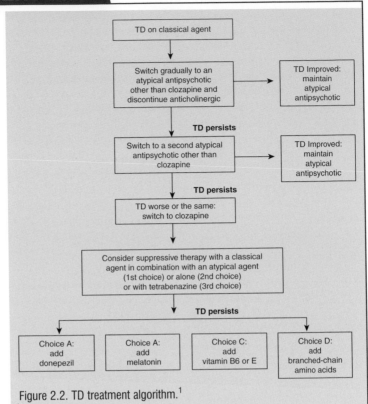

Figure 2.2. TD treatment algorithm.[1]

Posttest self-assessment question and answer

Which of the following are approved treatments for PME of existing depressive disorders?

A. Fluoxetine

B. Sertraline

C. Desvenlafaxine

D. Bupropion

E. A and B

F. None of the above

Answer: F

Fluoxetine and sertraline are approved for PMDD, and there are no current approvals for the clinical scenario of PME of existing depressive disorder.

[1] Margolese HC, Chouinard G, Kolivakis TT, et al. Tardive dyskinesia in the era of typical and atypical antipsychotics. Part 2: Incidence and management strategies in patients with schizophrenia. *Can J Psychiatry* 2005; 50:703–14.

In conclusion, the diagnostic criteria for PMDD, per the *DSM-V*, include:

1. In the majority of menstrual cycles, **at least five symptoms** must be present in the final week before the onset of menses, start to *improve* within a few days after the onset of menses, and become *minimal* or absent in the week after menses

2. One or more of the following symptoms must be present:
   - Marked affective lability (e.g., mood swings, feeling suddenly sad or tearful, or increased sensitivity to rejection)
   - Marked irritability or anger, or increased interpersonal conflicts
   - Marked depressed mood, feelings of hopelessness, or self-deprecating thoughts
   - Marked anxiety, tension, and/or feelings of being keyed up or on edge

3. One or more of the following symptoms must additionally be present, to reach a total of five symptoms when combined with the symptoms from #2:
   - Decreased interest in usual activities (e.g., work, school, friends, hobbies)
   - Subjective difficulty in concentration
   - Lethargy, easily fatigued, or marked lack of energy
   - Marked change in appetite, overeating, or specific food cravings
   - Hypersomnia or insomnia
   - A sense of being overwhelmed or out of control
   - Physical symptoms such as breast tenderness or swelling, joint or muscle pain, a sensation of "bloating" or weight gain

   These symptoms must have been met for most menstrual cycles that occurred in the preceding year

4. The symptoms are associated with clinically significant distress or inteference with work, school, usual social activities, or relationships with others (e.g., avoidance of social activities; decreased productivity and efficiency at work, school, or home)

5. The disturbance is not merely an exacerbation of the symptoms of another disorder such as MDD, panic disorder (PD), persistent depressive disorder (dysthymia), or a personality disorder (although it may co-occur with any of these disorders)

References

1. Stahl SM. Antidepressants. In: *Stahl's Essential Psychopharmacology*, 4th edn. New York, NY: Cambridge University Press, 2013; pp. 284–369.
2. Gupta S, Mosnik D, Black DW, Berry S, Masand PS. Tardive dyskinesia: review of treatments past, present, and future. *Ann Clin Psych* 1999; 11:257–66.

3. Margolese HC, Chouinard G, Kolivakis TT, et al. Tardive dyskinesia in the era of typical and atypical antipsychotics. Part 1: Pathophysiology and mechanism of induction. *Can J Psychiatry* 2005; 9:541–7.

4. Margolese HC, Chouinard G, Kolivakis TT, et al. Tardive dyskinesia in the era of typical and atypical antipsychotics. Part 2: Incidence and management strategies in patients with schizophrenia. *Can J Psychiatry* 2005; 50:703–14.

5. Stahl SM. Aripiprazole. In: *Stahl's Essential Psychopharmacology Prescriber's Guide*, 3rd edn. New York, NY: Cambridge University Press, 2009; pp. 45–50.

6. Steiner M, Pearlstein T, Cohen LS, et al. Expert guidelines for the treatment of severe PMS, PMDD, and comorbidities: the role of SSRIs. *J Womens Health (Larchmt)* 2006; 15:57–69.

7. American Psychiatric Association. *American Psychiatric Association Diagnostic and Statistical Manual of Mental Disorders*, 5th edn. Washington, DC: American Psychiatric Publishing, 2013.

8. Kornstein SG, Harvey AT, Rush AJ, et al. Self-reported premenstrual exacerbation of depressive symptoms in patients seeking treatment for major depression. *Psychol Med* 2005; 35:683–92.

9. Kim J, Donovan J, Schwartz T. Dextromethorphan for tardive dyskinesia. *Intern Neuropsychiatr Dis J* 2014; 2: 136–40.

The Case: The other lady with a moving jaw

The Question: How to determine the cause of movement disorder side effects?

The Psychopharmacological dilemma: Finding an effective regimen for depression while managing movement disorder side effects

Pretest self-assessment question (answer at the end of the case)

Which of the following may cause abnormal movement disorders?

A. Duloxetine
B. Mixed amphetamine salts
C. Aripiprazole
D. Lamotrigine
E. B and C
F. All of the above

Patient evaluation on intake

- 50-year-old woman with a chief complaint of unremitting depression for 30 years

Psychiatric history

- Onset of depression in late teens/early 20s
- MDEs sometimes due to stressful events, but most often occur regardless of adjustment stressors
- MDD became chronic in the patient's early 40s without any clear inter-episode recovery
- The patient likely has "double depression" where she meets dysthymic level (persistent depressive disorder in *DSM-V*) criteria with full MDEs superimposed intermittently
- History includes no hospitalizations. She had one suicide attempt as a teenager
  - Review of psychiatric systems revealed no formal anxiety disorder; however, she reports situational panic attacks at work when she feels overwhelmed with tasks
  - There is no evidence of schizophrenia or mania
  - History of AUD for which she went for rehabilitation and remains sober
    - There is no liver disease or damage from alcohol use
  - Previous psychiatric treatments included
    - Consistent supportive psychotherapy without formal PDP or CBT intervention

- ○ Amitriptyline (Elavil), a tricyclic antidepressant (TCA), was used for approximately 20 years, with partial response but no sustained remission
- ○ Fluoxetine (Prozac), a selective serotonin reuptake inhibitor (SSRI), up to 120 mg/d, allowed for a response but effect was lost over time
- ○ Sertraline (Zoloft), an SSRI, up to 100 mg/d and another SSRI, paroxetine (Paxil), 40 mg/d failed altogether

Social and personal history

- The patient is single, never married
- Is college-educated and works in management and has routinely been gainfully employed
- Grew up with alcoholic parents but without any abuse
- Grew up in relative poverty

Medical history

- Successful gastric bypass surgery allowing 100 16 of weight loss
- Gastroesophageal reflux disease (GERD)
- Type II diabetes (DM2)
- Hypertension (HTN)
- Asthma

Family history

- GAD and MDD in mother
- AUD in mother and father

Current psychiatric medications

- Duloxetine (Cymbalta) 60 mg/d (SNRI)
- Bupropion-SR (Wellbutrin-SR) 400 mg/d (NDRI)
- Buspirone (BuSpar) 60 mg/d (5-HT1A partial agonist)
- Trazodone (Desyrel) 50 mg/d (serotonin antagonist reuptake inhibitor [SARI])
- Clonazepam (Klonopin) 1 mg/d (BZ)

Current medical medications

- Metroprolol (Lopressor) 50 mg/d
- Omeprazole (Nexium) 40 mg/d
- Allopurinol (Aloprim) 300 mg/d
- Atorvastatin (Lipitor) 10 mg/d
- Advair Diskus (fluticasone–salmeterol)
- Albuterol (Ventolin inhaler)

PATIENT FILE

Question

Based on what you know about this patient's history and current symptoms, would you consider her to fall within the TRD spectrum?

- Yes
- No

Would you continue her SNRI duloxetine monotherapy?

- Yes, but increase the dose to the full approved 120 mg/d
- Yes, but add another augmentation or combination therapy
- No, taper off and try a new monotherapy
- No, taper off all medications and try a monoamine oxidase inhibitor (MAOI) or electroconvulsive therapy (ECT) treatment

Attending physician's mental notes: initial evaluation

- Nothing unexpected on mental status examination
- Because she has had chronic, unremitting symptoms without any full inter-episode recovery, this makes her depression chronic. She should also be considered resistant as she has failed antidepressants from at least three different classes (TCA, SSRI, NDRI) and augmentation strategies as well
- The best diagnosis for this patient may be chronic MDD
- During ongoing care, will need to better assess for personality disorder, and observe for an AUD relapse
- Increasing duloxetine (Cymbalta) to the 120 mg/d FDA limit seems reasonable in that it is more similar to her previous successful TCA trial than her failed SSRI trials. Duloxetine also likely increases NRI at higher doses that may be more effective in her case. Finally, it would be a definitive, full-dose clinical SNRI trial
- Medically, she reports her liver is fine despite her past history of excessive alcohol use, but laboratory specimens should be sent for analysis regardless when duloxetine is used on AUD patients
- In this case, she would be on maximal SNRI, NDRI, and 5-HT1A partial receptor agonist rational polypharmacy with the full-dose duloxetine being utilized
  - *Rational polypharmacy* occurs when drugs are added together to maximize their positives and complementary mechanisms of action *and* ideally when drugs can mitigate each others' side effects as well
    - In this case there is some redundancy in NRI that could result in HTN, dry mouth, nausea, or activating side effects, which is not rationale but rather a calculated risk that must be monitored

- ○ Alternatively, the NDRI might mitigate sexual dysfunction and weight gain from the SNRI and provide unique dopaminergic facilitation for better antidepressant effectiveness overall
- ○ The 5-HT1A receptor partial agonist may facilitate greater activity of the SNRI and may mitigate sexual dysfunction of the same SNRI

Further investigation

Is there anything else you would especially like to know about this patient?

- What about details concerning this patient's personality style or diagnostic and routine rating scale information?
- Upon entering into patient practice, she was given diagnostic questionnaires regarding psychiatric disorders. Clinically significant scores were noted for MDD, persistent depressive disorder, social anxiety disorder (SAD), bulimia nervosa (BN), drug and alcohol misuse
- These findings triggered the clinician to investigate further. The SAD symptoms seem to be more longitudinal and consistent with avoidant personality traits. The elevated score for BN seems relevant to past history where she was a comfort eater and gained weight. She is sensitive about weight-gain status post successful bariatric surgery. She clinically does not have an eating disorder now. The patient admits to two years of sobriety but answered questions based upon urges to use alcohol. Urine toxicology was negative
- At admission, she was given diagnostic questionnaires regarding personality disorders. This revealed elevated schizoid, avoidant, and borderline traits but not necessarily disorders
- In practice, utilizing routine outcomes-based rating scales is becoming more routine and is highly suggested in MDD treatment guidelines. She was given the Inventory of Depressive Symptomatology (IDS) and scored in the moderate range for MDD as well

Question

Based on what you know about this patient's history, current symptoms, and treatment responses, do you think that a bona fide, formal trial of an established evidence-based psychotherapy is warranted?

- Yes, a referral for PDP is warranted
- Yes, a referral for CBT is warranted
- No, this patient has had many years of supportive, eclectic style psychotherapy and further psychotherapy intervention is unlikely to be effective

Attending physician's mental notes: initial evaluation (continued)

- The patient is obviously depressed and clearly has some personality traits that are likely to make her more resistant to medication treatment in general
- The patient does have some clear strengths in that she is consistently gainfully employed and has had the ability to maintain successful relationships with significant others, peers, and those in authority. She seems to be in a solid recovery from her substance misuse. She is thoroughly compliant with medication management visits and taking medications as prescribed. Given these things, the use of ECT may not be warranted as it would disrupt her work, which she views as a positive and protective factor against further depressive decline
- There is a history of compliance to antidepressant trials where full, therapeutic dosing has been utilized
- Given her lack of formal outcome-based psychotherapy, this may be warranted at this time as well as maximizing the dose range of the medications she was on at the time of admission
- It would make sense to discontinue her potentially dependence-forming BZ and her ineffective buspirone (BuSpar) and trazodone (Desyrel) agents

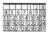

Case outcome: interim follow-ups through four months

- Full dose, 120 mg duloxetine (Cymbalta) SNRI treatment failed to lead to symptom remission
- The patient declined weekly, formal psychotherapy due to her busy work schedule
- She agreed to streamline her medications and proceed with a new augmentation strategy. Her bupropion-SR (Wellbutrin-SR) was lowered by converting to a single bupropion-XL (Wellbutrin-XL) 300 mg dose. She tapered off buspirone (BuSpar) but continued trazodone (Desyrel) for insomnia. Her duloxetine (Cymbalta) was continued. The depression augmentation atypical antipsychotic aripiprazole (Abilify) was next titrated from 2 mg/d to 15 mg/d over the course of four months

Question

Considering her current medication regimen, what types of clinical monitoring might you utilize in the outpatient office setting?

- Routine measurement of weight and abdominal girth due to the initiation of an atypical antipsychotic
- Routine blood pressure monitoring due to the use of noradrenergic antidepressants and due to the initiation of an atypical antipsychotic

- Intermittent blood draws to evaluate if there are elevations in blood glucose or lipids due to initiation of an atypical antipsychotic
- Given her bariatric surgery, monitoring of any available blood levels is warranted to determine if there is a malabsorption issue

Attending physician's mental notes: nine months

- The patient had failed to achieve remission with multiple SSRIs, combination SNRI/NDRI, augmentation with 5-HT1A partial receptor agonism, and augmentation with a BZ
- Starting an atypical antipsychotic is reasonable, based on available treatment guidelines, regulatory approvals, and randomized controlled trial empirical evidence
- The atypical antipsychotics do carry TD and metabolic risks (HTN, hyperglucosemia, hyperlipidemia, weight gain) over long-term use, which should not be taken lightly as other augmentation/combination strategies may have more favorable tolerability profiles
- Additionally, remember this patient was obese and required bariatric surgery and will be quite sensitive to any weight gain. Special attention should be paid to which atypical antipsychotic is chosen, not only based upon randomized controlled data but also based upon theoretical antidepressant activity and known metabolic profile
- Clinically, aripiprazole (Abilify), quetiapine (Seroquel), quetiapine-XR (Seroquel-XR), lurasidone (Latuda), olanzapine (Zyprexa) have varying approvals and indications in treating depression
- In this group, aripiprazole (Abilify) appears to have the most favorable metabolic profile (lurasidone was not available at the time), which minimizes comparative risk of weight gain, elevated blood glucose, elevated lipids, and elevated blood pressure
- Other atypical antipsychotics have yet to be empirically proven as antidepressants. However, pharmacodynamically, asenapine (Saphris) has a molecular structure very similar to the antidepressant mirtazapine (Remeron). Lurasidone (Latuda) gained approval later, likely due to its serotonergic potential (5-HT2A, 5-HT1A, 5-HT7 receptor manipulation) making them theoretical antidepressant treatments as alternatives for this patient
  - They also appear to be clinically less metabolically challenging than some of the aforementioned atypical antipsychotics

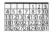

Case outcome: interim follow-ups through nine months

- The patient reports that aripiprazole (Abilify) has removed all of her passive suicidal thinking, which has not resolved with any prior treatment over many years. She is very happy with this clinical outcome but still admits to a moderate amount of depressive symptoms

- Her chief complaint is of fatigue and relative amotivation despite being on therapeutic SNRI, NDRI, and an atypical antipsychotic
- She has no TD/EPS, metabolic or acute side effects, and is tolerating her regimen well

Question

What would you do next?

- Increase the aripiprazole (Abilify) upward to 30 mg /d despite the average dose for MDD patients being 11 mg/d
- Augment the current regimen with a stimulant medication to treat fatigue and amotivation specifically
- As she is still a partial responder only, remove all medications and convert to an MAOI

Attending physician's mental notes: 9–12 month follow-ups

- Despite being still a partial responder and non-remitted, this patient is better than her usual baseline. It may be risky to remove any of her three main antidepressant agents. Adding another medication increases cost and side-effect burden
- In targeting her remaining vegetative symptoms, her current medications enhance norepinephrine (NE) by using an SNRI plus an NDRI effectively, and therefore, improving DA neurotransmission may be an important next step
- To increase DA activity, classic stimulants might be used but carry addiction risk for this patient. New generation wakefulness-promoting agents such as modafinil (Provigil) or armodafinil (Nuvigil) have less addiction risk and more empirical evidence for treating fatigue symptoms. Direct D2 receptor agonists such as pramipexole (Mirapex) or ropinirole (Requip) might be used but tend to have some sedating side effects
- Washing out her medications in order to utilize an MAOI might risk full recurrence of depression and thwart our current gains
  - Interestingly, some MAOI antidepressants have amphetamine-based metabolites, which may better target and improve fatigue

Question

How much do you weigh this patient's previous addiction to alcohol when determining the next step?

- Very much, she will likely become addicted to any controlled substance
- Somewhat, her addiction to alcohol may be triggered more by BZ use than stimulant or other controlled drug use as other agents are dissimilar to alcohol pharmacodynamics (GABA-A receptor PAM)
- Not much as addiction risk is minimal and can be monitored with pill counts, urine drug screens, and breathalyzer testing, if needed

Case outcome: interim follow-ups through 12 months

- Bupropion-XL (Wellbutrin-XL) is discontinued and modafinil (Provigil) is started, as it is less addicting than a formal stimulant and may facilitate wakefulness through the DA system to a greater extent than bupropion, but also theoretically via downstream histamine and orexin pathway facilitation. However, her insurance refuses to cover modafinil
- Therefore, the patient is issued the isomer product armodafinil (Nuvigil) due to availability of voucher coupons that enables a therapeutic trial to occur
  - Therapeutically, it was in the patient's interest to fight for access to modafinil
  - Therapeutically, it was in the patient's interest for the prescriber to meet with a sales team and procure samples
- Armodafinil (Nuvigil) is titrated throughout a full dose range up to 250 mg/d without an antidepressant response and with minimal improvement in her vegetative symptoms. She did not misuse this product
- Armodafinil is discontinued and methylphenidate-LA (Ritalin-LA) is started
  - In this manner, the prescriber switches from a less addictive product to a slightly more addictive product
  - Utilizing a slow release preparation of a stimulant allows for slower absorption and less likelihood of withdrawal or intoxication
  - These pharmacokinetic properties allow for less drug-liking properties from the stimulant and theoretically could lower addiction risk overall in this patient
- Methylphenidate-LA (Ritalin-LA) is titrated upward to 30 mg/d with very little effect, but again with good tolerability
- Blood pressure remains normal, and likely the use of stimulant medication acts as an appetite suppressant minimizing long-term weight gain from her other antidepressants
- No abnormal movements are observed and no acute side effects from her complex medication regimen are reported

Case outcome: multiple interim follow-ups through 16 months

- The patient is converted to a different stimulant, mixed amphetamine salts-XR (Adderall-XR) and titrated gradually to 60 mg/d for effect
- With each increase, the patient reports less depression and at the higher dose, she records her lowest depression rating scale score, which is near remission
- Motivation is improved and fatigue lessened. She is well focused at work. The patient reports she is very happy with the complex, yet effective medication regimen of SNRI, atypical antipsychotic, stimulant, and trazodone

- As the patient had a dramatic response to the stimulant medication, it was decided to discontinue some of her medications, which were deemed to be minimally effective. The aripiprazole (Abilify), given its longer-term metabolic and extrapyramidal risks, is gradually tapered without any return in her suicidal ideation
- Several weeks later, the patient developed bilateral recurrent masseter muscle spasms that were not alleviated by anticholinergic therapy, and therefore, judged not to be dystonia or EPS
- The patient states that she is quite anxious at work now due to new job descriptions and that she felt these were "nervous tics." However, she fails to respond to the non-addictive anxiolytic hydroxyzine (Vistaril), and the BZ are avoided due to her previous alcohol misuse history
- TD/withdrawal dyskinesia is now the working diagnosis, which seems to be triggered by the withdrawal of aripiprazole (Abilify)
  - Previous AIMS scores were all negative
- The aripiprazole (Abilify) is restarted at a low dose to stop the withdrawal dyskinesia and the abnormal movements dissipate. Next, she is more gradually and slowly tapered off this atypical antipsychotic in hopes of avoiding withdrawal dyskinesia albeit at some increased risk for TD permanence
- Simultaneously, her mixed amphetamine salts-XR (Adderall-XR) is also gradually lowered as it was felt her dyskinesia could be from D2 receptor toxicity due to stimulant use (i.e., motor tics)
- At this point, removing her therapeutically effective stimulant may risk depressive relapse, which is problematic, but this risk is weighed against worsening her possible TD

Attending physician's mental notes: 16-month follow-ups

- This patient was in near remission and now she has a possible, irreversible movement disorder, although many patients improve over time from their withdrawal dyskinesias
- Removal of all potentially offending agents is needed to lower the risk of TD permanence
- Best case scenario is that this dyskinesia is stimulant-induced motor tics, which should reverse
- Patient will likely relapse into depression

Case debrief

- The patient has a lengthy history of chronic depression, substance misuse, and mild personality disorder traits. Her MDD appears unipolar in nature, and had been partially responsive at best to antidepressant treatments in the past but she has never fully remitted

- This case was complicated in that she did achieve near remission for the first time in many years with the addition of an atypical antipsychotic and a stimulant to her SNRI
- Unfortunately, both classes of agents are clinically utilized in the treatment of depression but carry the risk for movement disorder development, which ultimately occurred
- Over the next few months, the patient had her trazodone discontinued due to ineffectiveness in treating insomnia and was placed on doxepin (Sinequan) and titrated to 200 mg/d to help the insomnia but also to act as a fully dosed TCA as well. The SNRI, duloxetine (Cymbalta), was discontinued
- She became slightly more depressed, but did not fully relapse to her admission baseline of full MDD symptoms
- The patient's stimulant was also discontinued while she was titrated onto the doxepin, and one week after the final 10 mg/d of mixed amphetamine salts (Adderall-XR) was discontinued, all of her abnormal jaw movements ceased

Take-home points

- This case emphasizes the need for full therapeutic trials of antidepressant treatments, augmentations, combinations
- This case emphasizes the need to continually evaluate if medications are effective and warranted, and that streamlining of medications is sometimes prudent
- This case emphasizes utilizing each medication, in combination, to complement the next with regard to maximizing the monoamine systems, in that there was very little overlap of pharmacodynamic mechanisms among the combined agents utilized to treat the depression
  - For example, when the TCA was started, the SNRI was removed
  - Alternatively, when the stimulant was added, the NDRI was removed
  - The rational polypharmacy goal here is to avoid combining identical, redundant antidepressant pharmacodynamic mechanisms of action
- This case emphasizes that use of rating scales can detect underlying comorbidities and better pinpoint response versus remission
  - In this case, stimulants were used and escalated as successive ratings showed a clear dose–response curve for this patient
- Finally, manipulating monoamine neural circuits may provide for depression relief, but at the same time cause serious side effects. The clinician must think carefully about the additive or synergistic effects of adding agents together with regard to both efficacy and tolerability

Performance in practice: confessions of a psychopharmacologist

- *What could have been done better here?*
  - Was the patient on too many medications?
  - Should the patient have been directed more toward MAOI monotherapy, or use of ECT, or psychotherapy?
- *Does it make sense to antagonize D2 receptors with an atypical antipsychotic while agonizing them with a stimulant?*
- *Possible action items for improvement in practice*
  - Make sure that augmentation with atypical antipsychotics is not the only option offered, or the only option offered early, as these drugs can be expensive and can have notable and sometimes permanent side effects
  - Be aware of the pharmacodynamic mechanisms of action of all agents utilized with regard to combining them for efficacy, but also be aware of potential toxicity and side effects

Tips and pearls

- Atypical antipsychotics have a solid evidence base in the treatment of MDD
- They may also carry distinct risk of metabolic disorder and movement disorder, which should clearly be incorporated into the informed consent process and also should be considered while prescribing in a rational polypharmacy approach
- Other approaches for TRD have much less definitive evidence to support their use but may actually have fewer risks

Two-minute tutorial *(four-minute foray…if you combine two tutorials)*

Part 1: Combining stimulants and atypical antipsychotics in TRD

- This type of combination is often used in children and adolescents who suffer from attention deficit hyperactivity disorder (ADHD), oppositional defiant disorder (ODD), and intellectual disability or autism spectrum disorder (ASD)
- The stimulants are felt to promote DA activity in the cortex and throughout the brain. This promotes better attention, concentration, vigilance, and motivation
- Stimulants often do not treat the affective lability and dyscontrol in these disorders and atypical antipsychotics are often added to help these residual symptom clusters
- Some atypical antipsychotics actually facilitate DA and NE release in the dorsolateral prefrontal cortex (DLPFC) to help cognitive and executive function symptoms
- Atypical antipsychotics that antagonize 5-HT2C receptors in the brainstem theoretically allow for a reduction in GABA interneuron tone there,

secondarily allowing the locus coeruleus (LC) and the ventral tegmental area (VTA) to promote greater NE and DA projection activity into the cortex

- Combining atypical antipsychotics and stimulants therefore may have a mechanistic rationale in that this combination may better maximize DA activity through multiple mechanisms
- A similar approach may be used in TRD where vegetative, amotivated, and executively dysfunctioned patients may benefit from stimulants, atypical antipsychotics, or both
- Unfortunately, there are negatives to this combination
- The atypical antipsychotics have a risk for TD and this patient did appear to have a withdrawal dyskinesia when her atypical antipsychotic was stopped
- The stimulants may cause motor tics and dyskinesias due to dopaminergic toxicity instead of D2 receptor blockade. Tics are more often noted in children and adolescents who are treated with stimulants for ADHD and are reversible, whereas TD may not be
- Theoretically, this patient's aripiprazole (Abilify) had the ability to promote DA activity through its novel partial agonist activities at the D3 receptor. This could increase tonic DA tone in the frontal cortex, which is believed to be beneficial in treating certain depression symptoms. This drug also blocks DA activity at the D2 receptor in the basal ganglia, which may lead to EPS/TD symptoms
- The mixed amphetamine salts (Adderall-XR) product has the ability to block the DA reuptake pump, reverse this pump, and reverse the vesicular monoamine transporter activity, providing a robust, high level of DA availability and neurotransmission
- In this case, this patient's basal ganglia had one drug blocking DA transmission, while the other was promoting it, setting up a conflict where movement disorder could occur. Depending upon which drug was more effective at manipulating the neurocircuit, too little DA could cause TD or too much could cause a toxicity based dyskinesia
- In removing the patient's aripiprazole (Abilify) initially, the patient was left with elevated hyperdopaminergic tone likely providing DA excess and resultant dyskinesia. This scenario is not unlike a Parkinson's disease patient developing dyskinesia if taking too much levodopa (Sinemet)
- The clinician tried to re-establish DA transmission balance by restarting aripiprazole (Abilify) at a low dose while slowly tapering the mixed amphetamine salt (Adderall-XR)
- This minimized the movement disorder when the atypical antipsychotic was removed and only a small dose of stimulant remained
- Upon total stimulant removal, all movement disorder symptoms resolved, suggesting that the patient's jaw movements, tics or dyskinesias were likely caused by the stimulant use, especially in the face of D2 receptor blockade from the atypical antipsychotic

Part 2: Monitoring for TD

Abnormal Involuntary Movement Scale (AIMS)

- This scale was developed initially for use in patients suffering from schizophrenia who often developed TD while utilizing first-generation, typical antipsychotics. In some institutions it is considered the standard of care to perform this evaluation annually if the patient is on an antipsychotic, with the intention to detect TD in its early stages when it is less likely to become permanent
- The risk for developing TD is the greatest for those who have accumulated the most days on active antipsychotic therapy. Furthermore, the elderly and those with affective disorder components are likely at greater risk
- With the introduction of the second-generation atypical antipsychotics, it appears that the TD rates are lower, but as noted in the first two cases in this book, it is still possible to develop TD with use of atypical antipsychotics
- Following is an example of how the AIMS scale is administered. Furthermore, it is scored objectively and can be used as a diagnostic tool and as an outcome measure to determine if TD is worsening or improving
- Perhaps this scale should be more readily utilized with the increased use of atypical antipsychotics in non-schizophrenia-based illnesses

AIMS instructions

1. Ask patient to remove shoes and socks
2. Ask patient if there is anything in his/her mouth (e.g., gum, candy); if there is, to remove it
3. Ask patient about the *current* condition of his/her teeth. Ask patient if he/she wears dentures. Do teeth or dentures bother the patient now?
4. Ask patient whether he/she notices any movements in mouth, face, hands, or feet. If yes, ask to describe and to what extent
   ○ They currently bother patient or interfere with his/her activities
5. Have patient sit in a chair with hands on knees, legs slightly apart, and feet flat on the floor
   ○ (Look at entire body for movements while in this position)
6. Ask patient to sit with hands hanging unsupported; if male, between legs, if female and wearing a dress, hanging over knees
   ○ (Observe hands and other body areas)
7. Ask patient to open mouth
   ○ (Observe tongue at rest in mouth)
   ○ Do this twice
8. Ask patient to protrude tongue
   ○ (Observe abnormalities of tongue movement)
   ○ Do this twice

9. Ask patient to tap thumb, with each finger, as rapidly as possible for 10–15 s; separately with right hand, then with left hand
   ○ (Observe facial and leg movements)
10. Flex and extend patient's left and right arms (one at a time)
   ○ (Note any rigidity)
11. Ask patient to stand up
   ○ (Observe in profile. Observe all body areas again, hip included)

– – –

- Finally, many of the psychiatric medications that clinicians prescribe may cause abnormal movements
- Clinicians most often think of TD but our antipsychotics may also induce dystonia or parkinsonism's resting tremor
- Antidepressants may induce a fine, intention tremor
- Mood stabilizing, epilepsy medications may induce a similar tremor, dysarthria, ataxia, or dysmetria
- Stimulant medications may also induce an intention tremor, but more prominently, may induce tic disorders

Part 3: Rating scale rant (a six-minute seminar now. . .)

Treatment guidelines are numerous for MDD. The American Psychiatric Association's guidelines suggest routine rating scale use in MDD. This case may be used to highlight some of their suggestions. The third edition American Psychiatric Association treatment guidelines for major depressive disorder of November 2010 also suggests

- Maintain therapeutic alliance, complete a full axis I/II assessment (published prior to *DSM-V*), provide for patient safety, evaluate patient's functional status and level of treatment acuity
- *Utilize outcome measures routinely*
- Coordinate care with all providers and include family members when possible; educate all parties
- Foster appointment and medication adherence
- Maximize monotherapy antidepressant for dose and duration of treatment
- For partial response, consider augmentation with lithium, thyroid hormone, anticonvulsants, stimulants, second-generation antipsychotics (atypical antipsychotics)
- Utilize depression-focused psychotherapies such as CBT, IPT, problem-solving psychotherapy

There are several full treatment guidelines that may be reviewed for further information. Most guidelines suggest the approaches simplified here.

These guidelines become very specific with regard to the management of depressive disorder in the acute phase, continuation phase, and after remission occurs.

It is also important to consider how long the patient has been depressed, how many depressive episodes the patient has been through, and if they have been suicidal.

This type of patient history is important when considering how aggressively to treat a patient with psychotropic medication. In general, mild depression is treated with psychotherapy whereas more moderate to severe depression and recurrent or chronic depression is more often treated with medications, psychotherapy, or both modalities.

Generally speaking, the longer a patient has been depressed, the more recurrences they have, and the more medications they have taken, the more likely they are to be considered to have more TRD. In these cases, once remission is obtained, the medication regimen is often continued over the long term, as a recurrence or relapse is highly probable.

Case outcome: use of outcome measures

- The IDS and the QIDS are two public domain rating scales (www.ids-qids.org) for depression. They were used in this particular case

- There are many other depression rating scales available, such as the Beck Depression Inventory, the Zung Depression Self Rating Scale, etc., that may also be utilized. The PHQ-9 (Patient Health Questionnaire, www.ncbi.nim.nih.gov/pubmed/11556941) is likely the most widely used in clinical practice and in primary care practice

- Routine use of rating scales in psychopharmacological practice may be similar to a PCP always measuring weight and blood pressure in each patient. It is even more similar to the routine use of blood glucose, renal, or blood pressure monitoring techniques in the diabetic patient

- In this TRD scenario, the clinician is acutely aware if the patient is better, worse, or the same at each visit. The clinician can also predict pending worsening or relapse of symptoms, or medication noncompliance based on ratings outcomes at each visit. As the patient enters the office after completing the ratings, the clinician has about 30 symptom data points already apparent before any questioning starts in the session. Theoretically, before the patient enters the psychopharmacologist's office, it is known what percent the patient is better or worse. This actually frees up clinician time to further investigate social stressors, maladaptive personality symptoms, or provide better education and informed consent. Interestingly, use of rating scales may make you a better therapist.

- An abnormal value on these types of routine outcome measures likely triggers a reaction from the clinician to re-evaluate the patient and consider more aggressive treatment in order to obtain a better remission of symptoms

- In the case of diabetes, this may decrease comorbidities, improve social functioning, and decrease healthcare utilization rates. In terms of MDD, rating scales likely orient the clinician that the patient, indeed, is not in remission, thus triggering more comprehensive and more aggressive care with regard to psychotherapy, medication management, and collaboration with other providers and family members. The end result likely is improved outcomes over the long term
- Finally, there are many public domain, short, and simple rating scales that may be utilized for each psychiatric disorder whether it is PD, obsessive compulsive disorder (OCD), post-traumatic stress disorder (PTSD), BN, AUD. Many of these could be simply incorporated into practice as a PCP might incorporate the taking of the blood pressure
- Rating scales:
  - Can save clinicians time if automated
  - May allow a clinician to stay within APA guidelines
  - May allow better detection of comorbidities and residual symptoms
  - May create pivotal treatment decision points as if these were abnormal laboratory values that require action
  - May free up more session time to address non-pharmacologic issues

Posttest self-assessment question and answer

Which of the following may cause abnormal movement disorders?

A. Duloxetine
B. Mixed amphetamine salts
C. Aripiprazole
D. Lamotrigine
E. B and C
F. All of the above

Answer: F

Duloxetine is associated with intention tremor. Mixed amphetamine salts are associated with intention tremor and tics. Aripiprazole is associated with resting tremor, akathisia, dystonia, and dyskinetic movements. Lamotrigine is associated with intention tremor, dysmetria, dysarthria, and ataxia.

References

1. Stahl SM. *Stahl's Essential Psychopharmacology*, 4th edn. New York, NY: Cambridge University Press, 2013.
2. Stahl SM. *Stahl's Essential Psychopharmacology: The Prescriber's Guide*, 4th edn. New York, NY: Cambridge University Press, 2011.

3. American Psychiatric Association. *Practice Guideline for the Treatment of Patients with Major Depressive Disorder*, 3rd edn. Washington, DC: American Psychiatric Association Press, 2010.

4. American Psychiatric Association. *Handbook of Psychiatric Measures*, 2nd edn, Rush JA Jr., First MB, Blacker D, eds. Washington, DC: American Psychiatric Publishing, 2008.

5. Inventory of Depressive Symptomatology (IDS) and Quick Inventory of Depressive Symptomatology (QIDS). http://www.ids-qids.org. Accessed November 2014.

6. Schwartz TL, Stahl SM. Treatment strategies for dosing the second generation antipsychotics. *CNS Neurosci Ther* 2011; 17:110–17.

7. Zimmerman M, McGlinchey JB, Chelminski I. Measurement-based care and outcome measures: implications for practice. In: Schwartz TL, Petersen T, eds. *Depression: Treatment Strategies and Management*, 2nd edn. New York, NY: Informa, 2009; Ch. 6.

8. Topel M, Zajecka J, Goldstein C, Siddiqui U, Schwartz TL. Using what we have: combining medications to achieve remission. *Clin Neuropsychiatry* 2011; 8:4–27.

9. Zimmerman M, Chelminski I, Young D, Dalrymple K. Using outcome measures to promote better outcomes. *Clin Neuropsychiatry* 2011; 8:28–36.

10. Guy W. *ECDEU* Assessment Manual for Psychopharmacology: Revised *(DHEW publication number ADM 76–338)*. Rockville, MD: US Department of Health, Education and Welfare, Public Health Service, Alcohol, Drug Abuse and Mental Health Administration, NIMH Psychopharmacology Research Branch, Division of Extramural Research Programs, 1976; pp. 534–7.

11. Stahl SM, Mignon L. *Stahl's Illustrated Antipsychotics: Treating Psychosis, Mania and Depression*, 2nd edn. New York, NY: Cambridge University Press, 2010.

12. Ishibashi T, Horisawa T, Tokuda K, et al. Pharmacological profile of lurasidone, a novel antipsychotic agent with potent 5-hydroxytryptamine 7 (5-HT7) and 5-HT1A receptor activity. *Pharmacol Exp Ther* 2010; 334:171–81.

13. Citrome L. Iloperidone, asenapine, and lurasidone: a brief overview of 3 new second-generation antipsychotics. *Postgrad Med* 2011; 123:153–62.

The Case: The lady with major depressive disorder who bought an RV.

The Question: What is a therapeutic dose and duration for vagus nerve stimulation therapy in depression?

The Psychopharmacological dilemma: Finding an effective treatment for chronic treatment-resistant or refractory depression while managing a severely ill patient

Pretest self-assessment question (answer at the end of the case)

Which of the following is not an invasive surgical treatment for resistant depression?

A. TMS
B. VNS
C. ECT
D. DBS
E. EpCS
F. A and C
G. B and D
H. All of the above

Patient evaluation on intake

- 55-year-old woman with a chief complaint of unremitting depression for 30+ years

Psychiatric history

- Onset of depression in her 20s
- Questionable recurrent depressive episodes versus a single, chronic unremitting episode. Patient cannot recollect a two-month symptom-free period or any clear inter-episode recovery
- MDD symptoms have never been mild enough to allow gainful employment, likely ruling out persistent depressive disorder plus MDD, which is often called "double depression"
- Meets melancholic MDD specifiers with severe anhedonia (patient was housebound and essentially bedridden), worse symptoms in the morning, marked psychomotor retardation (a simple depression symptom screening took 15 minutes to complete due to thought slowing), and weight loss (patient's weight was 90 lbs)
- History includes at least two psychiatric hospitalizations. She has had no suicide attempts
- Review of psychiatric systems revealed no formal anxiety disorder, psychosis, mania, eating disorder, SUD

- She has received eclectic, supportive psychotherapy in the past, but her mental state at this presentation made reciprocal talk therapy almost impossible
- There is no evidence of clear personality disorder
- Failed to respond to adequately dosed
  - Fluoxetine (Prozac) 60 mg/d and sertraline (Zoloft) 200 mg/d SSRI monotherapies
  - Venlafaxine-XR (Effexor-XR) 225 mg/d SNRI therapy
  - Bupropion-SR (Wellbutrin-SR) 400 mg/d NDRI therapy
  - Mirtazapine (Remeron) 45 mg/d NaSSA therapy
  - TCA trials in distant past
  - Course of ECT (electroconvulsive therapy)

Social and personal history

- Married and has a son
- High school educated and has not been gainfully employed outside raising children
- Grew up with outside relatives as both parents died when she was younger
- Does not drink alcohol, smoke cigarettes, or use addictive drugs

Medical history

- Coronary artery disease (CAD)
- Irritable bowel syndrome (IBS)
- GERD
- Hyperlipidemia

Family history

- Eating disorder (likely anorexia nervosa [AN]) in a sibling

Current psychiatric medications

- Citalopram (Celexa) 60 mg/d (SSRI)
- Olanzapine (Zyprexa) 30 mg/d (atypical antipsychotic)
- Dextroamphetamine (Dextrostat)10 mg/d (stimulant)
- Topiramate (Topamax) 100 mg/d (antiepileptic, anti-migraine, weight-loss agent)

Current medical medications

- Lansoprazole (Prevacid) 15 mg/d
- Diphenoxylate plus atropine (Lomotil) four tablets/d
- Cholestyramine (Questran) two packets/d

PATIENT FILE

Question

Based on what you know about this patient's history and current symptoms, would you consider her to be suffering from TRD or do you think she would be refractory (will never respond) to treatment altogether?

What conventional antidepressant-type treatments might you suggest?

- Lithium augmentation
- Thyroid augmentation
- Taper off medications and use an MAOI
- Try ECT again
- Try ketamine infusion therapy
- Try transcranial magnetic stimulation (TMS)
- Try vagus nerve stimulation (VNS)
- Try deep brain stimulation (DBS)
- Try magnetic seizure therapy (MST)

Attending physician's mental notes: initial evaluation

- The patient has melancholic MDD that is chronic and surprisingly has no other psychiatric comorbidities, which is relatively uncommon in this patient population
- Patient has marked psychomotor slowing: a symptom of melancholia or subtle psychotic depression? Could this be considered "psychiatric parkinsonism"?
- As she has had more than two years of unremitting symptoms without any full inter-episode recovery, this makes her depression chronic
- She should also be considered resistant as she has failed antidepressants from several different classes (TCA, SSRI, NDRI, SNRI, ECT) and augmentation strategies (olanzapine, dextroamphetamine, topiramate)
- She is treatment resistant so far, but she has not had some of the leading empirical augmentation strategies (lithium, thyroid) or an MAOI trial
- She also has utilized supportive psychotherapy well, but not formal CBT, IPT, or PDP
- Her regimen at her first outpatient visit is complicated and minimally effective. The prescriber could streamline her medications and discontinue ineffective medications as the current medications seem to be fairly well maximized
- She could be sent for neurostimulation treatment (VNS, DBS, TMS) given her medication failures and high treatment resistance, but ECT has already failed

Further investigation

Is there anything else you would especially like to know about this patient?

- What medical details about this patient are you concerned about?
- At the first visit, her weight was very low. Is she medically stable? Could she tolerate ECT or other neurostimulation treatments?
- Her medications seem contradictory in that she is on a weight gaining olanzapine (Zyprexa), but weight-losing topiramate (Topamax) and dextroamphetamine (Dextrostat)
- She has hyperlipidemia and CAD for which she is being treated. (Of note is that these were medications upon admission to author's service in 2000 and many of the warnings and guidelines about the atypical antipsychotic inducing metabolic disorders were not available until 2003–2004.)
- She has a family history of eating disorders and collateral information about her typical eating habits and body habitus should be collected
  - Preliminarily, she does not appear to suffer from AN
- Obtaining a nutrition or dietary consultation might be warranted as she is mostly immobile, bedridden, and her caloric intake is low
  - This may also help to determine if the patient is in a "failure to thrive" situation where an inpatient admission might be warranted
- Obtaining routine blood laboratory analyses and a discussion with her PCP is warranted, to determine medical stability for future treatment with psychotropics, neurostimulation techniques, and also to rule out medical causes of her depression

Question

Based on what you know about this patient's history, current symptoms, and treatment responses, do you think that a bona fide, formal trial of established psychotherapy is warranted?

- Yes, a referral for PDP is warranted
- Yes, a referral for CBT is warranted
- No, this patient has had many years of supportive, eclectic style psychotherapy and further psychotherapy intervention is unlikely to be effective
- No, specific psychotherapies are no better than eclectic psychotherapies in treating MDD
- No, this patient's cognitive impairment and psychomotor slowing would likely make psychotherapy ineffective

PATIENT FILE

Attending physician's mental notes: initial evaluation (continued)

- The patient is clearly depressed and seems to have had no clear benefit to monotherapy antidepressant treatments nor to her current aggressive augmentation regimen
- The patient may be psychotic given her marked cognitive impairment, but the current high-dose olanzapine (Zyprexa) use and past ECT trial likely rules out depressive psychosis, leaving her profound thought slowing and vegetative symptoms likely due to severe MDD without psychosis but with melancholic features
- She has a history of thorough antidepressant trial follow-through where full, therapeutic dosing has been utilized. Her husband is supportive and a good historian about her medical interventions
- Pharmacy records confirm her medication trials
  - Note that in the absence of a good historian or available medical records from previous providers, most pharmacies can print out medications dispensed, going back several years. This is often an easy way to tabulate how treatment resistant a patient is while confirming their medication trial history
- The patient really needs to be evaluated medically before more aggressive treatment is prescribed

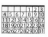

Case outcome: interim follow-ups through three months

- The patient is medically cleared without any concerns
  - Lipids are well controlled
  - Cardiac state is stable
  - Laboratory test results are normal
  - Nutritionally, she is meeting her minimal requirements despite her current weight and stature
- Psychotherapy was halted due to psychomotor and cognitive impairment
- A second trial of ECT was attempted. It was unclear if first trial was bilateral and conducted for at least 12 sessions. This second trial was also ineffective
- A reduction and streamlining of medications was refused as patient and spouse felt the medications were helpful to some degree, and feared a clinical worsening despite her current severe symptoms
- An inpatient stay was considered but her medical health was stable and she was not a danger to herself as her spouse is able to meet her instrumental activity needs
- TMS and DBS options were experimental and not readily available at the time. However, VNS was available at a local study site and this was more vigorously considered

Question

Considering her current medication regimen, what types of clinical monitoring might you utilize in the outpatient office setting?

- Routine measurement of weight and abdominal girth due to the use of an atypical antipsychotic
- Routine blood pressure monitoring due to the use of noradrenergic stimulant medication and the atypical antipsychotic
- An understanding with the primary care clinician that they will help monitor these as well and be responsible for continued treatment and monitoring of the patient's pre-existing hyperlipidemia. If not, independent monitoring of laboratory test results should occur in the psychiatric setting
- Topiramate (Topamax) has warnings about acidosis and requires blood draws to establish good renal function and then an absence of bicarbonate wasting over time. Patients on this medication should also be warned about acute eye pain and vision changes due to glaucoma, and about a loss of sweating (oligohydrosis) and risk of heat stroke and further weight loss

Attending physician's mental notes: four months

- Much collateral clinical information has been collected but no treatment changes issued as yet
- She has failed to achieve remission with multiple antidepressants, psychotherapy, and ECT
- Informed consent regarding lithium or thyroid augmentation was provided versus an experimental course of VNS
- At the time, VNS was not an approved treatment and two experimental open-label pilot studies showed good tolerability and reasonable effectiveness in highly treatment-resistant MDD patients
- Clinically, the patient perceived the offered medication augmentations to have end organ damage issues and the MAOI medications to have too many drug interaction issues. She was despondent that her previous medications had manipulated her brain monoamines excessively and to no avail. Hence, she had lost faith in pharmacotherapy
- The patient visited a VNS study team and was felt to be a good candidate for VNS given that
  - VNS is indicated for the adjunctive long-term treatment of chronic or recurrent depression for adult patients who experience MDEs and have not had an adequate response to four or more adequate antidepressant treatments
  - These four trials could be medications, psychotherapies, or ECT. This patient has had more than double the amount of qualifying treatment trials

– Present data would suggest that patients who have failed four medications (even with ECT) have very poor chances of achieving remission and then maintaining it, making experimental VNS a more viable option

Question

What would you do next?

- Allow patient to go for VNS
- Insist on an MAOI or other augmentation strategy

Case outcome: interim follow-ups through six months

- The patient enrolls in a trial, is implanted with the VNS pacemaker device, and allowed to heal for two weeks
- The device is started and titrated to a reasonable, suspected therapeutic dose (0.75–1.5 mA charge every 5 min)
- As the device sends small electrical currents afferently through the left vagus nerve, some charge dissipates toward the recurrent laryngeal nerve en route to the brainstem's nucleus tractus solitarius, causing temporary voice changes and hoarseness when the device activates every five minutes. This side effect lasts for 30 s, which the patient states she will be able to tolerate
- Other psychotropic medications continue as it is given that VNS is an adjunctive treatment and not studied as a monotherapy
- There is no effect two to three months after starting VNS and her acute VNS treatment is considered a failure

How long is a therapeutic trial of VNS?

- At the time of her enrollment in the study, this was unknown, but 8–10 weeks of treatment failed to separate from sham VNS treatments ultimately
- Therapeutic dosing was estimated to occur at 0.75–1.5 mA with the VNS device sending this charge to the brain every five minutes
- As this was an ongoing trial, the patient was allowed to continue VNS stimulation, despite its apparent acute failure, in a continuing manner while being evaluated for symptom reduction and tolerability over several years

Attending physician's mental notes: interim follow-up, nine months (continued)

- Patient is continued on the same medications
- Patient continues to be depressed to the same degree
- VNS continues at the same settings
- VNS is again considered to be ineffective but is allowed to continue as the device is permanently implanted and being evaluated by the FDA

Case outcome and multiple interim follow-ups to 12–120 months

- After one year of VNS treatment, the patient is unchanged and still depressed
- The VNS study team and prescribing clinician feel that the patient has failed to respond and are disappointed in this VNS therapy outcome. VNS follow-up now is for safety monitoring and occurs every three months, and the patient is asked to consider removing the ineffective device
- At 15 months of VNS treatment, the patient arrives with her spouse. Her hair is done and she is wearing makeup, which has not occurred in previous visits
- Her psychomotor impairment is moderately better to the degree in which the study team can engage her in a reciprocal conversation. She is deemed to be 30% better based on Hamilton Depression Rating Scale (HDRS) analysis
- After 18 months of VNS she is felt to be 70%–80% better, has no psychomotor or cognitive impairment, and informs the study team that she and her husband have purchased an RV camper, and they have planned several trips
- Her medications are continued as she is tolerating them well. Her metabolic parameters are controlled and there is no TD/EPS. It is unclear if she is responding to VNS alone, VNS plus her complex medication regimen, or if her depression remitted on its own after three decades
- Over a 10-year period of treatment with VNS
  - There has been no relapse into a full depression
  - The VNS dosing has increased in response to minor depression (threatened relapses detected as slight increases in scores on the HDRS) to where her device activates every 1.8 min, more than doubling her cumulative dose
  - The voice altering side effects gradually dissipated to the point of being undetectable by a layperson

Case debrief

- The patient has a lengthy history of chronic MDD that was not comorbid with other psychiatric or medical conditions, which is quite rare. This made her a good candidate for a VNS study focusing on TRD
- She failed to respond to many medications and solid psychotherapy attempts. Albeit, her psychotherapy did not give her formal CBT or PDP approaches
- She likely represents the most optimal, and by no means typical, response to long-term VNS. The study team and the prescribing clinician reported that they saw little hope of response given her chronic treatment history and ECT failure

- The learning curve in this case involved dosing VNS effectively and to wait out its longer therapeutic duration needed for effectiveness when compared to medication and psychotherapy trials
- Given the typically poor outcomes of sustaining a remission after successful treatment with medication or ECT, her VNS and all of her medications were continued over the long term. It appears that this patient meets the endpoint whereby those patients who achieve a remission by VNS tend to maintain remission for at least two years (69%). In this case, it has been 10 years
- This patient also fell into the category where one out of six patients is expected to achieve a remission that is based on less stringent open-label regulatory trial data
- However, her remission via VNS occurred well after a year of treatment where many patients see effects after three months but within one year

Take-home points

- This case emphasizes the need for full therapeutic trials of antidepressant treatments, augmentations, combinations, psychotherapy, *and VNS*
- VNS generally takes weeks or months to become effective
- Therapeutic dosing should be considered at 1–1.5 mA electrical charge with device activation every 1.8–5 min
- Cumulative dosing (dosing charge times frequency) seems to be a determining factor as well as longitudinal use over time. This is a newer finding
- VNS, when effective, appears to maintain its response equal to or better than medications alone
- VNS was FDA approved based upon long-term, open-label data and its comparison to an equally ill, depressed cohort not receiving VNS treatment. The VNS TRD patient has a 2:1 response rate over patients who received non-VNS but otherwise treatment as usual
- These data appear to have been compelling to the FDA, who deemed it approved for treating depression in 2005, but many insurance companies consider it experimental as there was never a long-term trial of VNS versus a sham control proving the device may become effective over a one-year period
- As a counterargument, investigators felt that giving a severely depressed patient a sham placebo treatment over 12–18 months would be unethical. The controversy about this treatment and adequate insurance coverage continues

Performance in practice: confessions of a psychopharmacologist

- *What could have been done better here?*
  - Was the patient on too many medications at the time of VNS?
  - Should the patient have been directed more toward the MAOI monotherapy, or use of more classic augmentations?
- *Possible action items for improvement in practice*
  - Make sure that augmentation/combination strategies are all considered and weighed against device-based treatments
  - Discussing options outside medications is always warranted. Psychotherapy or device-based treatments offer a way to treat MDD outside the norm and likely utilizes different mechanisms of action compared to our usual monoamine facilitation strategies. Sometimes this makes a difference in outcome
  - Of course, this means pushing the clinician's clinical envelope with regard to knowledge base. Outside being up-to-date on new medications, clinicians have to be aware of the indications, risks, and benefits of new device-based treatments

Tips and pearls

- VNS is FDA approved for TRD after four antidepression treatment failures, which include medications, psychotherapy, or ECT
- Many insurance carriers deny this treatment in their policy despite FDA approval, likely due to the up-front cost, although will consider it upon appeal on a case-by-case basis
- It has been studied in relatively non-comorbid, treatment-resistant patients. Therefore, to obtain outcomes seen in trials, similar patient selection is warranted
- It takes a long time, comparatively, for VNS to become effective and must be dosed judiciously, similar to strategies employed in administering medications or even psychotherapy

Mechanism of action moment

How does VNS theoretically work?

- Of course, there is no clear mechanism, but theoretically, it has preclinical evidence of antidepressant activity in several ways
- Medications manipulate neurotransmitters and receptors to change neurochemical activity, which often changes neuronal electrical firing. VNS may actually use electricity to change neuronal firing directly, thus changing neurochemical activity
  - Antidepressants are known to increase chemical neurotransmitter concentrations and these change electrical neuronal firing

- VNS appears to increase electrical neuronal firing with a resultant change in chemical neurotransmitter concentrations
- As a net result from either approach, brain neurocircuitry functioning changes, and ideally, symptoms are alleviated
- The left vagus nerve terminates in the brainstem and has secondary neural connections with brain areas associated with depression, such as the dorsal raphe (DR), LC, amygdala, insula, hypothalamus, and thalamus
- Increased DR and LC firing rates have been noted during VNS use, suggesting facilitation of 5-HT and NE, similar to antidepressant effects
- VNS promotes increases in neurotrophic factors that promote neuronal health and synaptic formation. This may allow for improved neurocircuitry function and alleviation of symptoms
- VNS increases in brain activity were found in the bilateral orbitofrontal cortex (OFC), bilateral anterior cingulate cortex (ACC), and right superior and medial frontal cortex. Decreases were found in the bilateral temporal cortex and right parietal area. Regions of change were consistent with brain structures associated with MDD symptomatology and the afferent pathways of the vagus nerve
- VNS therapy is associated with ventromedial prefrontal cortex (VMPFC) deactivation and produced greater right insula activation, which are similar to other antidepressant treatment findings
- Finally, VNS may allow for deactivation in the VMPFC, which correlates with the antidepressant response to VNS therapy

These preclinical and human model studies suggest VNS has properties similar to other FDA-approved depression treatments and facilitates brain activity in areas of the brain noted to be dysfunctional in major depression.

Two-minute tutorial

VNS side effects

- According to studies, during the first three months of VNS stimulation, adverse effects are no greater than 1.3%
- The most common side effects are VNS stimulation-related
  - voice alteration (59%)
  - increased cough (24%)
  - neck pain (16%)
  - dyspnea (14%)
  - dysphagia (13%)
  - paresthesia (11%)
  - laryngismus (10%)
- These side effects may dissipate over one year in up to 70% of patients
- VNS is not associated with weight gain or sexual problems and has no drug–drug interactions

- Surgical complications may include infection, general anesthesia reactions, and permanent left vocal cord paralysis
- The device may be turned off via a computer in the office setting or by use of a magnet by the patient in the home setting, in order to stop stimulation and lower side effects
- VNS device settings may be changed to lower side effects
  - The overall charge or its pulse width may be reduced to dampen the amount of electrical current reaching tissues in the neck and therefore lowering side-effect burden
  - The charge may be lowered to avoid side effects but dosing may be maintained by having the device activate every one to three minutes instead of every five minutes. This cumulative dosing may be used in patients who cannot tolerate higher charge doses to facilitate better VNS effectiveness
- Programing the device is pain free. A hand-held computer sends programing signals via a radio frequency wand that transmits the new settings to the internal pacemaker, which sits internally below the scapula and medial of the axilla
- Patients with VNS must avoid certain forms of high-dose ultrasound, lithotripsy, and magnetic resonance imaging (MRI) scans, as the device may malfunction or the VNS wires may overheat theoretically causing nerve damage

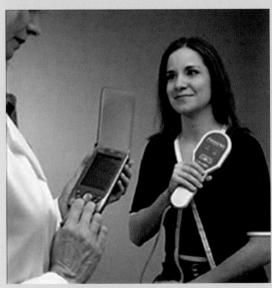

Figure 4.1. The VNS hand-held device and programing wand.

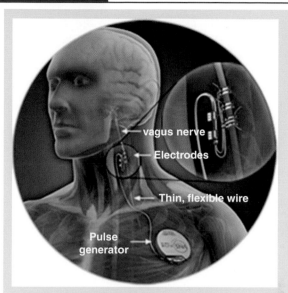

Figure 4.2. The VNS device placement, VNS generator, and wire leads.

Neurostimulation and neuromodulatory devices other than VNS

Electroconvulsive therapy (ECT)

- Is non-surgical
- FDA approved for depression although currently the FDA is discussing revising its FDA-approved device status as many devices were grandfathered an approval for MDD treatment
- Generally is accepted as very effective for the acute treatment of resistant depression, psychotic depression
- Works in the acute setting (whereas VNS works chronically) but long-term maintenance ECT may not be as effective

Transcranial magnetic stimulation (TMS)

- Is non-surgical
- FDA approved since 2008 for depression that is resistant to initial antidepressant therapy or for patients who cannot tolerate an initial antidepressant. (Patients failing four or more antidepressants were not part of regulatory trials, although many insurances insist on four trials)
- Works acutely over four to six weeks of treatment
- Magnetic coil is placed over the left DLPFC and stimulation is given every day
- Magnet creates electrical cortical impulses and neuronal activity in a focused brain area that may be associated with generating depressive symptoms when hypoactive

- Side effects are minimal: headache, toothache, ear pain. Rarely may induce a seizure

Deep brain stimulation (DBS)

- FDA approved to treat intractable tremors and for compassionate use in refractory obsessive compulsive disorder (OCD). Is being actively studied in TRD and has prior approvals for Parkinson's disease tremors and dyskinesias
- Requires more invasive, sterotactic insertion of two electrodes in deeper brain areas (i.e., Brodmann Area 25) and implantation of a pacemaker/generator device (similar to VNS)
- Stimulation side effects may include dizziness, insomnia, or hypomania. Acute clinical antidepressant effects appear to be rapid and within minutes of activating electrodes in some cases

Magnetic seizure therapy (MST)

- Is non-surgical
- Is experimental and not FDA approved
- Uses a device similar to TMS but with a stronger magnet and the ability to stimulate the cortex to a focal seizure (instead of generalized seizure, like those in ECT)
- May avoid the cognitive side effects of ECT

Transcranial direct current stimulation

- Is non-surgical
- Limited FDA approval with limited data available, this noninvasive brain stimulation technique involves the application of a low-amplitude direct current by two small electrodes placed on the scalp skin surface for up to 20 minutes at a time
- A small amount of current passes through the scalp where it induces changes in cortical excitability
- Modulation of neuronal resting membrane potentials appears to be the antidepressant mechanism. Alterations in glutamate NMDA receptor efficacy have also been noted

Epidural prefrontal cortical stimulation (EpCS)

- In this application, a Band-Aid size electrode is placed underneath the skull but on the surface of the prefrontal cortex. This is more invasive than TMS, MST, and VNS but less invasive than DBS, as EpCS electrodes are not placed into brain matter. These electrodes are also stimulated by a pacemaker/generator-type device

Posttest self-assessment question and answer

Which of the following is (are) not an invasive surgical treatment for resistant depression?

A. TMS

B. VNS

C. ECT
D. DBS
E. EpCS
F. A and C
G. B and D
H. All of the above

Answer: F

TMS and ECT are treatments that are not invasive and rendered at or near to the surface of the scalp. VNS, DNS, EpCS all require invasive surgeries.

References

1. http://dynamic.cyberonics.com/depression/hcp/THESYNAPSE/conway .htm. Accessed March 25, 2011.
2. Stahl SM. *Stahl's Essential Psychopharmacology*, 4th edn, New York, NY: Cambridge University Press, 2013; Ch. 12.
3. Stahl SM. *Stahl's Essential Psychopharmacology: The Prescriber's Guide*, 5th edn. New York, NY: Cambridge University Press, 2014.
4. American Psychiatric Association. *Practice Guideline for the Treatment of Patients with Major Depressive Disorder*, 3rd edn. Washington, DC: American Psychiatric Association Press, 2010.
5. George MS, Rush AJ, Marangell LB, et al. A one-year comparison of vagus nerve stimulation with treatment as usual for treatment-resistant depression. *Biol Psychiatry* 2005; 58:364–73.
6. Dorr AE, Debonnel G. Effect of vagus nerve stimulation on serotonergic and noradrenergic transmission. *J Pharmacol Exp Ther* 2006; 318:890–8.
7. Follesa P, Biggio F, Gorini G, et al. Vagus nerve stimulation increases norepinephrine concentration and the gene expression of BDNF and bFGF in the rat brain. *Brain Res* 2007; 1179:28–34.
8. Henry TR. Therapeutic mechanisms of vagus nerve stimulation. *Neurology* 2002; 59:S3–14.
9. Huynh N, McIntyre R. Algorithms: STAR*D, positives, negatives and implications for clinical practice. In: Schwartz TL, Petersen T, eds. *Depression Treatment Strategies and Management*, 2nd edn. New York, NY: Informa, 2009; Ch. 5.
10. Conway CR, Sheline YI, Chibnall JT, et al. Cerebral blood flow changes during vagus nerve stimulation for depression. *Psychiatry Res Neuroimaging* 2006; 146:179–84.
11. Zimmerman M, Chelminski I, Young D, Dalrymple K. Using outcome measures to promote better outcomes. *Clin Neuropsychiatry* 2011; 8:21–36.
12. Nahas Z, Teneback C, Chae JH, et al. Serial vagus nerve stimulation functional MRI in treatment-resistant depression. *Neuropsychopharmacology* 2007;32:1649–60.

13. Carpenter LL, Philip NS, O'Reardon J. Advances in neurostimulation for depression: electroconvulsive therapy, transcranial magnetic stimulation, vagus nerve stimulation and deep brain stimulation. In: Schwartz TL, Petersen T, eds. *Depression Treatment Strategies and Management*, 2nd edn. New York, NY: Informa, 2009; Ch. 9.

14. Carpenter LL, Megna JL, Herrera-Rojas M, Siddiqui UA. When medications fail. Neurostimulation therapies for depression. *Clin Neuropsychiatry* 2011; 8:61–80.

15. Rush AJ, Trivedi MH, Wisniewski SR, et al. Acute and longer-term outcomes in depressed outpatients requiring one or several treatment steps: a STAR*D report. *Am J Psychiatry* 2006; 163:1905–17.

The Case: The primary care physician who went the prescribing distance but came up short

The Question: Do atypical antipsychotics treat generalized anxiety?

The Psychopharmacological dilemma: Finding an effective treatment for chronic treatment-resistant generalized anxiety in an elderly patient

Pretest self-assessment question (answer at the end of the case)

What pharmacologic properties of quetiapine (Seroquel) lend themselves to providing clinical antidepressant and anxiolytic properties?

A. 5-HT1A partial receptor agonism (similar to buspirone [BuSpar], vilazodone [Viibryd])

B. Norepinephrine reuptake inhibition (NRI) properties (similar to bupropion-XL [Wellbutrin-XL])

C. Histamine-1 (H1) receptor antagonism (similar to hydroxyzine [Vistaril], doxepin [Silenor])

D. Selective serotonin reuptake inhibitor (SSRI) properties similar to fluoxetine (Prozac)

E. GABA-A receptor modulating properties similar to diazepam (Valium)

F. A, B, and C

G. All of the above

Patient evaluation on intake

- 83-year-old man states he has been anxious for at least 40 years and is not getting better in the primary care setting

Psychiatric history

- Onset of GAD in his 40s. Has fluctuating course of GAD ranging from mild to incapacitating. He states he has always had some level of anxiety and cannot recollect a substantial anxiety-free period
- He was actually doing well per his standards until about 18 months prior to the first office visit and felt his medications "controlled" his anxiety but did not alleviate it
- Has had increasing medical problems with age and has developed a hypochondriacal component to his GAD. He has become increasingly concerned about death and dying as a result of his medical issues, which is felt to be adjustment-based and somewhat set in reality, but he also has marked anxiety about medications and their possible side effects shortening his life further
- A review of psychiatric symptoms surprisingly shows no depression, psychosis, mania, other anxiety disorder, SUD, or personality disorder

- He had two to three voluntary, private psychiatric hospitalizations in the 1970s due to insomnia and worry. He states insomnia is a chief complaint again now. He has had no suicide attempts
  - In the past he has gone to eclectic, supportive psychotherapy but has had no formal CBT or PDP interventions
  - He has been treated pharmacologically by his PCP
- Previous medication trials included:
  - Diazepam (Valium) 30–60 mg/d, lorazepam (Ativan) 1–4 mg/d for many years effectively and without misuse or side effects
  - Paroxetine (Paxil) [SSRI] 30–40 mg/d, zolpidem (Ambien) [BZRA] 10 mg/d were used more recently with good effect and without misuse or side effects

Social and personal history

- Is married
- Gainfully employed in the engineering field for 50 years and is now retired and financially stable
- Was once very active but his medical problems have now precluded him from many of his usual activities
- Does not drink alcohol, smoke cigarettes, or take drugs of abuse

Medical history

- Has survived prostate cancer
- Myelodysplastic syndrome requires transfusions with transient iron toxicity
- Osteoporosis
- HTN

Family history

- Denies significant family mental health issues

Current psychiatric medications

- Escitalopram (Lexapro) 20 mg/d (SSRI)
- Mirtazapine (Remeron) 45 mg/d (NaSSA)
- Doxepin (Sinequan) 50 mg /d (TCA, low dose)

Current medical medications

- Nebivolol (Bystolic) 20 mg/d
- Zoledronic acid (Reclast) 5 mg/yr
- Epoetin (Procrit) 100 unit/kg/3 wk
- Darbepoetin alfa (Aranesp) 0.45 mcg/kg/2 wk

Question

Based on what you know about this patient's history and current symptoms, would you consider him to be suffering from treatment-resistant anxiety (TRA)?

- Yes
- No

What type of treatment might you suggest next?

- Maximize his doxepin (Sinequan) to full TCA therapeutic dosing
- Add a BZ–sedative in combination
- Add or switch to buspirone (BuSpar), a 5-HT1A partial agonist anxiolytic
- Switch to an SNRI like: venlafaxine-XR (Effexor-XR), duloxetine (Cymbalta), desvenlafaxine (Effexor-XR), levomilnacipran (Fetzima)
- Refer for CBT

Attending physician's mental notes: initial evaluation

- Patient has marked chronic history of non-comorbid GAD. He has never been symptom free but has had relatively long periods of well-controlled symptoms that are mild in nature
- Patient had 10–20 years of effective care with moderate-dose BZ sedatives. Why were these stopped? Addiction? Ataxia? Apnea?
- TRD is gaining ground as a clinical entity and approvals exist for TRD (olanzapine–fluoxetine combination [Symbyax], VNS, TMS, quetiapine [Seroquel])
  - Perhaps this patient has TRA as he has clearly failed two SSRIs (paroxetine and now escitalopram), two sedatives, and an NaSSA antidepressant (mirtazapine), supportive psychotherapy, and currently is failing a full dose of an SSRI plus NaSSA combination with low-dose TCA
- He appears to have much hypochondriacal thought, which may make prescribing side effect-prone medications tenuous and hurt compliance
- Collaboration with primary care and/or hematology is warranted
- Geriatric age may make dosing psychotropics proceed slowly and cautiously

Further investigation

Is there anything else you would especially like to know about this patient?

- Does he really have no psychiatric comorbidity, and does his medical history contribute to his anxiety?
  - Hypochondriasis (illness anxiety disorder in the *DSM-5*) is defined as a preoccupation with fears of having, or the idea that one has, serious disease based on the person's misinterpretation of bodily symptoms

This type of anxiety must persist despite appropriate medical evaluation and reassurance. In addition, it cannot be better accounted for by GAD. This patient reports that his anxiety symptoms regarding medical health really began a few years back when he started to have significant medical problems such as cancer. Prior to this, he reports that he was not preoccupied with his medical conditions or symptoms

- Primary insomnia occurs when the predominant complaint is difficulty initiating or maintaining sleep, or having non-restorative sleep. The insomnia must cause significant distress or impairment. Previously, it was felt that insomnia must not occur exclusively during the course of another mental disorder such as MDD or GAD
  - However, the *DSM-5* allows insomnia to be a stand-alone, comorbid psychiatric entity if it is a focus of clinical attention. It may not need to be declared if insomnia is primary, or secondary to another psychiatric or medical disorder
  - This patient reports classic "clock-watching" fear and phobia at nighttime. He reports these symptoms began after reading a report that patients who sleep less than eight hours are more likely to die of cardiac arrest
- Adjustment disorder is the development of an emotional or behavioral set of symptoms in response to an identifiable stressor. These symptoms are clinically significant in that the patient shows marked distress that is in excess of what would be expected from exposure to the stressor or that the patient has significant impairment in functioning. Again, for this *DSM-5* diagnosis, the adjustment does not meet criteria for MDD, anxiety disorder, etc. This patient's GAD symptoms have been ongoing for many years, but they seem to be exacerbated by adjustment-related issues due to his age, more severe medical conditions, threat of mortality. His insomnia and illness anxiety seem to fit under the rubric of generalized anxiety, but chronologically seem to be fueled by real-world stressful issues causing an exacerbation of GAD symptoms
- Iron deficiency/iron toxicity: iron deficiency often results in anemia and a clinical picture more consistent with depression or dementia. Iron toxicity, however, is mostly asymptomatic. Nonspecific early symptoms (such as abdominal discomfort and fatigue) may delay diagnosis until severe damage to the heart or liver produces clinically apparent symptoms. Anxiety exacerbation is not typical

Question

Based on what you know about this patient's history, current symptoms, and treatment responses, do you think that a bona fide, formal trial of established psychotherapy is warranted?

- Yes, a referral for PDP is warranted

- Yes, a referral for CBT is warranted
- No, this patient has had many years of supportive, eclectic style psychotherapy and further psychotherapy intervention is unlikely to be effective
- No, this patient's anxiety levels would likely make psychotherapy ineffective

Attending physician's mental notes: initial evaluation (continued)

- The patient is clearly suffering from a baseline of moderate to severe GAD, which appears to be complicated by adjustment disorder. He is reaching the end of his life span and is having pertinent medical issues that have increased his anxiety about mortality. As a result, he is much more functionally fixated about bodily sensations, side effects, and minor medical issues, which makes him appear to have illness anxiety
- The patient also seems very fixated about obtaining adequate sleep and has developed intense fear about a lack of sleep and the impact it will have on his life span. Insomnia is clearly part of GAD, but this patient's intense fear may need to be addressed clinically in a similar manner as the phobia associated with primary insomnia
- The recent PCP has done an excellent job of escalating two antidepressant agents and adding a third antidepressant that is known for inducing sleep. He has "gone the distance" likely as much as a primary care clinician can for treating this TRA. The patient, therefore, is currently on a therapeutic and reasonably aggressive psychopharmacology regimen, but without a response
- Again, if the combination of SSRI plus a BZ has been effective in the past, why have BZs not been used recently? There is no history of obstructive apnea, gait instability, cognitive impairment, addiction, etc.

Case outcome: interim follow-ups through one month

- The patient is medically cleared in that there is no obvious contribution of his medical problems with regard to causing his psychiatric problems. His red cell count and iron levels are adequately monitored and treated. His blood pressure is well controlled. There is no evidence of metabolic disorder
- The patient was offered a formal trial of CBT to address his generalized anxiety and phobia issues but he declined
- As the patient seemed relatively comfortable on his current set of medications with regard to tolerability, knowing that he would have anxious difficulty changing medications or adding new medications, it was decided to keep him on the current medications

- However, augmentation with the previously tried "as needed only" BZ, lorazepam (Ativan), was discussed. The patient states that he had no issues with the sedatives outside becoming aware that they were possibly addictive, which made him and his wife worried; therefore, he stopped them. With permission, this was also discussed with his spouse who corroborated his story
- Lorazepam (Ativan) 0.5 mg/d was initiated as a standing dose and added to the current medication regimen

Question

If the patient responds dramatically to the addition of this BZ, what would you consider next?

- Continue all four medications. He has treatment-resistant GAD and this pharmacodynamic regimen of complex polypharmacy is likely required to prevent relapse
- As he was minimally responsive to maximal doses of escitalopram (Lexapro) and mirtazapine (Remeron), his marked recovery on the BZ suggests that the antidepressant treatments are no longer needed and they should be systematically tapered off
- Continue the fully dosed, therapeutic escitalopram (Lexapro) and mirtazapine (Remeron) but discontinue the subtherapeutically dosed doxepin (Sinequan) in order to streamline his medications

Case outcome: interim follow-ups through two months

- The patient called the office several times reporting that his remarkable insomnia continued
- The patient called the office several times in the middle of his transfusions where he was watching his pulse and blood pressure readings and reported they went higher and higher. He states he had to utilize some of his BZ to lower his pulse and blood pressure. He states he was very worried about dying, based upon reading his vital signs in real time
- If the patient did not receive a return call in somewhat short order, he would contact support staff, also on multiple occasions
- He was not having overt panic attacks but genuinely appeared concerned about these issues, which he equated to serious medical problems associated with premature mortality
- His lorazepam (Ativan) was increased to 0.5 mg twice a day, which he admitted worked adequately for him in the past

Case outcome: interim follow-ups through three months

- As before, the patient called the office several times reporting that his marked insomnia and medical problems continued

- Additionally, as before, if the patient did not receive a return call in somewhat short order, he would contact support staff on multiple occasions.
- His lorazepam (Ativan) was increased to 1 mg twice a day

Question

What would you do next?

- Continue to titrate his BZ sedative standing dose as needed to treat anxiety to remission
- Consider changing his current antidepressant regimen to an SNRI such as venlafaxine-ER (Effexor-XR) or duloxetine (Cymbalta), as both have GAD approvals
- Consider removing ineffective TCA, doxepin (Sinequan), and augmenting his current antidepressant regimen with an atypical antipsychotic
- Consider removing ineffective doxepin (Sinequan) and augmenting his current antidepressant regimen with a calcium channel blocking epilepsy medication such as gabapentin (Neurontin)
- Consider removing all three to four ineffective medications and utilize atypical antipsychotic monotherapy

Attending physician's mental notes: four-month follow-ups

- Escalating the BZ lorazepam (Ativan) seemingly has no significant benefit initially
- The patient began to utilize it in more of an as-needed fashion, and repeatedly called for increasing doses, suggesting a penchant toward overuse
- Given these factors, it must be strictly utilized in twice-a-day fashion without flexibility on the patient's behalf to use as needed
- The patient then calls for escalations in doxepin (Sinequan) or mirtazapine (Remeron) to treat his anxiety flare-ups during the day and his insomnia at night

Question

What do you consider next?

- Continue escalating the BZ systematically but without any privileges of an as-needed basis
- Streamline medication regimen by removing ineffective products and augmenting remaining products

Case outcome: interim follow-ups through four months (continued)

- Patient again refuses formal CBT
- Now is anxious about his escalation of BZ use and refuses any systematic titration but prefers to leave the dose as it is because it is providing some anxiolytic relief
- After full informed consent, is agreeable to streamlining his medications as follows
  - Tapering off of doxepin (Sinequan) as it is not helping his sleep and he is already on the highly H1 receptor antagonizing NaSSA antidepressant mirtazapine (Remeron)
  - Continuing his mirtazapine (Remeron), escitalopram (Lexapro)
  - Augmenting with the atypical antipsychotic quetiapine (Seroquel) with the prospect of tapering off the BZ once this atypical antipsychotic becomes effective

Attending physician's mental notes: interim follow-ups through four months

- As this patient has failed to respond to differing antidepressants, or a low-dose BZ, the use of an augmenting agent with a different pharmacodynamic mechanism of action seems warranted
- He will need to be monitored for metabolic disorder more closely, onset of EPS, TD, development of vision change, if an atypical antipsychotic is started

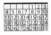

Case outcome and multiple interim follow-ups to six months

- Quetiapine (Seroquel) is titrated slowly from 25 mg/d up to 150 mg/d
- Appreciates its sedating quality at night and reports that he does not need doxepin (Sinequan) at all
- Reports that he is still anxious throughout the day and continues to require 1 mg of lorazepam (Ativan) standing dose as a result
- Instructed to take 25 mg of quetiapine (Seroquel) twice during the daytime and to leave the remaining 100 mg to bedtime to continue treating his insomnia
- Reports some success. However, now complains of significant daytime fatigue and requests to lower his quetiapine (Seroquel) and to again increase use of lorazepam (Ativan)
- Patient is told not to escalate his BZ, and is asked to visit the office in order to discuss future treatment options. At this session he is offered
  - Another atypical antipsychotic with less sedation such as aripiprazole (Abilify)
  - Removal of all medications as being ineffective/intolerable and proceed with a GAD approved SNRI monotherapy such as venlafaxine (Effexor-XR) or duloxetine (Cymbalta)

- Consideration of changing his Seroquel (quetiapine) to the slow-release version quetiapine-XR (Seroquel-XR)
- This patient chose the latter and was switched to 150 mg of quetiapine-XR (Seroquel-XR) while he was maintained on his usual mirtazapine (Remeron) and escitalopram (Lexapro)
- However, he called back a few weeks later to report that his GAD symptoms were gradually abating on the quetiapine-XR preparation, but his ability to fall asleep diminished and his insomnia was returning
- Instead of manipulating his medication regimen at this point, he chose a CBT psychotherapy approach for his residual insomnia

Case debrief

- The patient has a lengthy history of chronic GAD, which has been exacerbated by adjustment disorder issues and possibly complicated by legitimate primary insomnia. He initially responded to BZ monotherapy many years ago and more recently failed to respond to several initial antidepressant treatments
- The antidepressants were maximized in the primary care setting prior to referral to psychiatric practice for further augmentation. Here, he was augmented with low-dose BZ but with some risk of misuse and inconsistent use. This approach was abandoned for the augmentation strategy of utilizing an atypical antipsychotic, which ultimately was effective for his TRA
- Eventually, the patient did accept CBT for the treatment of his primary insomnia-like symptoms, which diminished over time
- As the addition of the atypical antipsychotic became remarkably more helpful, his medications were streamlined, where the BZ and his antidepressant doses were halved
- He gained 10 lb of weight but overall remained metabolically stable and without any abnormal movement disorder

Take-home points

- This case emphasizes the need for full therapeutic trials of antidepressant treatments, augmentations, combinations, psychotherapy, and liaison with primary care and other specialty providers
- This case also illustrates how some generally anxious patients with hypochondriacal thinking can be very difficult to manage given their high medical service utilization rates and difficulty tolerating medication regimens
- Many psychotropic agents are now available in immediate-release and slow-release preparations. Typically, slow-release preparations maintain lower plasma levels of drug concentration and theoretically yield less side-effect burden

- In this patient's case, the side effect of somnolence was actually a positive therapeutic effect. While trying to mitigate daytime fatigue by using a slow-release preparation, there was a loss of clinical effectiveness in treating his insomnia. These pharmacokinetics must be weighed when choosing a psychotropic, and sometimes combining an immediate-release and a slow-release preparation of the same psychotropic may be quite effective and clinically warranted
  - Some prescribers consider using both immediate-release and slow-release preparations in the same patient, but for different clinical reasons
    - The immediate-release quetiapine has a faster peak plasma level that is clinically associated with greater sedation and somnolence. It may peak within an hour and work as an off-label hypnotic for some patients
    - The slow-release preparation may not be sedating enough within its first three hours after ingestion to induce sleep, but it may therapeutically last longer throughout the day to provide less sedating anxiolysis
    - The immediate-release version is used to improve sleep and the slow release for anxiolysis
- FDA approval for GAD include some of the BZs, buspirone (BuSpar), venlafaxine-XR (Effexor-XR), and duloxetine (Cymbalta), and some of the SSRIs. Although none of these agents were utilized in this case, it is important to know which agents are formally approved for use and to advise the patient when off-label approaches are utilized

Performance in practice: confessions of a psychopharmacologist

- *What could have been done better here?*
  - The lorazepam (Ativan) dosing was limited due to fear of its misuse. In this case, the fear of misuse was not about addiction but more toward ataxia or fall potential. It certainly could have been maximized further
  - The use of antihistamine products to promote better sleep is reasonable. In this case, both mirtazapine (Remeron) and doxepin (Sinequan) were utilized but with limited results. Possibly, utilizing more BZ sedative at night may have improved sleep or use of a more formal BZ receptor agonist (BZRA) such as zolpidem (Ambien) or zaleplon (Sonata) might have been more effective
- *Possible action items for improvement in practice*
  - Instead of escalating polypharmacy in this geriatric but fairly medically stable patient, perhaps streamlining medications back to an FDA-approved SNRI would make sense. In this case, venlafaxine-XR (Effexor-XR) would be approved and also have a minimum of drug–drug interactions

– Discussing options outside of medications is always warranted. Psychotherapy, CBT in this case, may ultimately be helpful and relatively side effect free

Tips and pearls

- The SNRI class of antidepressants is approved for the treatment of MDD and also a myriad of anxiety disorders
- Each SNRI (except for levomilnacipran) appears to be more serotonergic at low doses, and more noradrenergic at higher doses, allowing the clinician to tailor treatment based upon how much of each neurotransmitter is desired
- It may be possible to create SNRI-like mechanisms of action or facilitate both neurotransmitters through rational polypharmacy approaches when one starts with an SSRI monotherapy
- Classically, a clinician may add a predominant NRI TCA such as desipramine (Norpramin) or the NDRI bupropion-XL (Wellbutrin-XL) to an SSRI
  - A more novel approach would be to augment with certain atypical antipsychotics that have NRI potential (quetiapine [Seroquel]), ziprasidone (Geodon), stimulants, or the ADHD medication atomoxetine in order to convert an SSRI into an SNRI-similar mechanism of action. Mirtazapine (Remeron) does not have an NRI component but can facilitate NET through alpha-2a receptor antagonism

Two-minute tutorial

Is quetiapine (Seroquel) an antipsychotic, anti-manic, antidepressant, anxiolytic, or a hypnotic?

- Quetiapine (Seroquel) and its slow-release preparation quetiapine-XR (Seroquel-XR) are multifactorial drugs. The parent drug and its metabolite, norquetiapine, both have complicated, multimodal pharmacodynamic profiles, which lend themselves to treating a myriad of psychiatric symptoms
- These two products carry approvals for the treatment of schizophrenia, manic or mixed states associated with bipolar disorder, as monotherapy or as adjunctive treatment to lithium or divalproex, bipolar depression, maintenance treatment in bipolar disorder in conjunction with those patients already taking lithium or divalproex, as adjunctive therapy in patients with MDD who have failed to respond to initial antidepressant therapy, and have published data currently suggesting its use for GAD. Clinically, quetiapine (Seroquel) and quetiapine-XR (Seroquel-XR) are often used in an off-label manner to treat the symptom of insomnia

- These drugs may exhibit different pharmacological properties at different dosing levels. For example, these two agents appear to be better at treating MDD at lower doses, mania at moderate doses, and psychosis at high doses. In the literature, dosing strategies range from 50 mg/d to 1500 mg/d
- Although many of the atypical antipsychotics appear to be effective in treating affective disorder symptoms, the risks and benefits must be weighed by both the clinician and the patient equally, given the ability of atypical antipsychotics to cause metabolic and movement disorders

Pharmacodynamics of quetiapine and norquetiapine

- Higher doses (400–800 mg/d) are required to control the symptoms associated with mania or psychosis, as its D2 receptor antagonism is quite weak due to low affinity compared to all other atypical antipsychotics. Doses greater than 800 mg/d and up to 2400 mg/d have been noted in anecdotal reports
- This does not suggest it has low effectiveness, but rather requires more dosing milligrams to maintain at least 60% D2 receptor occupancy to stop psychosis or mania. This low affinity may allow for quetiapine to maintain a lower EPS side-effect profile as a benefit
- Quetiapine is approved as a monotherapy for bipolar depression, and also as an augmentation strategy when added to SSRI or SNRI antidepressants in unipolar MDD. D2 antagonism cannot explain its antidepressant effectiveness
- Multiple, confirmative, regulatory studies have consistently shown that lower doses of quetiapine are effective in treating depressive states (150–600 mg/d). Quetiapine also has some limited data in the treatment of GAD at doses starting at 50 mg/d
- Treating depression or anxiety at these lower doses likely does not inhibit DA transmission compared to higher doses used in mania or schizophrenia
- Its antidepressant effects may come from several different mechanisms of action
  - This drug has marked H1 receptor antagonism (antihistamine properties), which promotes sedation and weight gain. H1 receptor antagonism is also the theoretical mechanism of anxiolysis utilized by the approved anxiolytic agent, hydroxyzine (Vistaril/Atarax), and a mechanism for hypnosis utilized by over the counter diphenhydramine (Benadryl) products and the prescription sleep-inducing agent doxepin (Silenor). Therefore, H1 receptor blockade in certain patients causes sedation and somnolence as adverse effects, but in others may be regarded as providing the positive clinical effects of anxiolysis and hypnosis, which are beneficial in those with MDD or GAD

- Quetiapine also has 5-HT2A and 2C receptor antagonism. The former lowers EPS risk and also allows more cortical noradrenergic transmission to occur. The 5-HT2C blockade hypothetically allows for loss of interneuronal GABA inhibition in the brainstem, with resultant increases in cortical DA transmission from the VTA and NE from the LC. Facilitation of these two monoamines may improve mood, drive, motivation, concentration, and vigilance
- Finally, 5-HT2C antagonism may allow for improved sleep architecture, sleep efficiency, and greater slow wave sleep capacity. The antihistamine and promonoamine properties are suggestive of an antidepressant profile
- Specifically, the active norquetiapine metabolite has two interesting features
    ○ It allows for 5-HT1A receptor partial agonism similar to the approved anxiolytic buspirone (BuSpar) and the recently approved novel antidepressant vilazodone (Viibryd)
    ○ It has NRI properties similar to properties possessed by approved unipolar antidepressants such as venlafaxine-XR (Effexor-XR), duloxetine (Cymbalta), bupropion-XL (Wellbutrin-XL), and nortriptyline (Pamelor)
- In summary, the quetiapine products possess several defined anxiolytic and antidepressant pharmacodynamic properties:
    - 5-HT2A and 2C receptor antagonism (similar to nefazodone [Serzone], mirtazapine [Remeron], and trazodone [Desyrel])
    - 5-HT1A partial receptor antagonism (similar to buspirone [BuSpar], vilazodone [Viibryd], and vortioxetine [Brintellix])
    - NRI properties (similar to bupropion-XL [Wellbutrin-XL], and atomoxetine [Strattera])
    - H1 receptor antagonism (similar to hydroxyzine [Vistaril], and doxepin [Silenor])
- These five distinct properties may lend to the ability of this drug to treat depression and/or anxiety as a monotherapy or augmentation strategy

Posttest self-assessment question and answer

What pharmacologic properties of quetiapine (Seroquel) lend themselves to providing clinical antidepressant and anxiolytic properties?

A. 5-HT1A partial receptor agonism (similar to buspirone [BuSpar], vilazodone [Viibryd])

B. NRI properties (similar to bupropion-XL [Wellbutrin-XL])

C. H1 receptor antagonism (similar to hydroxyzine [Vistaril], doxepin [Silenor])

D. SSRI properties similar to fluoxetine (Prozac)

E. GABA-A receptor modulating properties similar to diazepam (Valium)

F. A, B, and C
G. All of the above
Answer: F
Quetiapine possesses 5-HT1A receptor partial agonism and NRI properties, both via its active metabolite norquetiapine. It also has antihistaminergic properties allowing for sedation, anxiolysis, and hypnosis. It does not possess SSRI or BZ-like qualities.

References

1. American Psychiatric Association. *Diagnostic and Statistical Manual of Mental Disorders, Revised*, 5th edn. Washington, DC: American Psychiatric Association Press, 2013.
2. Stahl SM. *Stahl's Essential Psychopharmacology*, 4th edn. New York, NY: Cambridge University Press, 2013.
3. Stahl SM. *Stahl's Essential Psychopharmacology: The Prescriber's Guide*, 5th edn. New York, NY: Cambridge University Press, 2014.
4. Malcovati L, Della Porta MG, Pascutto C, et al. Prognostic factors and life expectancy in myelodysplastic syndromes classified according to WHO criteria: a basis for clinical decision making. *J Clin Oncol* 2005; 23:7594–603.
5. Rickels K, Pollack MH, Sheehan DV, Haskins JT. Efficacy of venlafaxine extended-release (XR) capsules in non-depressed outpatients with generalized anxiety disorder. *Am J Psychiatry* 2000; 57:968–74.
6. Schwartz TL, Stahl SM. Treatment strategies for dosing the second generation antipsychotics. *CNS Neurosci Ther* 2011; 17:110–17.
7. Kroeze WK, Roth BL. The molecular biology of serotonin receptors: therapeutic implications for the interface of mood and psychosis. *Biol Psychiatry* 1988; 44:1128–42.
8. Stahl SM. Enhancing outcomes from major depression: using antidepressant combination therapies with multifunctional pharmacologic mechanisms from the initiation of treatment. *CNS Spectr* 2010; 15:79–94.
9. Stahl SM. *Essential Psychopharmacology: The Prescriber's Guide*, 4th edn. New York, NY: Cambridge University Press, 2011.
10. Schwartz TL, Stahl SM. Optimizing antidepressant management of depression: current status and future perspectives. In: Cryan JF, Leonard BE, eds. *Depression: From Psychopathology to Pharmacotherapy*. Basel: Karger, 2010; pp. 254–67.
11. Sorbera LA, Rabasseda X., Silvestre J, Castaner J. Vilazodone hydrochloride–antidepressant–5-HT1A partial agonist–5-HT reuptake inhibitor. *Drugs Future* 2001; 26:247–52.

12. Katzman MA, Vermani M, Jacobs L, et al. Quetiapine as an adjunctive pharmacotherapy for the treatment of non-remitting generalized anxiety disorder: a flexible-dose, open-label pilot trial. *J Anxiety Disord* 2008; 8:1480–6.

13. Wang Z, Kemp DE, Chan PK, et al. Comparisons of the tolerability and sensitivity of quetiapine-XR in the acute treatment of schizophrenia, bipolar mania, bipolar depression, major depressive disorder, and generalized anxiety disorder. *Intern J Neuropsychopharmacol* 2011; 14:131–42.

14. Katzman MA, Brawman-Mintzer O, Reyes EB, et al. Extended release quetiapine fumarate (quetiapine XR) monotherapy as maintenance treatment for generalized anxiety disorder: a long-term, randomized, placebo-controlled trial. *Intern Clin Psychopharmacol* 2011; 26:11–24.

The Case: Interruptions, ammonia, and dyskinesias, oh my!

The Question: Can stimulants complicate bipolar presentations?

The Psychopharmacological dilemma: Finding an effective treatment for mania and mixed features without exacerbating symptoms and side effects

Pretest self-assessment question (answer at the end of the case)

What is the evidence to support the use of clonazepam (Klonopin) in manic patients?

A. It is not approved but meta-analysis studies show effectiveness
B. It is not approved but small-scale studies show effectiveness
C. It is not approved but case series and case studies show effectiveness
D. It is approved, based on large-scale regulatory studies
E. A, B, and C

Patient evaluation on intake

* 35-year-old woman with a chief complaint of difficulty coping at her job

Psychiatric history

* The patient has had psychiatric symptoms since her 20s. She reports depression and agitation as her predominant, albeit fluctuating symptoms
* States that she has alienated friends and co-workers by being verbally intrusive at times
* Cannot complete work assignments and feels depressed
* Admits full MDD symptoms now but is not suicidal
* Simultaneously is agitated, has rapid speech, intrusive behaviors, condescending demeanor, distractibility, and appears thought disorganized with blocking
* States that she also suffers interruptions
  - These are described initially as her own thoughts taking over her brain, or as her own thoughts making their own comments to her, but never defined as other voices or hallucinations. These events cause her thought blocking
* History includes at least two psychiatric hospitalizations for depression She has had no suicide attempts
  - A review of psychiatric systems revealed no formal anxiety disorder, eating disorder, SUD over the last decade. She states the only addictive drugs she has used are those provided by her previous psychiatrist (d/l-mixed amphetamine salts [Adderall])
  - Attended eclectic, supportive psychotherapy in the past but has not had formal CBT or PDP
  - There is no evidence of marked personality disorder

- Patient states that she suffers from ADHD per her previous prescriber and has utilized stimulants more recently as a result. Her inability to focus right now is a main concern as she cannot get tasks completed
- Presents with no medications as her previous psychiatrist has terminated with her
- Previously failed to respond to adequately dosed SSRIs (escitalopram [Lexapro] 30 mg/d, fluoxetine [Prozac] 40 mg/d, paroxetine [Paxil] 40 mg/d) and SNRIs (venlafaxine-XR [Effexor-XR] 300 mg/d) in the past
- Responded to typical antipsychotics (thiothixene [Navane] 40 mg/d, haloperidol [Haldol] 10–20 mg/d), and atypical antipsychotics (risperidone [Risperdal] 4 mg/d), but has had abnormal movements, which she states were TD, as a result
- Has responded to divalproex sodium (Depakote) 1500 mg/d but developed elevated ammonia levels with an altered mental state
- Lamotrigine (Lamictal) was not therapeutic as she developed a non-serious rash at low doses and had to discontinue it
- Most recently has been taking mixed amphetamine salts (Adderall) 50 mg/d and subsequently lisdexamfetamine (Vyvanse) 60 mg/d in order to improve energy, concentration, and focus, but has run out of medications between providers

Social and personal history

- Married and has no children
- Is college educated, works as a social worker at a local hospital
- Does not drink alcohol, smoke cigarettes, or take illegal drugs

Medical history

- Asthma
- Migraines
- Possible history of drug-induced dyskinesia

Family history

- None

Current psychiatric medications

- None as she has been off her stimulant and SSRI for two weeks

Current medical medications

- None

PATIENT FILE

Question

Based on what you know about this patient's history and current symptoms, what would you consider her working diagnosis to be?

- Psychotic MDD
- Bipolar mania
- Bipolar or MDD with mixed features
- Stimulant intoxication
- Borderline personality

What would you do first?

- Obtain information from previous provider
- Obtain information from previous inpatient stays
- Obtain information from her pharmacy regarding medications filled to better assess the completeness of her medication trials and to corroborate her fragmented history
- Add an antidepressant
- Add lithium or divalproex sodium (Depakote) or carbamazepine (Equetro)
- Add an atypical antipsychotic

Attending physician's mental notes: initial evaluation

- Patient is 100% dysphoric overall, appears to be distraught, agitated, and has some subsyndromal manic symptoms and psychotic thought disorder (versus hallucinations)
  - Per *DSM-5*, once psychosis occurs, the patient is declared fully manic and a bipolar 1
  - Per new entity in *DSM-5*, this could be a (if bipolarity is being considered) "with mixed features specifiers" scenario
    - This specifier may occur in bipolar *or* MDD patients
    - In this case, three MANIA criteria must be met in presence of MDD
- Obtaining an accurate history is difficult given her mental state
- Could be an agitated depression, mixed features, borderline personality or stimulant intoxication
- Key is initially to confirm with her family that patient is safe to be at home, given her lability and thought disorder
- Then will need to corroborate her history by obtaining records
- Patient also reports she has had marked side effects
  - To most antidepressants
  - May have had TD but reports many of these movements occurred more while taking stimulants

- Has had problems with mood stabilizers increasing ammonia levels and causing rashes
- Has had marked serotonin side effects
- Will need to consider these symptoms as possibly hypochondriacal, legitimate, or that patient has a p450 isoenzyme deficiency causing marked side effects
- She is on no medications now; she ideally needs a monotherapy with low side effects, benign p450 isoenzyme profile, with inherent ability to treat depression/mania, mixed features, and psychosis all in one
- In case this is bipolar mixed features, unipolar mixed features, or iatrogenic escalated mania, her stimulants and antidepressants likely should be avoided and not restarted

Further investigation

Is there anything else you would especially like to know about this patient?

- What is her longitudinal history?
  - She has been gainfully employed
  - She is intelligent
  - She is successfully married with a supportive spouse
  - She has clear exacerbations of her psychiatric symptoms and has required inpatient stays but apparently without suicidal ideas, intentions, or attempts
  - She appears to function well with inter-episode recovery
  - Almost every medication has caused side effects
  - Her exacerbation currently seems to involve increased irritability, intact self-esteem, and thought disorder, which is a novel presentation per the patient
  - She states typically she would be depressed with agitation and insomnia, but not with these possible psychotic features, which are alarming to her and a novel presentation

Attending physician's mental notes: initial evaluation (continued)

- The patient is clearly distressed and is overly focused on improving her ability to concentrate and function better
- Stimulants increase the DA/NE activity of her brain and could make her lability or thought disorder worse
- At the initial session, it is impossible to obtain old records and a decision to mitigate symptoms has to be made now
- She appears to have mixed features and is minimally psychotic, although it is possible these have been iatrogenically started by use of stimulants without an appropriate mood stabilizer in place

- As she has had difficulty on most medications and this history is sparse and complicated, a trial of an atypical antipsychotic is best positioned to cover all clinical scenarios: psychosis, mania, mixed features, agitation, intoxication, depression, and should avoid any further manic escalation
- A mood stabilizer (carbamazepine[Equetro] or divalproex[Depakote]) will not cover psychosis or help her depression
- Lithium cannot easily be loaded and utilized quickly due to toxicity and a narrow therapeutic window
- Adding a stimulant may cause psychosis
- Adding an antidepressant may cause more mixed–manic features
- Choice of medication should include an agent that requires little CYP450 hepatic metabolism
- The patient does not wish to gain weight

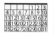

Case outcome: interim follow-ups through one month

- The patient is seen weekly because of her symptoms
  - Records are requested but do not arrive
  - Several medications are presented and the patient states she has a negative tolerability history with many of them
  - States divalproex sodium (Depakote) has worked well but she fears re-emergence of hyperammonemia
  - Feels that risperidone (Risperdal) was helpful too but caused weight gain and movement disorder
- After the following informed consent she agrees to a trial of paliperidone (Invega)
  - Is the atypical in the class that least requires p450 metabolism
  - Is primarily renally excreted
  - Can be titrated easily to allow adequate monitoring and treatment of emergent extrapyramidal symptoms
  - She is at risk for TD again, but this can be monitored closely and removed if needed
  - Has 52 weeks of data showing minimal metabolic impact
  - It is approved to treat schizophrenia but its D2 receptor antagonism might alleviate mania and mixed features
- Paliperidone (Invega) 3 mg/d is initiated, which is subtherapeutic but should limit adverse effects initially. On day 4, the patient states she has more insomnia and dysphoric lability post dose, but is better able to focus and concentrate during the daytime
- Dosed next at 6 mg/d, which is not tolerated due to agitation and gastrointestinal (GI) issues. There were no EPS side effects, however
- Patient states that the typical antipsychotic thiothixene (Navane) had helped at one hospitalization and asked to try this instead, and it was dosed now at 5–10 mg/d

- Now allowed to take diphenhydramine (Benadryl) 50mg for insomnia or emergent EPS as needed

Considering her current use of a typical antipsychotic, what clinical monitoring would you suggest?

- Routine monitoring for treatment-emergent TD/EPS is needed as she reports a history of movement disorder, which appears to include dystonias and dyskinesias involving tic-like features
  - Consider AIMS testing frequently
  - Provide clear informed consent regarding emergence of TD and its possible permanence
- Is routine measurement of weight, abdominal girth, blood pressure, blood lipids, and glucose warranted due to metabolic risks?
  - The typical antipsychotics do not carry metabolic risk warnings like the atypical antipsychotics
  - Thiothixene (Navane) and other high-potency typicals are not clinically well documented to cause AAWG; therefore, this type of monitoring may not be necessary
  - If lower-potency typicals (chlorpromazine [Thorazine], thioridazine [Mellaril]) are to be used, they clearly promote weight gain and likely metabolic disorder, and monitoring similar to that utilized during atypical antipsychotic use should occur
- If records can be obtained and if her EPS
  - Appear more dystonic, then prophylactic use of anticholinergics (diphenhydramine [Benadryl], benztropine [Cogentin]) are warranted
  - Appear more akathisia-based, then as needed-or even prophylactic beta-blocker or BZ use may be warranted
- This patient has a tenuous history of tolerating medications
  - Being diligent about side, effect monitoring is worthwhile clinically
  - Utilizing antidotes for side effects is imperative
  - Additionally, being patient and supportive with numerous complaints may be good for rapport building, medication compliance, and ultimately allow better outcomes due to the ability to obtain better dosing

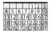

Case outcome: interim follow-ups through two months

- After two weeks of thiothixene (Navane) 10 mg/d, patient is showing global, gradual improvement, but calls with fever, rash, and upper respiratory tract infection (URI) symptoms
- There is a fine intention tremor noted, but no leadpipe muscle rigidity or vital sign changes, and neuroleptic malignant syndrome (NMS) is ruled out
- The URI resolves and the patient continues the typical antipsychotic and the nightly diphenhydramine (Benadryl)

- Gradually there is no more thought disorder or other psychotic symptoms
- Sadness is alleviated but irritability continues
- Sleep is improved
- Chief concern continues to be poor concentration and less productivity
- Patient asks for cognitive-enhancing agents, but is warned again that some of her previous prescription stimulant use may have caused her apparent mixed features/psychosis
- Collateral history obtained
  - Showing that the last stimulant use was several weeks before her presentation so that stimulant intoxication appears to be ruled out
  - However, it does appear that the stimulant use was chronologically related to the emergence of her mixed feature and psychotic symptoms noted earlier
  - It also appears to have led to tic-like movements that the patient reported

Attending physician's mental notes: two months

- Given frequent appointments, concern for side effects and tolerability being emphasized over efficacy, clinician availability via phone between appointments is needed
- Patient appears content and willing to maintain monotherapy as long as empathic limits are set
- Patient affect can likely be contained while waiting for full effects of psychotropics to occur
- Residual symptoms will likely exist and quickly addressing the remaining irritability, depressive symptoms, and cognitive problems should help compliance and tolerability

Question

What would you do next?

- Continue to use the thiothixene monotherapy
- Continue the monotherapy discussed for a few months to clear all psychosis completely and then switch to a better mixed features, atypical antipsychotic
- Continue the typical antipsychotic monotherapy indefinitely but add an antidepressant as needed if there is a failure of full depressive symptoms to remit

Case outcome: interim follow-ups through two months

- Records continue to arrive and full medication trial history is elucidated chronologically as follows

- Fluoxetine (Prozac) 40 mg/d, sertraline (Zoloft) 100 mg/d, XL – escitalopram (Lexapro) 10 mg/d, bupropion (Wellbutrin) 300 mg/d, buspirone (BuSpar) 30 mg/d full trials now documented
- Methylphenidate (Ritalin) 30 mg/d trial noted
- Carbamazepine (Tegretol) caused increased impulsivity and hair loss
- Lithium caused GI upset
- Clonazepam (Klonopin) low dose was effective for mood lability and agitation
- Bilateral ECT treatment – short course only due to prolonged anterograde amnesia
- Olanzapine (Zyprexa) 10 mg/d helpful but metabolic problems occurred
  - Weight increased 30+ lbs, triglycerides went above 600 mg/dL, and a statin was required
  - Quetiapine (Seroquel) caused metabolic issues to continue after a switch from olanzapine
- Clozapine (Clozaril) 100 mg/d short trial caused threat of agranulocytosis
- At one point, records suggest she was taking several medications per day, equalling 20+ pills per day

How does this history support or change your differential diagnosis?
- It appears her initial working diagnosis was unipolar MDD perhaps with mixed features and/or psychosis
- Perhaps the evolution of her illness was a transition from unipolar to bipolar symptoms, given the progression to mood stabilizers and atypical antipsychotic use
- Perhaps the evolution of her illness was a transition from unipolar or bipolar illness toward a schizoaffective disorder (although she has no negative symptoms and mild psychosis at best)
- The use of major tranquilizer and mood stabilizer medications suggest that despite her current advanced education and degrees, she has been significantly impaired and likely will experience relapses as she has a severe and persistent mental illness (SPMI) or personality disorder
- She experienced relative stability on an SSRI, but addition of a stimulant appears to have activated the current mixed features and psychotic episode and caused movement disorder symptoms so that much of her symptoms appeared to be iatrogenic, and she is likely a unipolar depressive with mixed features or has a subtle personality disorder comorbidity

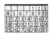

Case outcome: interim follow-ups through three months

- Patient develops lip puckering movements and a fine intention tremor on thiothixene (Navane) typical antipsychotic monotherapy

- Is fearful of permanent TD, has had poor experience on previous atypical antipsychotics, and is leery about data on newer atypical antipsychotics suggesting they are less metabolically adverse
- Previous mood stabilizers have been problematic
- Patient is relatively mood stable, not psychotic, and has returned to work
- Would like a medicine that can control mood and not escalate it
  - This is more psychologically minded compared to the "fix my cognition at all costs mentality" with the stimulants
- Is eventually agreeable to a new trial of lithium as previous trial only caused GI upset and no serious end organ side effects
- thiothixene (Navane) is tapered off and lithium 300 mg/d started without issue. Her fine intention tremor continues but lip puckering subsides
- With between 600–900 mg/d of lithium, GI side effects begin with a marked amount of weight loss (20 lbs)
- Patient attempts to tolerate these symptoms with therapeutic levels; is switched to slow-release lithium and then lithium citrate with continued poor tolerability, and lithium has to be stopped altogether

Question

Early in this case did you have a sense that the history of mounting side effects was hypochondriacal? Have you changed your opinion?

- Yes, as she has developed the same side effects again, in real time, with the repeated medication trials
- No, it is possible these are psychosomatic or psychogenic

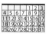

Case outcome and multiple interim follow-ups up to six months

- Agrees next to a trial of divalproex sodium (Depakote), despite previous history of hyperammonemia
- Has seen the benefits of mood stabilization while avoiding antidepressants and stimulants and wishes to continue mood stabilization but without risk of TD
- Despite slow titration and methodical use of laboratory testing, ammonia elevations occur again without transaminase elevations
- This was tolerated initially, but subtle cognitive issues began to emerge and divalproex sodium (Depakote) was discontinued
- Reviewing the patient's history
  - Has had side effects to all major approved mood stabilizers and many antipsychotics
  - Has used clonazepam (Klonopin) in the past for insomnia and agitation control without any side effects
  - Does not have a substance misuse problem
  - Clonazepam is started and utilized from 1 mg/d to 2 mg/d and she continued in an anti-manic state and non-mixed features state

- Unfortunately, several weeks later a depressive episode began
- Wishing to avoid mixed features or re-escalation of mania and the fact that SSRIs had not been helpful in the past, off-label use of modafinil (Provigil) was initiated and titrated to 200 mg/d, given its initial evidence base for successful use in bipolar depression. Its mechanism of action is similar to that of the classic stimulants, albeit with weaker dopamine reuptake inhibition, thus tolerability was expected to be better
- Full antidepressant effects were noted and patient remained in euthymic state for several weeks
- Mood stability was achieved with clonazepam (Klonopin) and modafinil (Provigil) after failures and retrials of other approved medications and with clear side effect recurrence

Case debrief

- The patient has a lengthy history of likely MDD with mixed features with clear iatrogenic exacerbation due to the stimulants and antidepressants
- She has a clear history of attempting to take and use approved mood stabilizers, antipsychotics, and antidepressants with some ability to reach euthymia, but also at the cost of many adverse effects
- Use of a BZ sedative and a non-approved wakefulness-promoting stimulant ultimately proved effective, but is also counterintuitive in a patient with a history of mixed features and psychosis
- The clonazepam (Klonopin) was tolerated well and without metabolic issues, tremors, EPS, TD, or laboratory abnormalities. All these factors thwarted her previous care and ability to sustain euthymia
- Modafinil (Provigil) had limited data in bipolar depression and could have been risky given her manic escalation and movement disorder on previous classic, high-dose amphetamine stimulants
- Modafinil (Provigil) was judged to be theoretically safer as its mechanism of action is less robust with regard to DA facilitation than a classic stimulant, and its isomer armodafinil (Nuvigil) also has published successful trials for use in bipolar depression

Take-home points

- This case emphasizes the need for obtaining information from previous providers to help delineate a complicated diagnosis and also determine what medications have been dosed in full therapeutic trials
- Guidelines suggest using mood stabilizers and atypical antipsychotics to treat all phases of bipolar disorder or those with mixed features of any kind
- Antidepressants and stimulants ideally should not be utilized in bipolar patients unless warranted and assuming that an adequate mood stabilizer or antipsychotic is therapeutically in place

- Guidelines for monitoring end organ damage should be heeded and followed. This patient developed movement disorder and blood laboratory abnormalities that were discovered through usual monitoring practices
- If patients are to be rechallenged on previously difficult-to-tolerate medications, adequate informed consent, increased follow-ups and monitoring should be considered. Slower titration schedules and perhaps slow-release preparations should be utilized
- When approved medications fail to help or are intolerable, referring to guidelines and the available literature is warranted when prescribing off-label medications
- In the absence of literature, consulting with colleagues, attending continuing medical education (CME) activities, or using theoretical mechanism of action, knowledge about off-label medications is warranted to help guide prescribing
  - Documentation in the medical record is needed regarding the clinical rationale of off-label use

Performance in practice: confessions of a psychopharmacologist

- *What could have been done better here?*
  - Was it inappropriate to retry divalproex (Depakote), thiothixene (Navane), or lithium carbonate?
    - Patient developed the same side effects compared to previous trials
    - However, in the current trials, attempts were made to monitor, minimize, and treat side effects as they emerged
    - Patient also achieved documented therapeutic levels on all agents, and documented euthymia was noted despite the adverse effects
    - Ultimately however, the agents were not tolerated and forced clinical decisions to lean toward the use of off-label approaches
    - The myriad of records actually showed good tolerability for clonazepam but risk of dependence, relatively less evidence base, and taboo of using sedatives to treat mixed features likely interfered with the decision to believe in the collected chart information
- *Possible action items for improvement in practice*
  - For diagnosis, in the absence of old records, consider using diagnostic rating scales such as the Mood Disorder Questionnaire (MDQ) or the Psychiatric Diagnostic Screening Questionnaire (PDSQ)

- Consult peer-reviewed practice guidelines when making real-time treatment decisions in these complex cases
- In the case of hypochondriacal, side effect-prone patients, sometimes believing the history is warranted and retrials may not be wise

Pharmacodynamic moment

- Consider modafinil (Provigil) and its isomer armodafinil (Nuvigil) not as classic stimulants, but as novel stimulants or wake-promoting agents as their mechanism of action is different than the true, classical stimulants
- These two wake promoters do require an intact DAT system, but it is unclear if they block this transporter, reverse the transporter, or facilitate vesicular monoamine transporter systems like the classic mixed amphetamine salts. Most likely the mechanism is of a DRI
- They also may promote wakefulness by promoting downstream histaminergic activity and orexin activity
- Currently, these two agents are approved for treating narcolepsy, obstructive sleep apnea (OSA) fatigue, or shift-work sleep disorder fatigue
- Evidence is mounting for their successful use in bipolar depression

Two-minute tutorial

What is worse in causing escalated mania or mixed features, antidepressants or stimulants?

- Recent reports suggest less risk of triggering bipolar disorder onset among stimulants and antidepressants than previously thought, particularly in adolescent patients who are thought to be prone to activation of bipolarity
- Smaller controlled trials in adolescents with ADHD and bipolar disorder support the notion that stimulants may also trigger less escalation to mania than antidepressants

Should unipolar antidepressants be used in bipolar disorder?

- Guidelines and data from the last few decades suggest that mania, mixed features, and rapid cycling may be induced in bipolar 1 patients when antidepressants are added to their medication regimens. Data regarding stimulant additions are relatively less well known
- The TCA and MAOI antidepressants appear to cause these bipolar exacerbations more often than the SSRI class or an NDRI (bupropion [Wellbutrin])
- The SNRI are suspected to be similar to the TCAs given that both classes involve dual reuptake inhibition and have similar mechanisms of action

- Guidelines suggest avoiding the use of unipolar antidepressants in bipolar depression unless an adequate mood stabilizer or atypical antipsychotic is already therapeutically dosed
- In the case of bipolar depression, approved treatments should be utilized first (olanzapine–fluoxetine combination [Symbyax], quetiapine [Seroquel], quetiapine [Seroquel-XR]), or lurasidone [Latuda])
- However, it should be noted that these agents have more serious adverse effects (metabolic disorder, movement disorders, sedation, EPS, and possibly agranulocytosis) and require laboratory monitoring and higher healthcare utilization. These agents, when used for depressive disorders, carry the risk of increasing suicidal symptoms in those younger than 25 years
- Considering that bipolar patients spend more time depressed and may accrue more cumulative disability from the depressed state, novel treatments without end organ damage risk are needed
- Certain unipolar antidepressants (SSRI, NDRI) offer an option for less medically risky treatment but with minor risks of worsening the principal bipolar illness at hand. This fact is more apparent in treating bipolar II patients

Does clonazepam (Klonopin) work in bipolar mania?

- It is not approved
- Data are available for this intervention, as follows:
  - APA guidelines for acute manic or mixed episodes suggest that BZs may make effective adjuncts while awaiting the effects of a primary anti-manic agent to become evident
  - APA guidelines recommend combination therapy for patients inadequately controlled within 10–14 days of optimized-dose first-line treatment as another instance where BZ intervention may be warranted
- Five randomized controlled studies of the BZ clonazepam for acute mania exist and were conducted in small patient populations
- Meta-analysis suggests that clonazepam reduced mania scores statistically
- Furthermore, there may be higher efficacy of clonazepam versus lorazepam (Ativan)
- Some case studies suggest that clonazepam is efficient in reducing symptoms of acute mania even when used as monotherapy
- Dosing in these trials ranged from 2–6 mg/d

Posttest self-assessment question and answer

What is the evidence to support the use of clonazepam (Klonopin) in manic patients?

A. It is not approved but meta-analysis studies show effectiveness

B. It is not approved but small-scale studies show effectiveness
C. It is not approved but case series and case studies show effectiveness
D. It is approved, based on large-scale regulatory studies
E. A, B, and C

Answer: E

As noted in the prior section, clonazepam (Klonopin) is not FDA approved but is suggested as an augmentation strategy per the APA guidelines. Its use as a monotherapy has supportive small clinical trials and case reports to condone its use, especially when other therapies fail or are not tolerated. Large, 200–300-patient, randomized and controlled regulatory trials are nonexistent, and therefore, no formal approval exists.

References

1. Emsley R, Berwaerts J, Eerdekens M, et al. Efficacy and safety of oral paliperidone extended-release tablets in the treatment of acute schizophrenia: pooled data from three 52-week open-label studies. *Int Clin Psychopharmacol* 2008; 23:343–56.

2. Stahl SM. *Stahl's Essential Psychopharmacology*, 4th edn. New York, NY: Cambridge University Press, 2013.

3. Stahl SM. *Stahl's Essential Psychopharmacology: The Prescriber's Guide*, 5th edn. New York, NY: Cambridge University Press, 2014.

4. American Psychiatric Association. *Practice Guideline for the Treatment of Patients with Bipolar Disorder*, 2nd edn. Washington, DC: American Psychiatric Association Press, 2002.

5. Twiss J, Jones S, Anderson I. Validation of the mood disorder questionnaire for screening for bipolar disorder in a UK sample. *J Affect Disord* 2008; 110:180–4.

6. Zimmerman M, Mattia JI. The psychiatric diagnostic screening questionnaire: development, reliability and validity. *Compr Psychiatry* 2001; 42:175–89.

7. Frye MA, Grunze H, Suppes T, et al. A placebo-controlled evaluation of adjunctive modafinil in the treatment of bipolar depression. *Am J Psychiatry* 2007; 164:1242–9.

8. Calabrese JR, Ketter TA, Youakim JM, et al. Adjunctive armodafinil for major depressive episodes associated with bipolar I disorder: a randomized, multicenter, double-blind, placebo-controlled, proof-of-concept study. *J Clin Psychiatry* 2010; 71:1363–70.

9. Chen J, Fang Y, Kemp DE, Calabrese JR, Gao K. Switching to hypomania and mania: differential neurochemical, neuropsychological, and pharmacologic triggers and their mechanisms. *Curr Psychiatry Rep* 2010; 12:512–21.

10. Shelton RC, Reddy R. Adjunctive use of modafinil in bipolar patients: just another stimulant or not? *Curr Psychiatry Rep* 2008; 10:520–4.

11. Pagano ME, Demeter CA, Faber JE, Calabrese JR, Findling RL. Initiation of stimulant and antidepressant medication and clinical presentation in juvenile bipolar I disorder. *Bipolar Disord* 2008; 10:334–41.

12. Lydon E, El-Mallakh RS. Naturalistic long-term use of methylphenidate in bipolar disorder. *J Clin Psychopharmacol* 2006; 26:516–18.

13. Scheffer RE, Kowatch RA, Carmody T, Rush AJ. Randomized, placebo-controlled trial of mixed amphetamine salts for symptoms of comorbid ADHD in pediatric bipolar disorder after mood stabilization with divalproex sodium. *Am J Psychiatry* 2005; 162:58–64.

14. Hellander M. Medication-induced mania: ethical issues and the need for more research. *J Child Adolesc Psychopharmacol* 2003; 13:199.

15. American Psychiatric Association. *Practice Guidelines for the Treatment of Patients with Bipolar Disorder.* http://www.psychiatry .org/psychiatrists/practice/clinical-practice-guidelines. Accessed March 26, 2011.

16. American Psychiatric Association. *Treating Bipolar Disorder. A Quick Reference Guide.* http://psychiatryonline.org/pb/assets/raw/sitewide/ practice_guidelines/guidelines/bipolar-guide.pdf. Accessed March 26, 2011.

17. Nardi AE, Perna G. Clonazepam in the treatment of psychiatric disorders: an update. *Intern Clin Psychopharmacol* 2006; 21:131–42.

18. Nihalani N, Schwartz TL, Siddiqui UA, Megna JL. Weight gain, obesity, and psychotropic prescribing. *J Obes* 2011; 2011:893629.

The Case: The lady and the man who sat on couches

The Question: Are the symptoms of apathy of an elderly man and woman due to depression, dementia, or side effects of medication?

The Dilemma: How to tell depression from vascular dementia (and everything in between as well)

Pretest self-assessment question (answer at the end of the case)

Which are correct regarding vascular depression?

A. There is evidence that cerebrovascular disease creates vulnerability to depression, as well as cognitive impairment and neurologic signs
B. Clinical presentation suggests a medial frontal lobe syndrome with psychomotor retardation, apathy, and marked disability
C. Cerebrovascular lesions on neuroimaging results in poor outcomes, including persistence of depression with unstable remission and increased risk for dementia
D. Depression–executive dysfunction syndrome (DED) is similar but may have multifactorial causes, that is, vascular disease, aging-related changes, degenerative brain disease, combined in a cumulative or synergistic effect
E. All of the above

Patient evaluation on intake

- Patient #1
  - 79-year-old woman whose chief complaint was of "feeling awful"
- Patient #2
  - 85-year-old man who had no chief complaint

Psychiatric history

- Each patient presents with family members
  - Patient #1 has a history of recurrent mild MDEs throughout her life
    - This latest MDE is more severe and more incapacitating than previous episodes
  - Patient #2 has no history of mental illness
    - Survived cancer and was robust and active until a recent pneumonia
    - Despite recovery, seems depressed and inactive
- Neither patient has any clear psychiatric comorbidity
  - Except that Patient #1 appears to have a phobia with an intense fear reaction that occurs only if her elderly husband leaves the house for too long
- Neither has any psychiatric inpatient admissions, nor suicide attempts
- Initially, Patient #2 was somewhat confused and/or thought disordered

- A delirium workup ensued and was negative
- Initial treatment with an antipsychotic cleared his symptoms

Outside of this, *both* patients admitted being depressed, down, fatigued, unable to concentrate, unable to sleep well. Both deny guilt, worthlessness feelings, or any suicidal thoughts.

- These patients are not related and not married to each other, but both families presented concerned that their once robust, energetic family members were now down, out, and despondent. In fact, the families chief complaint is that these patients "just sit on the couch all day"

Question

Of the following depression treatment choices, what would you do?

- Start an SSRI
- Start an SNRI
- Start an NDRI
- Start an NaSSA (mirtazapine [Remeron])
- Initiate or refer to psychotherapy

Case outcome

- Both patients are tried sequentially on therapeutically dosed SSRI, SNRI, NDRI, and NaSSA monotherapies
- Both were augmented with stimulants, atypical antipsychotics, and BZs
- Patient #1 now receives maintenance ECT
- Patient #2 is off all psychotropics as there was no benefit noticed during any medication trial
- Both declined psychotherapy
- Both had relief from sadness, insomnia, fatigue, anorexia within the first few months
- Both now still sit on their couches (in their separate houses) most of the day, with little motivation or concern for time and other interests
- Both are somewhat docile and dependent and have little interest in other pursuits
- When asked if they like and enjoy their lifestyles and their daily routine, the answer is "yes" with little relationship to the active lives they used to lead
- They are not upset by these losses
- They have short-term memory problems, which have become more pronounced with time
- Their treatment course was complicated
  - Patient #1: by oversedation and a fall while taking BZs
  - Patient #2: by onset of mild TD that has mostly remitted
  - Regardless of agents used, such as antidepressants, sedatives, stimulants, and antipsychotics, both patients' apathy did not worsen or lighten, suggesting that their apathy was not iatrogenic nor

side-effect driven. In fact, one of the patients who is off all medications remains the same

Case debrief

- Both patients were treated with the "start low, go slow" geriatric pharmacology mantra
- Both were given more monotherapies than polypharmacy approaches
- Both patients received psychotropics from all major classes
- Sadness and dysphoria seemed to be easily treated
- However, a docile indifference and apathy were left as residual symptoms that were untreated despite use of several classes of antidepressants, stimulants, and even ECT in one of the patients
- During the course of treatment, all laboratory values were normal
- CT, MRI, and positron emission tomography (PET) scans were also ordered
  - In Patient #1, findings revealed slight hypoactivity in temporal lobes and mild ventriculomegaly, suggesting a picture of early Alzheimer's disease and possible vascular disease versus age-associated degeneration
  - In Patient #2, generalized atrophy was also noted but no activity difference among various brain areas
  - Both patients had some subcortical infarcts and leukomalacia

Take-home points

- These imaging findings are not necessarily classic for vascular depression due to the absence of marked numbers of subcortical lacunar infarcts
- It is more likely that these patients suffer from DEFS as there were minimal subcortical lesions but overall atrophy instead
- Clinically, these two patients were not psychomotor impaired, suggesting less subcortical neurodegenerative damage, but felt to have more atrophy and cumulative disruptions of frontocortical tracts allowing for the clinical presentations noted
- Both patients exhibited executive dysfunction and had little familial genetic depression loading or risk
  - The absence of psychomotor slowing, presence of executive dysfunction, and lack of familial risk factors again suggests that DEFS might be a better working diagnosis than vascular depression or dementia
  - Often these vascular depression and DEFS patients are minimally responsive to serotonergic antidepressants, as was found in this case
  - However, they were also unresponsive to all antidepressants as well

Tips and pearls

- MDD, vascular depression, and DED all involve similar clinical presentations and symptomatology

- The following table suggests ways to better delineate each clinical entity
- The following images help to visualize how neurocircuitry, when degraded by infarcts, aging-related atrophy, and neurodegenerative dementia processes, may disrupt usual brain functioning and allow psychiatric symptoms to develop
  - Any breakage in this circuitry could allow for executive dysfunction symptoms. In these cases, apathy may have developed as the frontal cortex does not receive impulsive drive or initiative signals from subcortical structures due to neuronal tract disruption via aging-related atrophy

Table 7.1. Symptoms of major depression, vascular depression, and depression–executive dysfunction syndrome

Presentation	Major depression	Vascular depression	DED
Full *DSM* symptoms possible	+	+	+
Psychomotor slowing predominant	+/−	+	−
Indifference/apathy predominant	+/−	+	+
Executive dysfunction predominant	+/−	+	+
Caused by lacunar infarcts and medial frontal lobe dysfunction	−	+	−
Caused by brain atrophy, other etiologies, and frontocortical tracts dysfunction	−	−	+

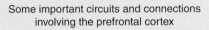

Some important circuits and connections involving the prefrontal cortex

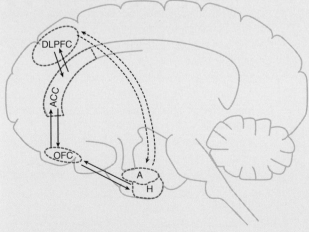

Figure 7.1. Key corticocortical circuits.

- Several important prefrontal corticocortical circuits are shown. The anterior cingulate cortex (ACC) has corticocortical interactions with the dorsolateral prefrontal cortex (DLPFC) and the orbital frontal cortex (OFC). The OFC, in turn, has corticocortical interactions with the hippocampus (H). The DLPFC has only sparse direct connections with the amygdala (A) and hippocampus.

DLPFC $\longrightarrow$ Striatum $\longrightarrow$ Thalamus $\longrightarrow$ DLPFC

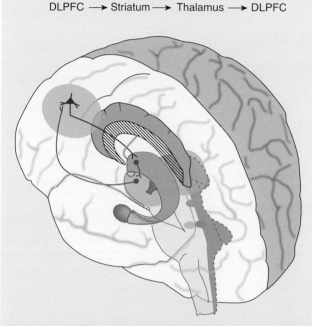

Figure 7.2. Hypothetical corticostriatal–thalamic–cortical loop for executive function.

- This three-dimensional figure depicts a hypothetical corticostriatal–thalamic–cortical (CSTC) neural loop, or circuit, for executive functions, which involves the DLPFC and the rostral (top) part of the caudate within the striatal complex
- There are many CSTC loops that also connect brain areas together, and when in balanced communication, psychiatric symptoms are not present
  - Again, if damage or atrophy occurs anywhere along these neural circuits (depending on which prefrontal region is involved), psychiatric symptoms may develop as one brain area may now be hypofunctioning while others are hyperfunctioning. This imbalance may allow for clinical psychiatric symptoms to manifest

– In these cases, the patients seemed to have no drive to move off their couches. If the depicted neural loop were disrupted, the patients may not have been aware that so much time had passed while sitting on the coach and may have developed an inability to plan and schedule their days as part of their executive dysfunction symptomatology

Posttest self-assessment question and answer

Which are correct regarding vascular depression?

A. There is evidence that cerebrovascular disease creates vulnerability to depression, as well as cognitive impairment and peripheral neurologic signs

B. Clinical presentation suggests a medial frontal lobe syndrome with psychomotor retardation, apathy, and marked disability

C. Cerebrovascular lesions on neuroimaging results in poor outcomes, including persistence of depression with unstable remission and increased risk for dementia

D. DED is similar but may have multifactorial causes, that is, vascular disease, aging-related changes, degenerative brain disease, combined in a cumulative or synergistic effect

E. All of the above

Answer: E

Vascular depression assumes that there are vascular insults in subcortical brain areas usually involving lacunar infarcts or leukomalacia around the ventricles. These injuries disrupt neural connections, most likely in mediofrontal areas, causing the symptoms noted in (B) and the clinical outcomes noted in (C). DED is similar but posits that there still may be frontocortical disruptions, but vascular insults are not necessarily required; rather atrophy and cell death may cause the disruptions alone. The final common pathway of neurocircuitry disruption may yield apathy, executive dysfunction, and psychomotor impairment, which appears similar to those symptoms noted in MDD. In both of the cases described here, the patients' affective depression symptoms responded somewhat. They were not sad. Their brain atrophy and its resultant apathy and executive dysfunction symptoms did not respond to treatment.

References

1. Stahl SM. *Stahl's Essential Psychopharmacology*, 4th edn. New York, NY: Cambridge University Press, 2013.

2. Stahl SM. *Stahl's Essential Psychopharmacology Prescriber's Guide*, 5th edn. New York, NY: Cambridge University Press, 2014.

3. Alexopoulos GS, Meyers BS, Young RC, et al. 'Vascular depression' hypothesis. *Arch Gen Psychiatry* 1997; 54:915–22.

4. Alexopoulos GS. The vascular depression hypothesis: 10 years later. *Biol Psychiatry* 2006; 60:1304–5.

The Case: The lady who had her diagnosis altered

The Question: When are symptoms psychotic or dissociative?

The Psychopharmacological dilemma: Finding an effective treatment for dissociative, depressed, psychotic patients while not ruining the outcomes of their previous bariatric weight-loss surgeries

Pretest self-assessment question (answer at the end of the case)

Which of the following approaches likely has the most evidence to support its use as a weight-loss strategy in patients suffering from antipsychotic-associated weight gain (AAWG)?

A. Orlistat (Xenical)
B. Sibutramine (Meridi 4)
C. Fenfluramine (Pondi Min)
D. Topiramate/phentermine combination (Q-Symia)
E. Metformin (Glucophage)
F. Naltrexone/bupropion combination (Contrave)
G. Lorcaserin (Belviq)
H. Bariatric surgery

Patient evaluation on intake

- 32-year-old woman with a chief complaint of unremitting depression for several years, who was transferred from another provider who had just retired

Psychiatric history

- The patient had onset of MDD in her 20s, which was likely predated by comorbid GAD
- Presents moderately depressed but is partially responding to medication now
- Depressive symptoms have fluctuated from mild to severe but have never remitted
- Sober from prior AUD for three years
- Despite these symptoms, has been gainfully employed at times and has been able to return to school for college credits on a part-time basis
- Exhibits classic symptoms of MDD but the depression is also vegetative in that she is not predominantly sad, but more anhedonic with blunted affect, and poor energy and concentration
- Admits to passive suicidal thoughts but has never acted on them
- Required no psychiatric hospitalizations in her lifetime
  - A review of psychiatric systems revealed no other formal anxiety disorder, psychosis, mania, eating disorder

- Has undergone eclectic, supportive psychotherapy in the past but her mental state at this presentation made reciprocal talk therapy almost impossible given her psychomotor slowing and lethargy
- There is no evidence of marked personality disorder
- Inherited from a previous psychiatrist, the patient currently takes an SNRI (duloxetine [Cymbalta]) and a stimulant (methylphenidate [Concerta])
- The stimulant is for depression augmentation and she only experiences dry mouth as a side effect
- States she is about 30% better on this regimen
- Previously, the patient failed to respond to
  - Two or three SSRIs prescribed in the primary care setting prior to being seen in psychiatry. She is unaware of the dose strength utilized but states she spent several months on each
  - Adequately dosed NaSSA, mirtazapine (Remeron) 45 mg/d
  - Patient had previous trials of a TCA but these appear to be low doses used for treating insomnia and pain only
- Continues to be seen weekly by a supportive psychotherapist with whom she has a good rapport

Social and personal history

- Divorced and has two children
- Is high school educated, working part-time and taking courses part-time
- Has supportive parents and siblings who help her with childcare
- Does not drink alcohol, smoke cigarettes, or take illegal drugs

Medical history

- Iron deficiency anemia treated with iron supplements
- Successful bariatric surgery, lost 70 lbs., and weighs 130 lbs.
- Is normotensive
- History of lower back pain

Family history

- SUD in parents and many relatives, largely AUD
- MDD in mother
- No history of schizophrenia or bipolar disorder in the family

Current psychiatric medications

- Duloxetine (Cymbalta) 60 mg/d (SNRI)
- Methylphenidate-ER (Concerta) 36 mg/d (stimulant)

Current medical medications

- Iron supplements 1500 mg/d
- Ibuprofen (Motrin) 600–1800 mg/d

Question

Based on this patient's history and the available evidence base, do you consider augmentation with stimulants to be a reasonable approach?

- Yes
- No

What makes, or would make you comfortable using a stimulant augmentation?

- Stimulants are not approved but are covered in many psychopharmacology texts as legitimate augmentations, and in many peer-reviewed journal review articles, and there are a few trials available in the literature supporting the practice
- Larger controlled trials seem to indicate that, if not a full antidepressant, stimulants have anti-fatigue and procognitive effects useful in treating MDD
- Stimulants often offset side effects induced by SSRI and SNRI, such as sedation, fatigue, executive dysfunction, and weight gain
- Stimulants often treat residual depressive symptoms not managed by SSRI, such as fatigue and poor concentration

What makes, or would make you uncomfortable with stimulant augmentation?

- A history of addiction
- A history of cardiac or hypertensive issues
- A history of tic or movement disorders
- A history of anxiety

Attending physician's mental notes: initial evaluation

- This patient seems to be typical of many patients referred for inadequate response to antidepressants in that she is in her 30s, moderately depressed, and has failed mostly SSRI treatment in primary care settings
- The previous psychiatrist changed classes of medications from the SSRI to an SNRI and achieved a partial response
  - This approach follows most MDD guidelines where, if there is a failure on initial SSRI montherapy, then a switch to a novel pharmacological class antidepressant is the next step
- A stimulant augmentation was added to promote more clinical symptom response and also likely to avoid side-effect weight gain in this case
- Unfortunately, she is not in remission, which requires further action and prescribing

- Common practice suggests looking at the current medication regimen, and if safe, reasonable, and rational, doses can be increased within approved limits to see if remission can occur before adding yet another medication
- She has minimal side effects and likes her current regimen, hence compliance looks to be favorable

Further investigation

Is there anything else you would especially like to know about this patient?

- What medical details concerning this patient are you concerned about?
  - She has a history of AUD but has been sober for three years. She is taking duloxetine (Cymbalta) now, which has warnings about its use in acute alcoholism due to liver damage issues
    - Her liver function tests are normal
  - She has a history of being overweight but underwent successful bariatric surgery
  - Does she have any history of BN?
    - No, psychiatric interview at present shows no eating disorder and psychological evaluation prior to bariatric surgery also showed no contraindication
  - She has chronic depression; therefore, is there a medical cause such as hypothyroidism or anemia?
    - Thyroid panel is normal. Cell count is normal and she is on iron replacement

Question

Based on what you know about this patient's history, current symptoms, and treatment responses, do you think that maximal doses of her antidepressant are warranted at this time?

- Yes, clinical experience dictates that increased doses work better in some patients
- Yes, psychopharmacology textbooks suggest that increased doses may work better in certain patients
- No, her doses are clinically adequate
- No, her dose is average and the FDA suggests no benefit from higher doses

Attending physician's mental notes: initial evaluation (continued)

- The patient is clearly depressed
- Her medications are well tolerated and have room to be maximized with regard to dose

- The patient has a good supportive psychotherapist and should continue with that, but perhaps consider augmenting this psychotherapy with group CBT
- She seems to be a typical treatment-resistant patient, but has good prognostic factors

Case outcome: interim follow-ups through three months

- The patient's duloxetine (Cymbalta) SNRI is maximized to 120 mg/d without clear benefit or improved partial response
- Methylphenidate-ER (Concerta) is next increased to 54 mg/d without clear benefit. There are no additional side effects
  - Blood pressure, heart rate, and weight are monitored
- Lamotrigine (Lamictal) is gaining popularity as a bipolar maintenance treatment and as an antidepressant augmentation as it has minimal day-to-day side effects
  - Less stringent unipolar depression augmentation trials have suggested effectiveness, whereas more stringent monotherapy trials suggest little benefit over placebo
  - Lamotrigine also has a purported mechanism of action that is novel (glutamate dampening by inhibiting the release of glutamate into the synapse) compared to the patient's current regimen, which uses a rational polypharmacy approach where each psychotropic contributes a novel mechanism of action to the regimen
  - Lamotrigine is known for minimal to no weight-gain effects, but does have serious, but rare rash adverse effects to consider. Given this, it must be titrated very slowly, which makes it an inopportune acute antidepressant treatment as it takes six to eight weeks to reach 200 mg/d
- Patient is mildly depressed now given the partial response noted earlier. Therefore, a slow titration is acceptable clinically. The lack of weight-based side effects is comforting in this case
- Fortunately, she gains no weight, has no side effects, but she has no mood stabilizer benefit despite dosing of lamotrigine up to 300 mg/d

Question

Considering her current medication failures (SSRI, SNRI, stimulant, and antiepileptic), what would you consider next?
- Discontinue current ineffective medications and
  - Start a new SNRI and consider combining with an NDRI such as bupropion-XL (Wellbutrin-XL), which all together continue to facilitate synaptic DA, NE, and serotonin (5-HT), albeit with a different combination of medications

- Remove lamotrigine (Lamictal), maintain the SNRI, and add mirtazapine (Remeron), a NaSSA, instead seeking a "California rocket fuel" combination to maximize synaptic NE and 5-HT
- Remove all agents, washout, start an MAOI
- Refer for ECT, VNS, TMS treatments
- Refer for a course of group CBT

Attending physician's mental notes: four months

- The patient has been compliant with visits and medications
- She now has several failed full medication trials where the drugs inhibit monoamine reuptake pumps
- Weight-gain potential medications like mirtazapine (Remeron), the TCAs, and the atypical antipsychotics will not be appreciated by the patient
- The newer MAOI transdermal patch selegiline (Emsam) has data suggesting minimal weight gain and utilizes a novel mechanism of action elevating all three monoamines in one monotherapy, and may be a rational choice

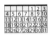

Case outcome: interim follow-ups through six months

- The patient accepts education and the risks of drug and diet interactions and starts this MAOI after appropriate washout of her previous antidepressants
  - An appropriate washout in this case was a gradual taper off of each medication to avoid withdrawal, followed by five half-life duration waiting periods specific to each agent prior to MAOI initiation
- Selegiline (Emsam) patch is escalated eventually to the full 12 mg/d maximal dose but without any clinical response
- This drug is discontinued and appropriate washout implemented
  - Two weeks must lapse prior to a contraindicated medication being started
  - This allows for adequate replenishment of MAO enzymes to be synthesized and return of drug metabolism to normal capability
- She elects, despite some weight-gain potential, to take a TCA and is titrated to therapeutic doses and levels of nortriptyline (Pamelor), but also without clinical response
- Weight begins to increase
- Metformin (Glucophage) is a diabetes medicine known to cause weight loss and is initiated and titrated to 2000 mg/d, and weight gain is halted but not reversed
  - There is a reasonable evidence base to support the use of metformin prophylactically or after the fact to lower or inhibit AAWG
- She has gained 15 lbs

- Laboratory blood samples are drawn and renal function is normal and there is no acidosis with metformin use. Blood glucose is normal
- The wakefulness-promoting agent modafinil (Provigil) is added now to her current TCA as a depression augmentation, and titrated eventually to 400 mg/d
- Her chief symptoms continue to be anhedonia, blunted affect, and low energy
- There was only a minimal response and weight starts to increase on this combination again
- Orlistat (Xenical) is an approved weight-loss medication, which patient agrees to start (360 mg/d). It is a fat-blocking (intraluminal lipase inhibitor) drug with two-year regulatory effectiveness in overweight patients but has a minimum of evidence for its use in iatrogenic weight gain from psychotropic administration

Case outcome: interim follow-ups through nine months

- The patient's therapist makes contact and states that patient became increasingly suicidal due to social stress and was admitted to an inpatient facility with superficial wrist cuts
- The inpatient psychiatrist calls to inquire about the patient's previous psychotic history
  - None of which she exhibited in sessions, nor admitted to at initial evaluation
  - Patient currently states that she "feels like other people"
  - She will act like a "little girl" or an "angry big girl"
  - She is deemed to have dissociative identity disorder (DID) and placed on risperidone (Risperdal) up to 4 mg/d and these symptoms resolve while in the inpatient unit

Question

What would you do when the patient returns to your office?

- Continue risperidone (Risperdal) despite its AAWG and relatively poor metabolic profile
- Switch to a more metabolically friendly atypical antipsychotic
- Refer to an appropriate therapist with experience reuniting dissociative personality alters
- Discuss with the patient why she did not confide in you regarding her alter personalities

Attending physician's mental notes: nine-month follow-ups

- This is tough as somehow this dissociative process was missed in the initial presentation

- The inpatient team has possibly undone rapport with this prescription and attempts to minimize this patient's AAWG by using a metabolically unfriendly atypical antipsychotic
- Wonder if the patient is actually depressed and psychotic instead of DID? *How can one tell dissociative symptoms from psychotic symptoms?*
- Dissociative symptoms often do not remit with antipsychotic treatment, but psychotic symptoms do!
- Dissociative symptoms are often predated by childhood, or even more recent trauma, and may be associated with PTSD and borderline personality
- Dissociative symptoms tend to be associated with time losses where patients may be unaware of their behavior or "wake up" in different places

Attending physician's mental notes: interim follow-up, nine months (continued)

- This patient has no clear trauma, PTSD, or personality disorder conditions after re-evaluation
- She had a fairly robust response to the atypical antipsychotic
- However, when interviewed, she stated that she was "hearing voices" of a little girl or a grownup girl and the voices were telling her to act in certain ways
- She denied time losses and there were no reports, even on the inpatient unit, of her regressing, acting like a little girl or taking on a new distinct personality
- Conclusion: she is not DID, but unfortunately in some ways has become more severely depressed and with psychotic symptoms
- Her new atypical antipsychotic medication is effective, but will likely cause more weight-gain issues in the future

Case outcome and multiple interim follow-ups to 24 months

- The patient does gain another 15 lbs, but the use of the atypical antipsychotic helps the depression resolve back to her baseline moderate levels, although she still has the same residual vegetative symptoms
- We agree to a washout of her ineffective medications and to "start over"
- The TCA nortriptyline (Pamelor) is tapered off and she is titrated to 300 mg/d of the SNRI, desvenlafaxine (Pristiq)
- Augmentation with tri-iodothyronine (Cytomel) is initiated in the hope of lowering her weight gain and finally treating her residual vegetative depression symptoms, as SNRI monotherapy is failing again
- The risperidone (Risperdal) dose is also lowered as her psychosis associated with her depression has solidly remitted

- Unfortunately, her depression and some minimal hallucinations return. Risperidone (Risperdal) is cross-titrated to the approved antipsychotic/ antidepressant augmentation aripiprazole (Abilify) up to 30 mg/d
- The SNRI plus thyroid augmentation plus atypical antipsychotic augmentation resolves her psychosis. Her depression returns to its partially responded, baseline state
- After treatment now with SSRI, SNRI, TCA, stimulants, thyroid hormone, atypical antipsychotics, and an MAOI, the patient has not improved over her baseline partial response
- She starts and completes a one-year course of dialectical behavior therapy (DBT) to improve her coping and stress management as these were felt to play a part in inducing her depressive psychosis
- This helps alleviate social stress but she continues with her vegetative presentation
- Develops orofacial TD on the atypical antipsychotic aripiprazole (Abilify) and it is systematically lowered
- This time with the antipsychotic tapering off, there is no return of psychosis
- ECT is offered for the residual symptoms, which is declined
- She next agrees to lithium carbonate augmentation and is titrated to 1200 mg/d allowing for a therapeutic level of 1.1 mEq/l
- Affective range changes from blunted to minimally constricted. Her motivation increases and she starts dating
- She continues with low energy and poor concentration
- This partial response is not at the remission stage but is now improved from her baseline at her first appointment
- Currently, she takes
  - lithium 1200 mg/d, desvenlafaxine (Pristiq) 300 mg/d, metformin (Glucophage) 2000 mg/d, orlistat (Xenical) 360 mg/d, and ramelteon (Rozerem) 8 mg as needed for insomnia, which is transient
  - AAWG halted and she experienced a 10–15 lbs weight loss

Case debrief

- The patient has a history of chronic MDD that ultimately became more treatment resistant and more complicated with the evolution of psychotic symptoms
- Psychotic symptoms had to be differentiated from dissociative symptoms
- Developed iatrogenic weight gain from her psychotropics that had to be aggressively managed in order to avoid undoing her bariatric surgery effects
- Gained 30 lbs at one point, but half of this was ultimately lost due to pharmacological interventions noted earlier

- This attention to side-effect mitigation allowed for a positive clinician–patient maintenance of rapport and compliance with medication polypharmacy
- Developed TD after exposure to two different atypical antipsychotics that resolved completely after full antipsychotic discontinuation
- This patient failed the more modern augmentation strategies where atypical antipsychotics, mood stabilizers, and stimulants were utilized
- She failed psychotherapy combination treatment (supportive plus DBT strategies)
- She failed one classic thyroid augmentation but has started to respond to a classic lithium augmentation
- ECT would have been a reasonable acute treatment, but the patient declined
- VNS or TMS might be a reasonable long-term option if lithium fails to provide complete remission in the future

Take-home points

- This case emphasizes the need for full therapeutic trials of antidepressant treatments, augmentations, combinations, and psychotherapy
- This case seems reasonable in that an MAOI was started after only a few antidepressant trial failures instead of waiting for several failures to occur. In this manner, the patient spent less time in a depressed state prior to MAOI therapy being utilized
- Both novel and classic antidepressant augmentation strategies should be used
- Rational polypharmacy is essential
  - Medications that were used serially did not overlap with regard to the antidepressant class. A mixture of trials using SNRI, MAOI, and TCA were employed
  - Augmentation strategies included drugs that operate outside the usual monoamine-enhancing agents
    - Lamotrigine (Lamictal) dampened glutamate
    - Thyroid hormone improved metabolism and perhaps provided trimonoamine facilitation, as it is theorized that this drug may increase production of NE, DA, and 5-HT in the midbrain
    - Lithium "did what lithium does," which is largely unknown
      - Lithium might be a trimonoamine modulator and facilitate neuronal increases in available monoamines
      - It might stabilize neuronal membranes or second messenger systems via the inositol second messenger pathways
      - It might provide an increase in neurotrophic factors for better neural connectivity, improved brain circuitry, and communication with regard to its antidepressant mechanism of action

Performance in practice: confessions of a psychopharmacologist

- *What could have been done better here?*
  - As the psychopharmacologist, seeing the patient every four to eight weeks may not have been adequate
    - ∘ She seemed to collect social stressors and become more depressed and even psychotic very quickly
    - ∘ Secondarily, increased contact with the therapist may also have provided a better alert to the pending full relapse
    - ∘ Finally, as antidepressant regimens are cross-titrated, there likely exists a time frame when overall antidepressant plasma levels are low, predisposing the patient to a depressive relapse
- *Possible action items for improvement in practice*
  - Make sure that augmentation/combination strategies are all considered and weighed against potential for side effects, especially weight gain in this patient [pun intended]
    - ∘ Keeping this patient's wishes to avoid weight gain in mind and having open discussions about these risks and benefits allowed her to stay involved in treatment, and even to take medications with some metabolic risks
    - ∘ The patient was more willing to maintain her medications and having achieve therapeutic dosing based on rapport developed in this manner

Tips and pearls

- There are no approved weight-loss strategies in cases like this where psychotropic treatment creates immense amounts of weight gain
- Metformin (Glucophage) likely has the most evidence for reversal of AAWG but is not actually approved for weight loss
- Orlistat (Xenical), amantadine (Symmetrel), topiramate (Topamax), topiramate–phentermine combination (Q-Symia), lorcaserin (Belviq), naltrexone–bupropion combination (Contrave), zonisamide (Zonegran) have less available data for treating psychotropic-induced weight gain but some are approved for weight loss in general
  - Interestingly, if one were to postulate that increasing serotonin or specifically antagonizing the 5-HT2C receptor is the cause of AAWG, then lorcaserin (Belviq), which agonizes the 5-HT2C receptor, may have the theoretical pharmacodynamic rationale for future study as it may most likely reverse the serotonergic cause of the weight gain in the first place
- All of these agents carry side-effect risks, where you might develop side effects while trying to treat side effects. This could be a lose–lose situation
- Portion-control dietary instructions are easy to give and easy-to-follow for patients and should be attempted

- Using safer metabolic drugs at treatment initiation or switching to them makes clinical sense in the outpatient practice setting
- In inpatient units, the focus is often on fast symptom control rather than long-term side-effect management or patient rapport and compliance development
- Different practitioners will utilize different medication approaches, depending upon their experience and practice settings

Two-minute tutorial

What drugs appear to have less risk of weight gain?

- Typical antipsychotics
  - High-potency agents, i.e., haloperidol (Haldol), fluphenazine (Prolixin)
- Atypical antipsychotics
  - Lurasidone (Latuda), ziprasidone (Geodon), aripiprazole (Abilify), paliperidone (Invega), brexpiprazole (Rexulti)
  - Possibly asenapine (Saphris)
- Mood stabilizers
  - Lamotrigine (Lamictal)
- Antidepressants
  - Bupropion (Wellbutrin), vilazodone (Viibryd), Trazodone-ER (Oleptro), selegiline (Emsam), vortioxetine (Brintellix)
- Stimulants
  - All
- Sedative/hypnotics (BZs)
  - All

What drugs appear to be more weight promoting?

- Typical antipsychotics
  - Low-potency agents, i.e., chlorpromazine (Thorazine), thioridazine (Mellaril)
- Atypical antipsychotics
  - Clozapine (Clozaril), olanzapine (Zyprexa), quetiapine-XR (Seroquel-XR), iloperidone (Fanapt), risperidone (Risperdal)
  - Possibly asenapine (Saphris)
- Mood stabilizers
  - Carbamazepine (Equetro), divalproex sodium-ER (Depakote-ER), lithium
- Antidepressants
  - Mirtazapine (Remeron)
  - Most TCAs
  - Most MAOIs

- Most SSRIs
- Possibly SNRIs
- Sedative/hypnotics (antihistamine-based)
  - Possibly trazodone (Desyrel), doxepin (Silenor)

Treating AAWG with metformin

- Possibly the greatest evidence base for treating AAWG exists for metformin
- This drug is known to cause weight loss in its approved use for DM2
- It typically will not lower blood glucose to levels associated with hypoglycemic shock
- It may be associated rarely with acidosis side effects due to renal bicarbonate wasting
  - A baseline basic metabolic panel is warranted
  - Follow-up panels every 6–12 mo can evaluate for low bicarbonate level development
  - Typical side effects include nausea and diarrhea
- It is dosed at 500 mg twice a day and if no weight loss is noted in 6–8 wk, it can be maximized to 1000 mg twice a day
- If no weight loss is noted several weeks later, it should be discontinued as ineffective
- As of 2008
  - Multiple trials have evaluated the effect of metformin on weight and other metabolic parameters in adults and adolescents without diabetes as their primary illness
    - ○ Five of 12 trials in adults evaluated weight loss as a primary endpoint
    - ○ Significant weight reduction was found in four of these studies
    - ○ Weight reduction was significant in five of the six adolescent trials
    - ○ Metabolic parameters (blood pressure, waist circumference, cholesterol parameters, insulin/glucose levels) often showed varying results

Posttest self-assessment question and answer

Which of the following approaches likely has the most evidence to support its use as a weight-loss strategy in patients suffering from AAWG?

A. Orlistat (Xenicol)
B. Sibutramine (Meridin)
C. Fenfluramine (Pondimin)
D. Topiramate/phentermine combination (Q-Symia)
E. Metformin (Glucophage)

F. Naltrexone/bupropion combination (Contrave)

G. Lorcaserin (Belviq)

H. Bariatric surgery

Answer: E

Orlistat is approved for weight loss in general and has minimal evidence in psychiatric conditions. Sibutramine and fenfluramine have been removed from the market due to cardiac side effects, and were relatively contraindicated in patients taking antidepressants due to serotonin syndrome risks, thus limiting their use. Topiramate has a reasonable evidence base to support its use, but likely has less effectiveness and greater side effects compared to metformin. However, more recently, it was approved as a combination (with phentermine) weight-loss product called Q-Symia. Metformin likely has the most controlled data and a reasonably benign side-effect profile. Contrave was also recently approved for general weight loss and uses the combination of naltrexone to curb appetite reward and the noradrenergic potential of bupropion to curb appetite itself. Lorcaserin (Belviq) agonizes the 5-HT2C receptor. In animal models, antagonism here allows for marked weight gain. Some of the atypical antipsychotics with greater AAWG potential antagonize this receptor as well (e.g., clozapine [Clozaril], olanzapine [Zyprexa]). This theoretically gives lorcaserin the ability to pharmacodynamically counteract the offending pharmacologic property that causes AAWG. Bariatric surgery for AAWG is supported by small case studies, but often, mentally ill patients are screened out as not stable enough to participate in the rigorous eating pattern retraining that most bariatric programs enforce to obtain optimal postsurgical results.

References

1. Barowsky J, Schwartz TL. An evidence-based approach to augmentation and combination strategies for treatment resistant depression. *Psychiatry* 2006; 3:42–61.

2. Stahl SM. *Stahl's Essential Psychopharmacology*, 5th edn. New York, NY: Cambridge University Press, 2014.

3. Stahl SM. *Stahl's Essential Psychopharmacology: The Prescriber's Guide*, 4th edn. New York, NY: Cambridge University Press, 2013.

4. American Psychiatric Association. *Practice Guideline for the Treatment of Patients with Major Depressive Disorder*, 3rd edn. Washington, DC: American Psychiatric Association Press, 2010.

5. Topel ME, Zajecka JM, Goldstein CN, Siddiqui UA, Schwartz, TL. Using what we have: combining medications to achieve remission. *Clin Neuropsychiatry* 2011; 8:4–27.

6. Schwartz TL, Petersen T, eds. *Depression: Treatment Strategies and Management*, 2nd edn. New York, NY: Informa, 2009.

7. Megna JL, Schwartz TL, Siddiqui UA, Herrera Rojas M. Obesity in adults with serious and persistent mental illness: a review of postulated mechanisms and current interventions. *Ann Clin Psychiatry* 2011; 23:131–40.
8. Gokcel A, Gumurdulu Y, Karakose H, et al. Evaluation of the safety and efficacy of sibutramine, orlistat and metformin in the treatment of obesity. *Diabetes Obes Metab* 2002; 4:49–55.
9. Wu RR, Zhao JP, Jin H, et al. Lifestyle intervention and metformin for treatment of antipsychotic-induced weight gain a randomized controlled trial. *JAMA* 2008; 299:185–93.
10. Golay A. Metformin and body weight. *Intern J Obes* 2008; 32:61–72.
11. Ahmed AT, Blair TR, McIntyre RS. Surgical treatment of morbid obesity among patients with bipolar disorder: a research agenda. *Adv Ther* 2011; 28:389–400.
12. Desilets AR, Dhakal-Karki S, Dunican KC. Role of metformin for weight management in patients without type 2 diabetes. *Ann Pharmacother* 2008; 42:817–26.
13. Hahn MK, Cohn T, Remington G. Efficacy of metformin and topiramate in prevention and treatment of second-generation antipsychotic–induced weight. *Ann Pharmacother* 2010; 44.1349–50.
14. van der Loos ML, Mulder PG, Hartong EG, et al. Efficacy and safety of lamotrigine as add-on treatment to lithium in bipolar depression: a multicenter, double-blind, placebo-controlled trial. *J Clin Psychiatry* 2009; 70:223–31.
15. Calabrese JR, Huffman RF, White RL, et al. Lamotrigine in the acute treatment of bipolar depression: results of five double-blind, placebo-controlled clinical trials. *Bipolar Disord* 2008; 10:323–33.
16. Sadock BJ, Sadock VA. *Kaplan and Sadock's Synopsis of Psychiatry: Behavioral Sciences/Clinical Psychiatry*, 10th edn. Philadelphia, PA: Lipincott Williams & Wilkins, 2007.
17. Machado-Vieira R, Manji HK, Zarate CA Jr. The role of lithium in the treatment of bipolar disorder: convergent evidence for neurotrophic effects as a unifying hypothesis. *Bipolar Disord* 2009; 11:92–109.

The Case: The man who picked things up

The Question: How many antipsychotics can a patient take?

The Psychopharmacological dilemma: Finding an effective antipsychotic monotherapy and treating side effects simultaneously

Pretest self-assessment question (answer at the end of the case)

Which of the following is true regarding QTc prolongation and antipsychotics?

A. Thioridazine (Mellaril) has a warning
B. Ziprasidone (Geodon) has a warning
C. Iloperidone (Fanapt) has a warning
D. Electrocardiogram (EKG) monitoring should occur in cardiac risk patients, or those on antipsychotic polypharmacy, or those on super-dosed monotherapies
E. Only the antipsychotics in A, B, C should have EKG monitoring
F. All antipsychotics should have EKG monitoring
G. B and C
H. A, B, C, and D

Patient evaluation on intake

- 42-year-old man with a chief complaint of depression and family stress

Psychiatric history

- Was doing well until he became stressed with household issues and family issues
- Remains gainfully employed as an assembly line worker despite his stress
- When seen by a previous provider, was diagnosed with minor depression/adjustment disorder and placed on a minimal dose trial of an SSRI
- Goes to weekly supportive psychotherapy
- His psychiatrist moved and he presented for admission with minor depressive symptoms as noted
- However, this initial psychiatric interview revealed poor sleep, irritable and low mood, poor concentration, affect constriction, loss of speech prosody, and concrete thoughts
- Furthermore, when asked about psychotic symptoms, the patient nonchalantly stated that he did in fact receive messages from the TV, radio, and the assembly line at work. He admitted to "picking things up" all the time
- Outside picking up messages from the TV

- If a car drove by, he could hear people talking in the car even if they were miles away
- He would also pick up images in mirrors
- These took the form of hallucinations with which he has interacted
- The messages he received from these were mostly neutral and not affective laden, although some are derogatory
- These have been present for at least a year
- He is not distressed over these occurrences
- Currently takes only an SSRI from the previous provider
  - Sertraline (Zoloft) 50 mg/d
- No other previous medication trials
- No psychiatric admission history
- No suicide attempts

Social and personal history

- Married and has four adult children
- High school educated and is working full time
- Has a supportive wife, but they have had difficulties in the past
- Does not drink alcohol, smoke cigarettes, or abuse drugs
- There are no legal issues and he gets along well in the community and at work

Medical history

- There are no acute and no chronic medical problems
- Normal with regard to height, weight, and vitals
- There are no abnormal movements

Family history

- MDD in mother
- SUD throughout extended family
- ADHD in grandson

Current psychiatric medications

- Sertraline (Zoloft) 50 mg/d (SSRI)

Current medical medications

- None

Question

Based on this patient's history and the available evidence, what do you consider his diagnosis to be?

- MDD with psychotic features
- Adjustment disorder

- Schizophrenia
- Schizoaffective disorder
- Schizotypal personality

What would your next treatment likely be?

- Increase the SSRI, as sometimes this alleviates depressive psychosis
- Add an atypical antipsychotic
- Switch to an atypical antipsychotic
- Better delineate his diagnosis
- Refer for CBT or family therapy

Attending physician's mental notes: initial evaluation

- This patient is psychotic, which was apparently missed by the previous providers
- He is not guarded. Perhaps this was missed as he appears normal to most people, has a family, is gainfully employed, is older, and does not "look schizophrenic"
- Perhaps these symptoms have started in last few months and these did not exist when he started treatment with the prior provider
- Perhaps these symptoms have been present for several years regardless of his stress and depression levels and he has learned to live with them
- His depression is mild at best and does not appear severe enough to fuel psychotic symptoms
- Will need to see if he is psychotic even when fully euthymic, which suggests the differential diagnosis of schizoaffective disorder versus schizophrenia
- Will need to rule out substance-induced psychosis, although his history suggests no drug abuse
- Will need to rule out medically induced psychosis as he is a bit older with regard to developing schizophrenia

Further investigation

Is there anything else you would especially like to know about this patient?

- His history does need further clarification
  - Family members eventually present with the patient and confirm his history
    - They have seen the patient stressed and depressed but never to the degree where he missed work
    - They have not witnessed overt psychotic behavior where he has been seen interacting with his hallucinations (although he was moved from one assembly line to another the previous year).

Patient confirms he asked to move as the hallucinations were distracting

○ They deny that he abuses drugs or alcohol
○ They deny any previous family history consistent with an SPMI
○ The family reports that the patient has been more concrete and less emotional over the years. His loss of facial expression and bland speech has been felt to be due to depression. The patient does not see himself as depressed
○ The patient states that he has had these hallucinations for some time but has not recognized them as foreign. They occur regardless of mood
○ Medical workup shows no laboratory test abnormalities and his physical and neurological examination is normal

Question

Based on what you know about this patient's history and current symptoms, what would you do now?

- Increase the SSRI as sometimes this alleviates depressive psychosis
- Add an atypical antipsychotic
- Switch to an atypical antipsychotic
- Better delineate his diagnosis
- Order neuroimaging such as a brain MRI or computerized tomography (CT)
- Order an electroencephalogram (EEG)
- Order psychological testing
- Refer for CBT or family therapy

Attending physician's mental notes: initial evaluation (continued)

- The patient is consistently psychotic now. He has negative symptoms that were prodromal, and this appears to be late-onset schizophrenia
- Medical workup is negative
- He should have brain imaging to prove he has no mass lesion, given the late-age onset of symptoms
- There are no neurological changes, confusion, altered states of consciousness (delirium), and no seizure activity, thus an EEG is not warranted
- He is clearly psychotic; therefore, psychological testing is not warranted

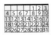

Case outcome: interim follow-ups through six months

- The patient is started and titrated slowly onto risperidone (Risperdal) without issue, and is left on 4 mg/d for several weeks
- This is partially effective in treating his positive symptoms. Dose is escalated to 6 mg/d

- The hallucinations resolve and the mild negative symptoms continue. He continues to work without any issues
- Toward the end of this period, his ideas of reference (IOR) begin to return
  - Higher dosing (8 mg/d) causes mild parkinsonism-like extrapyramidal symptoms, noted as resting tremor in one arm/hand
- Next he is switched to the only other atypical antipsychotic, olanzapine (Zyprexa), available at the time and is titrated to the recommended 10 mg/d, which alleviates his psychosis
- Psychosis returns after several more weeks
  - The atypical antipsychotic is increased to the maximum approved dose of 20 mg/d with resolution of the positive symptoms
- Again psychosis returns; olanzapine (Zyprexa) is increased above the approved norm to 30 mg/d
  - Positive symptoms resolve. He remains psychosis free for many months and continues to work
  - 15 lbs of AAWG occurs and there is a recurrence of mild parkinsonism. He tolerates both of these side effects without immediate concern
- Brain MRI is negative

Considering his current medication side effects, do you have any concerns?

- The weight gain might coexist with a metabolic disorder and laboratory samples should be sent for analysis
- The EPS is mild and tolerated, but he should be offered antiparkinsonian medication
- This early EPS is a poor prognostic indicator and TD is more likely to develop
- Need to make sure to monitor EPS closely and frequently
- Given the difficulty managing his psychosis and his initial propensity to side effects, a referral for family therapy may be warranted to keep his stress levels and expressed emotion levels in the home low

Attending physician's mental notes: six months

- At the time of this treatment, metabolic disorder was not well understood or appreciated, guidelines did not exist, and laboratory blood samples were not drawn for monitoring very often
- Initially, this patient looked easy to treat as his initial atypical antipsychotic was effective at usual dosing guidelines
- Now, he is looking more treatment resistant as his second atypical antipsychotic is requiring very high doses to alleviate his psychosis
- Olanzapine (Zyprexa) was approved at doses up to 20 mg/d
  - The use of 30 mg/d is off-label
  - There is little available data to support this practice but he is responding

- Theoretically, his dose must now be blocking enough D2 receptors to provide antipsychotic effects
- What were the causes of his relapses on risperidone (Risperdal) and lower dose olanzapine (Zyprexa)?
  - Treatment resistance and his more severe illness
  - An artifact of switching his medications and a window of undertreated psychosis during the cross-titration when both atypical antipsychotic doses were relatively low
- He is being very compliant despite weight gain and EPS side effects
- Will need to convince him to stay on his medications over the long term to avoid a worsening prognosis and social downward drift

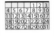

Case outcome: interim follow-ups through nine months

- EPS are easy to monitor and to treat
  - Patient is offered benztropine (Cogentin) 1 mg/d to control his EPS and this was effective without any burdensome anticholinergic side effects

Case outcome: interim follow-ups through 18 months

- Continues to see his supportive psychotherapist, who also intervenes more with family in sessions aimed at decreasing household stress and high expressed emotions
- Olanzapine (Zyprexa) 30 mg/d is continued
  - At the time of this treatment, metabolic disorder was not well understood, guidelines were not available, and laboratory blood samples were not analyzed, but his weight was followed sequentially. His weight gain did not progress past 15 lbs
- He continued to do well with only mild negative symptoms

Attending physician's mental notes: through 20 months

- Patient is doing very well
- Have to continue his simple medication regimen as long as possible
- It appears we began treatment in his first psychotic break
- His prognosis is promising

Question

How long should you treat this patient with his antipsychotic?
- After remission of psychosis, treat one year and then discontinue
- After remission of psychosis, treat five years and then discontinue
- After remission of psychosis, treat 10 years and then discontinue
- After remission of psychosis, treat indefinitely as only 10% of schizophrenics go on to maintain remission without medications and to lead relatively normal lives

- After remission of psychosis, treat indefinitely unless side effects complicate ongoing treatment

Case outcome: interim follow-ups through 24 months

- The patient gradually presents with difficulties
  - Increased stress due to issues with his family
  - Now has insomnia
  - He is not depressed, nor suicidal
  - Starts to have problems at work, which require intervention and moving to yet another assembly line
  - In session, he admits his psychosis is back to a moderate level. His hallucinations are mostly neutral but more now have negative and critical content
  - Mild IOR are back and they may be delusional, as he feels a local company's work trucks are following him around (this regional company has thousands of service trucks randomly around at any given time)

Question

What would you do now?

- Superdose the olanzapine (Zyprexa) up to 40 mg/d to recapture efficacy
- Add a typical antipsychotic as a combination therapy
- Switch to a new atypical antipsychotic
- Switch to a typical antipsychotic monotherapy

Attending physician's mental notes: 24-month follow-ups

- Life stress likely has caused his recurrence
- Need to make sure psychotherapy is in place and need to discuss with his work how to keep him employed without losing his job. Consider disability
- 40 mg/d of olanzapine (Zyprexa) seems high, but he did very well for many months on the 30 mg/d dose, and could temporarily use a higher dose until psychosis subsides
- Switching to the other, then currently available, a typical antipsychotic, quetiapine (Seroquel), is possible, but the cross-titration and its lower affinity may allow for more breakthrough psychosis to evolve
- Clozapine (Clozaril) is an option but perhaps his schizophrenia is not sufficiently resistant yet to require clozapine and its excessive side-effect burden

Does psychotherapy treat schizophrenia?

- The patient is getting supportive, intermittent family interventions but not formal family therapy in an ongoing manner. This type of therapy has an evidence base for treating schizophrenia

- CBT also has data to support its use in schizophrenia, more so for improving cognition and executive functioning
- Unfortunately, he likely needs more medication to lower his positive symptoms over the acute period to save his job in the short term

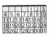

Case outcome: interim follow-up, 36 months

- Olanzapine (Zyprexa) monotherapy is increased to 40 mg/d to no avail and his psychosis continues
- Rather than cross-titrate over to the lower-potency quetiapine (Seroquel), use of a high-potency typical antipsychotic is used in combination with his olanzapine
  - Thiothixene (Navane) 5 mg/d is added to a reduced olanzapine (Zyprexa) dose (30 mg/d) to "top up" his failing atypical antipsychotic
  - This approach should make olanzapine seem more like a higher-potency antipsychotic with much more D2 receptor antagonism available
  - Psychosis resolves
- Parkinsonism increases
  - Benztropine (Cogentin) is increased to 2 mg/d with some mild anticholinergic constipation side effects emerging
- After a few months of combined antipsychotic therapy his psychosis resolved again
  - With the presence of moderate EPS and anticholinergic side effects, the patient complains of tolerability issues
    ○ Typical antipsychotic thiothixene (Navane) is lowered to avoid side-effect burden while olanzapine (Zyprexa) is continued
- Trazodone (Desyrel) 50 mg/d is given as needed to control insomnia flare-ups and to avoid future psychotic relapses
- He does well for a few more months with only residual negative symptoms present
- Unfortunately, lateral tongue movements develop and are noticed on routine annual AIMS examination. He is informed this may become permanent TD and is given treatment options
- The olanzapine (Zyprexa) is slowly discontinued. He is treated with vitamin E 800 IU to help alleviate the TD. The TD does gradually resolve
- Fearing for a relapse into psychosis, the patient chooses to start quetiapine (Seroquel)
  - Its lower D2 receptor affinity antagonism and its shorter half-life may benefit the patient due to a lower EPS risk profile
  - It is titrated to 600 mg/d
  - Higher doses are found to be too sedating
  - The psychosis begins to return

- Quetiapine (Seroquel) is topped up again with a different typical antipsychotic, perphenazine (Trilafon) 8 mg/d and the psychosis continues
- Quetiapine (Seroquel) is abandoned and tapered off while the typical perphenazine (Trilafon) is increased as a monotherapy to 40 mg/d
  - Psychosis continues
  - Parkinsonism increases
  - TD returns

Attending physician's mental notes: 48-month follow-ups

- This patient now has failed three atypical antipsychotics (risperidone, olanzapine, quetiapine), two typical augmentations (thiothixene, perphenazine), one typical antipsychotic monotherapy (perphenazine) at therapeutic doses, and yet his psychosis continues
- His prognosis now seems guarded as he is in another psychotic episode, and despite more aggressive treatment, his psychosis continues
- He has developed EPS, TD, and anticholinergic side effects, thus tolerability is becoming problematic
- He was taken out of work as his symptoms could cause a danger to self or others on the assembly line, which has put more stress on the family financially
- This is now a risky, complicated, and treatment-resistant case

Question

What would you do next?

- Continue to try a new monotherapy every one to two years as new atypical antipsychotics are approved and released to the market
- Use typical antipsychotics from different chemical families. Thus far, a thioxanthene (thiothixene) and a phenothiazine (perphenazine) have been tried. Consider a butyrophenone (haloperidol), dibenzoxazepine (Loxitane), or other chemical family
- Clozapine (Clozaril) is often more effective than other antipsychotics and can be used in more refractory cases or those with problematic movement disorders complicating treatment

Case outcome and multiple interim follow-ups to 48 months

- The patient elects to take clozapine (Clozaril)
- This trial escalates to 400 mg/d where side effects become problematic
  - Sedation ruins his quality of life
  - He developes enuresis
  - He begins drooling. At night, he chokes and aspirates
- This agent is lowered to a better tolerated 300 mg/d, albeit with subtheraputic levels (<0.3 mg/L)

- This prescriber obtained an informal consultation via email at this point to discuss refractory schizophrenia treatment options with two well-published colleagues in order to better delineate future treatment options for this patient
- Clozapine is now augmented with the typical antipsychotic loxapine (Loxitane) from the dibenzoxazepine chemical family up to 200 mg/d for a few months
  - Psychosis is less but still fluctuates
  - EPS continues but is treated with benztropine (Cogentin) 1–3 mg/d
  - TD is not apparent
  - EKG is obtained and shows some nonspecific changes and a slightly increased QTc that is not alarming but must be monitored
- A newer version of clozapine (Fazaclo) is released
  - It utilizes a dissolving oral preparation tablet with some preliminary evidence of less sedation and drooling effects
  - It replaces the patient's usual clozapine tablets but without a clinical or side-effect difference
  - Psychosis continues
- Weight gain now becomes problematic
  - 30 lbs of AAWG occurs gradually
  - Laboratory results are monitored and now suggest increased blood glucose levels (100–120 mg/dL), which is consistent with DM2
  - Prophylactically takes metformin (Glucophage) 1000 mg twice a day to lower his weight and keep blood glucose levels down
  - Lipid triglyceride levels later increase (200–250 mg/dL) and are controlled with omega-3-acid ethyl esters (Lovaza) 4 gm/d
- Clozapine is discontinued as ineffective and unable to be tolerated much past the therapeutic 300 mg/d dose
- Loxapine (Loxitane) is tapered off as ineffective
- Ziprasidone (Geodon) is started and ultimately dosed above approved levels to 200 mg/d
  - Is not effective
  - EKG shows cardiac changes (QTc prolongation above 450 ms) and he has clinical palpitations and dyspnea
  - It is stopped
- Paliperidone (Invega) is approved and tried next
  - Approved dose of 12 mg/d is not effective
  - Blood levels are measured now and are low despite excellent compliance
  - It is super-dosed to 18 mg/d
    - Plasma levels are obtained and found to be comparable to 12 mg risperidone
    - There is no antipsychotic response

- EPS continues and requires ongoing benztropine (Cogentin), which at 3 mg/d is moderately effective but dry mouth and constipation are problematic
- Asenapine (Saphris) is approved and the patient is switched to this agent and titrated to approved 10 mg twice a day sublingual dose, to no avail
  - 30 mg/d super-dosing is tried, also without psychosis relief
- Iloperidone (Fanapt) is approved and is administered next as monotherapy
  - Half-way through usual titration there is marked fatigue and orthostasis, thus it is discontinued
  - QTc was elevated, which would have limited further titration
  - Interestingly, his weight began to decrease with use of the last three atypical antipsychotics as clozapine was no longer being utilized
- Most recently, patient was placed on the latest atypical antipsychotic approved, lurasidone (Latuda) 40 mg/d
  - This was titrated to 120 mg/d, which was the highest approved dosing at the time, but without effect
  - It was next dosed to 160 mg/d without result
  - He continued on low-dose benztropine (Cogentin) for mild EPS
  - Since switching off olanzapine (Zyprexa), quetiapine (Seroquel), and clozapine (Clozaril), his weight, blood glucose, and lipids normalized
    - He lost his 30 lbs of AAWG
    - He does not require metformin
    - His EKG is normal
    - He does not have TD

Case debrief

- The patient has later-onset schizophrenia. It was actually caught in his first psychotic break
- After early remission of symptoms, he had a second break, which never truly remitted. He has continued with mild to moderate positive and mild negative symptoms throughout treatment
- He tried typical antipsychotics, atypical antipsychotics, clozapine (Clozaril) without remission
- He tried typical antipsychotics, atypical antipsychotics, clozapine (Clozaril) and developed EPS and TD
- He tried typical antipsychotics, atypical antipsychotics, clozapine (Clozaril) and developed metabolic disorder
- Finally, it was decided that his symptoms would likely be controllable but remain mild and that finding an agent with less EPS and metabolic side effects would be beneficial over the long term
- Almost every atypical antipsychotic (except aripiprazole [Abilify]) was tried, but finally dosed on an atypical antipsychotic with low EPS and low

metabolic risks (lurasidone [Latuda]), frankly as it was the most recently approved and released to the market at the time

- At the time of this book going to press, he was also tried on the new liquid preparation of clozapine (Versacloz), and again at 200–300 mg/d, developed excessive drooling, which was unresponsive to scopolamine and glycopyrrolate augmentation
- Given his previous TD and EKG changes, he is monitored closely
- This patient was discovered later to have mild Wolf–Parkinson–White arrhythmia, which was ablated by cardiology. Upon retrial with Versacloz, he did not experience cardiac tachyarrhythmia side effects again, although his QTc did suffer a 20 ms elongation limiting the use of the clozapine product line
- This patient has failed to respond to non-antipsychotic augmentation options: lamotrigine (Lamictal), minocycline (Minocin) [yes, the antibiotic], lithium carbonate
  - Interestingly, these ideas were obtained by attending a CME event where an expert panel discussed refractory schizophrenia cases
- ECT may be considered
- Despite his remaining symptoms, the patient works part-time as a store clerk and seems to be doing well psychosocially
- There are flare-ups in his symptoms, which are often dealt with by changing his environment and utilizing family therapy and job counseling
- He is maintained on the higher-potency typical antipsychotic trifluoperazine (Stelazine) at varying doses, on top of a low dose of clozapine
- This strategy appears to keep psychosis from worsening and minimizes his EPS, and he has less need for anticholinergics and their associated side effects

Take-home points

- This case emphasizes the need for full therapeutic trials of antipsychotic treatments
- Many guidelines suggest aggressive monotherapies versus polypharmacy approaches
- Use of approved medications at approved doses is warranted
- However, in more treatment-resistant cases, doses above those approved may be warranted, if monitored reasonably
  - Sometimes, patients metabolize antipsychotics aggressively and blood levels may be low
  - Measuring therapeutic drug levels, if available, may allow super-dosing strategies that actually bring the patient to therapeutic levels
  - Obtaining therapeutic drug levels may increase the clinician's confidence in dosing the antipsychotic to higher levels

- Finally, much consideration should be given to the patient's symptom severity, chronicity, and the ultimate side-effect burden as they will endure over a lifetime of treatment
- Choosing a lower side effect burden agent is preferred when possible
  - There are 11 different atypical antipsychotics (12 with clozapine) in the United States and all with differing side-effect profiles
- When side effects develop and must be endured, utilizing polypharmacy to reduce these side effects is often warranted
  - In this case, benztropine for EPS, metformin, and omega-3-acid ethyl esters for metabolic side effects were used

Performance in practice: confessions of a psychopharmacologist

- *What could have been done better here?*
  - Possibly using augmentation strategies sooner
  - Obtain a second opinion to see if any strategies were overlooked
  - More aggressive use of clozapine (Clozaril) despite side-effect burden and day-to-day intolerability issues may have been warranted
- *Possible action items for improvement in practice*
  - Read more review articles on treatment-refractory schizophrenia
  - Attend more educational events to develop new treatment ideas/plans and to increase confidence in prescribing rational off-label treatments
  - Be familiar with approved dosing strategies and also those super-dosing strategies outlined in the evidence-based literature

Tips and pearls

- At least three antipsychotics carry distinct warnings about QTc prolongation: ~20 ms for ziprasidone (Geodon), ~90 ms for thioridazine (Mellaril), ~9 ms for iloperdione (Fanapt)
- In practice, QTc prolongation has been seen with many of the atypical antipsychotics, some of the typical antipsychotics, and may be case specific
- More caution and EKG monitoring are warranted in those cases with cardiac histories, those who take other medications that prolong QTc (TCAs), those who are dosed above the approved limits, and those on antipsychotic polypharmacy
- EKG monitoring is not required specifically for any antipsychotic, but clinical rationale suggests monitoring similar to guidelines for TCA or lithium use

Two-minute tutorial

Switching atypical antipsychotics in this case?

- Early in this case, a classical titration switch strategy was utilized. The first or failing antipsychotic was tapered off gradually, while simultaneously the new antipsychotic was added at a roughly equal pace

- – Pros: The patient is never on two full-dosed antipsychotics at the same time
  - ○ This lowers risk of EPS and other side effects. This lowers cost
- – Cons: There may be a window, when both antipsychotics are subtherapeutic during the crossover
  - ○ This may leave the patient with lower levels of D2 antagonism and psychosis may worsen in the middle of the cross-titration
  - ○ This may make the clinician feel that the second agent is also failing
- • Later in this case, the current/failing antipsychotic was maintained at an approved, top antipsychotic dose while the new antipsychotic was added gradually. Once the second antipsychotic reached a minimally therapeutic dose, the initial, failing agent was discontinued
  - – Pros: In this strategy, essential therapeutic doses of two antipsychotics are reached before any drug tapering off
    - ○ This might allow for better psychosis control and no breakthrough psychosis window to occur
  - – Cons: Extra side-effect risks and increased cost, being on two medications at once
    - ○ Sometimes clinicians feel that the antipsychotic response was due to both agents. Both agents are maintained at full doses, gaining the prescriber the notoriety of being an atypical antipsychotic polypharmacist
    - ○ Again, this increases cost and side effect risk
    - ○ Guidelines and available data suggest this practice does not boost antipsychotic effects

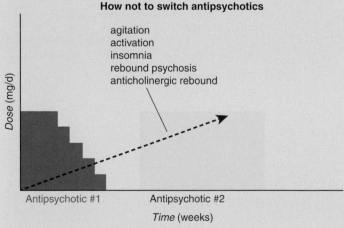

Figure 9.1. How not to switch antipsychotics.

Techniques for switching antipsychotics

- Converting patients from one antipsychotic to another requires great care in order to ensure that they do not develop withdrawal symptoms, rebound or breakthrough psychosis, or aggravation of side effects
- Generally, as shown in Figure 9.1, this means not precipitously discontinuing the first antipsychotic, therefore not allowing a true washout where subtherapeutic dosing gaps may occur between the administration of the two antipsychotics
- This approach was never utilized in this case

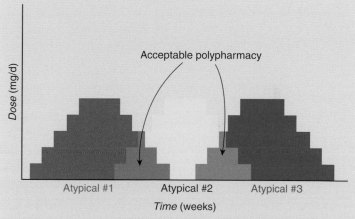

Figure 9.2. Switching from one antipsychotic to another.

- When switching from one antipsychotic to another, it is frequently prudent to "cross-titrate"; that is, to lower the dose of the first drug while building up the dose of the other in equal proportions or rations over a few days to a few weeks (Figure 9.2)
- This leads to transient administration of two drugs (polypharmacy) but is justified in order to reduce side effects and the risk of rebound symptoms, and to accelerate the successful transition to the second drug
- This approach was utilized initially for the first three monotherapies in this case

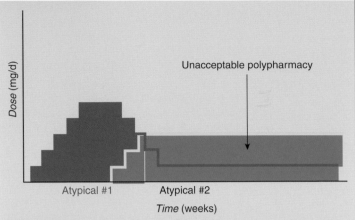

Figure 9.3. Getting caught in cross-titration.

- When switching from one atypical antipsychotic to another, the patient may improve in the middle of cross-titration
- Polypharmacy results if cross-titration is stopped at this point and the patient continues on both drugs indefinitely (Figure 9.3)
- It is generally better to complete the cross-titration ending with a solid monotherapy approach. This allows for the discontinuation of the first antipsychotic and use of an adequate monotherapy trial of the second antipsychotic before trying long-term polypharmacy
- One method for switching from one antipsychotic to another is to maintain the full dose of the initial failing antipsychotic agent until the second (new) antipsychotic agent is at its therapeutic dose
- This switching method may be best for patients who are switching due to lack of adequate control of symptoms on their initial antipsychotic rather than for those who are switching due to intolerability, as the temporary use of two fully dosed antipsychotic agents concomitantly may cause more side effects
- This approach was utilized later in this case when symptom control was minimal and even more breakthrough psychotic symptoms were feared

What are usual doses of the atypical antipsychotics in schizophrenia?

Risperidone (Risperdal)

- 1–8 mg/d approved dosing
- Usual dosing 4–6 mg/d

- Super-dosing up to 12 mg/d

Olanzapine (Zyprexa)

- 5–10 mg/d
- Usual dosing 15–20 mg/d
- Super-dosing up to 40+ mg/d

Quetiapine (Seroquel-XR)

- 50–800 mg/d
- Usual dosing 400–800 mg/d
- Super-dosing up to 1500 mg/d

Ziprasidone (Geodon)

- 40–160 mg/d
- Usual dosing 120–180 mg/d
- Super-dosing up to 320 mg/d

Aripiprazole (Abilify)

- 2–30 mg/d
- Usual dosing 15–30 mg/d
- Super-dosing 45–60 mg/d

Paliperidone (Invega)

- 3–12 mg/d
- Usual dosing 6–12 mg/d
- Super-dosing up to 18 mg/d

Asenapine (Saphris)

- 5–20 mg/d
- Usual dosing 10–20 mg/d
- Super-dosing up to 30+ mg/d

Iloperidone (Fanapt)

- 2–24 mg/d
- Usual dose 12–24 mg/d
- Super-dosing is poorly studied/reported

Lurasidone (Latuda)

- 40–120 mg/d
- Usual dosing 40–80 mg/d
- Super-dosing up to 240 mg/d in ongoing studies

Brexpiprazole (Rexult)

- 2–4 mg/d

Cariprazine (Vraylan)

- 1.5–6 mg/d

Posttest self-assessment question and answer

Which of the following is true regarding QTc prolongation and antipsychotics?

A. Thioridazine (Mellaril) has a warning
B. Ziprasidone (Geodon) has a warning

C. Iloperidone (Fanapt) has a warning
D. EKG monitoring should occur in cardiac risk patients, or those on antipsychotic polypharmacy, or those on super-dosed monotherapies
E. Only the antipsychotics in A, B, C should have EKG monitoring
F. All antipsychotics should have EKG monitoring
G. B and C
H. A, B, C, and D

Answer: H

Agents in A, B, C have QTc prolongation warnings from 9–90 ms and are true. D is accurate in that, clinically, this approach is warranted to prevent sudden cardiac death in at-risk patients. Therefore, A–D are correct, making H the best answer. G is false in that it leaves out thioridazine's 90 ms QTc warning that was levied some 40+ years after its approval. E and F are false in that more than A–C should be monitored, but that all patients treated with any antipsychotic should have an EKG every time is too stringent.

References

1. Rector NA, Beck AT. Cognitive behavioral therapy for schizophrenia: an empirical review. *J Nerv Ment Dis* 2001; 189:278–87.
2. McFarlane WR, Dixon L, Lukens E, Lucksted A. Family psychoeducation and schizophrenia: a review of the literature. *J Marital Fam Ther* 2003; 29:223–45.
3. Stahl SM. *Stahl's Essential Psychopharmacology*, 4th edn. New York, NY: Cambridge University Press, 2013.
4. Stahl SM. *Stahl's Essential Psychopharmacology: The Prescriber's Guide*, 5th edn. Cambridge University Press, New York, 2014.
5. Citrome L, Jaffe A, Levine J. Dosing of second generation antipsychotic medication in a state hospital system. *J Clin Psychopharm* 2005; 25:388–390.
6. Citrome L, Volavka J. Optimal dosing of atypical antipsychotics in adults: a review of the current evidence. *Harv Rev Psychiatry* 2002; 10:280–91.
7. Citrome L, Kantrowitz JT. Olanzapine dosing above the licensed range is more efficacious than lower doses: fact or fiction? *Expert Rev Neurother* 2009; 9:1045–58.
8. Citrome L, Stauffer VL, Kinon BJ, et al. Olanzapine plasma concentrations after treatment with 10, 20, 40 mg/d in patients with schizophrenia: an analysis of correlations with efficacy, weight gain, and prolactin concentration. *J Clin Psychopharmacol* 2009; 29:278–83.

9. Citrome L, Jaffe A, Levine J, Lindenmayer JP. Dosing of quetiapine in schizophrenia: how clinical practice differs from registration studies. *J Clin Psychiatry* 2005; 66:1512–16.

10. Citrome L, Jaffe A, Levine J. How dosing of ziprasidone in a state hospital system differs from product labeling. *J Clin Psychiatry* 2009; 70:975–82.

11. Milner KK, Valenstein M. A comparison of guidelines for the treatment of schizophrenia. *Psychiatr Serv* 2002; 53:888–90.

12. Schwartz TL, Stahl SM. Treatment strategies for dosing the second generation antipsychotics. *CNS Neurosci Ther* 2011; 17:110–17.

13. Golden G, Honigfeld G. Bioequivalence of clozapine orally disintegrating 100-mg tablets compared with clozapine solid oral 100-mg tablets after multiple doses in patients with schizophrenia. *Clin Drug Invest* 2008; 28:231–9.

14. Stahl SM, Grady MM. A critical review of atypical antipsychotic utilization: comparing monotherapy with polypharmacy and augmentation. *Curr Med Chem* 2004; 11:313–27.

15. Zhang XY, Zhou DF, Cao LY, et al. The effect of vitamin E treatment on tardive dyskinesia and blood superoxide dismutase: a double-blind placebo-controlled trial. *J Clin Psychopharmacol* 2004; 24:83–6.

16. Tiihonen J, Wahlbeck K, Kiviniemi V. The efficacy of lamotrigine in clozapine-resistant schizophrenia: a systematic review and meta-analysis. *Schizophr Res* 2009; 109:10–14.

17. Miyaoka T, Yasukawa R, Yasuda H, et al. Minocycline as adjunctive therapy for schizophrenia: an open-label study. *Clin Neuropharmacol* 2008; 31:287–92.

18. Leucht S, Kissling W, McGrath J. Lithium for schizophrenia revisited: a systematic review and meta-analysis of randomized controlled trials. *J Clin Psychiatry* 2004; 65:177–86.

19. Van Sant SP, Buckley PF. Pharmacotherapy for treatment refractory schizophrenia. *Expert Opin Pharmacother* 2011; 12:411–34.

The Case: It worked this time, but with a hitch

The Question: Can clozapine (Clozaril) work for patients without side effects?

The Dilemma: Using this medication in treatment-resistant schizophrenia frequently requires measures to make the drug better tolerated. Sialorrhea is often a stumbling block

Pretest self-assessment question (answer at the end of the case)

Clozapine (Clozaril)-induced sialorrhea (CIS), or excessive drooling, is caused by what theoretical pharmacologic mechanism?

A. Dopamine-2 receptor antagonism
B. Alpha-2 receptor antagonism
C. Serotonin-2A receptor antagonism
D. Muscarinic-3 receptor antagonism
E. B and D
F. A and C
G. All of the above

Patient evaluation on intake

- 26-year-old man met initially on an inpatient unit while paranoid

Psychiatric history

- This patient was admitted to a psychiatric inpatient unit in the middle of a second paranoid psychotic schizophrenia episode
- Symptoms consisted mainly of paranoid- and guilt-based delusions, thought blocking, and mild negative symptoms
- During his first psychotic break, he was released after successful inpatient treatment with haloperidol (Haldol) 10 mg/d
- Despite this treatment, the symptoms increased to the point of requiring a second inpatient stay where an increase in haloperidol (20 mg/d) was ineffective
- At this time, risperidone (Risperdal) was the only atypical antipsychotic available and he was switched and titrated to 6 mg/d with relief of psychosis, and discharged from the hospital
- Over the next year while followed in an outpatient setting, he was noted to be very compliant with his medication and appointments
- Family was supportive and involved in his care, and he wished to return to college to obtain an advanced degree
- Things were going well clinically and psychosocially; discussions were begun about long-term treatment, the risk of TD, and what his wishes were if he began a third psychotic break

- Unfortunately, the psychosis returned, and while an inpatient again
  - Risperidone (Risperdal) 10–12 mg/d was ineffective, and based upon previous discussions regarding the most effective and least TD-prone antipsychotic and with written advanced treatment, Psychiatric Advance Directives signed by the patient, he was started on clozapine (Clozaril), which was titrated to 400 mg/d
  - Psychosis resolved
  - Has been relatively symptom free for several years
  - Plasma levels are therapeutic at 500 ng/ml (levels >350 ng/ml have been shown to be clinically effective)
  - White blood cells have been stable (>3000/mL)
  - Mild sedation and moderate CIS are experienced

Question

Of the following choices, what would you do?

- Lower the clozapine (Clozaril) to lower CIS while trying to maintain a reasonable blood level to avoid breakthrough psychosis
- Lower the clozapine (Clozaril) to lower CIS while trying to maintain a reasonable blood level but combine with another atypical antipsychotic to maintain remission
- Lower the clozapine (Clozaril) to lower CIS while trying to maintain a reasonable blood level but combine with a typical antipsychotic to maintain remission
- Switch to oral, dissolving clozapine (FazaClo) tablets or liquid clozapine (Versacloz) to lower CIS
- Switch to an atypical antipsychotic monotherapy now that more are available
- Try to use an augmentation as an antidote to CIS while maintaining his effective current clozapine dose

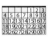

Case outcome

- Patient was very cautiously switched to aripiprazole (Abilify) over several weeks
  - There was a prompt relapse into psychosis
  - Switched back to clozapine (Clozaril) 400 mg/d with symptom resolution but with a return of CIS
- Eventually the clozapine dose was lowered to 300 mg/d and the CIS lowered partially
  - Plasma levels ranged from 200–350 ng/ml
- Later, a trial of oral dissolving clozapine (FazaClo) lowered his CIS to a mild and better-tolerated level
- He declined CIS antidotes as he felt he was able to tolerate his mild CIS as it is and did not want to have to take extra medication

- He remains positive symptom free, and has mild negative symptoms only
- He completed college and is gainfully employed in entry-level management at a local business

Case debrief

- This treatment-refractory schizophrenia case embraces the idea that schizophrenia is progressive and with each successive psychotic break, medication failure that more resistance develops
- This is contrary to the other treatment-resistant case where the schizophrenia patient was dosed on several typical and atypical antipsychotics for years prior to a trial of clozapine
- To counter this clinically, the theory was to use the most effective antipsychotic medication as soon as possible in this young adult's life
- The rationale was to offer the best chance of psychotic symptom remission with the hope of halting the progression of schizophrenia
- With advanced treatment planning, family consultation and proxy, written consent for the use of clozapine (Clozaril) early in treatment (he had only been on one typical and one atypical antipsychotic beforehand), he was placed on the most effective, albeit most side-effect prone, antipsychotic earlier in the course of his illness
- In this case, this was an excellent clinical decision as he had no TD/EPS or metabolic issues
- The mild sedation abated, and his CIS became much less problematic, avoiding the need for antidote-based polypharmacy, as clozapine dosing was refined to the lowest therapeutic dose in this particular patient
- Psychosocial decline was halted and actually reversed

Two-minute tutorial

Clozapine sialorrhea statistics and etiology

- CIS may occur in 10%–80% of patients taking clozapine
- The mechanism of CIS is poorly understood, but theoretically
  - Salivary flow is under parasympathetic control and mediated possibly by muscarinic M3 receptors
    - Agonism here produces more saliva output
  - Noradrenergically, alpha-2 receptor antagonism in salivary tissue may increase blood flow and saliva output. This blockade leaves beta-adrenergic receptors unopposed, causing salivary output as well

- Muscarinic receptor agonism and anticholinergic receptor antagonism (M1, M2, M3, M4)
  - M3 receptors are the most predominant receptors in salivary tissue and these are initially antagonized by clozapine (Clozaril)
    - Salivary secretions increase
    - M4 receptors are now unopposed and secondarily stimulated
    - This occurs to a lesser degree by clozapine, resulting in more predominant CIS

Possible antidotes for CIS

- Antidotes for CIS include
  - Alpha-2 agonists such as clonidine, lofexidine, guanfacine, alpha-methyldopa, and moxonidine
  - Anticholinergics such as pirenzepine, atropine, trihexiphenidyl, benztropine, procyclidine, biperiden, propantheline, scopolamine, glycopyrrolate, ipratropium (nasal)
  - Miscellaneous agents such as benztropine and terazocin combination, beta-blockers, and botulinum toxin injection

Posttest self-assessment question and answer

Clozapine (Clozaril)-induced sialorrhea (CIS), excessive drooling, is caused by what theoretical pharmacologic mechanism?

A. Dopamine-2 receptor antagonism
B. Alpha-2 receptor antagonism
C. Serotonin-2A receptor antagonism
D. Muscarinic-3 receptor antagonism
E. B and D
F. A and C
G. All of the above

Answer: E

CIS is felt to be initiated by (B) alpha-2 receptor agonism and (C) muscarinic-3 receptor antagonism, making answer E correct. Dopamine-2 receptor antagonism alleviates psychosis but does not contribute to salivary flow. Serotonin-2A receptor antagonism alleviates EPS but does not contribute to salivary flow.

References

1. Stahl SM. *Stahl's Essential Psychopharmacology*, 4th edn. New York, NY: Cambridge University Press, 2013.
2. Praharaj SK, Arora M, Gandotra S. Clozapine-induced sialorrhea: pathophysiology and management strategies. *Psychopharmacology* 2006; 185:265–73.

3. Iqbal A, Rahman MJL, Schwartz TL, et al. Therapeutic options in the treatment of clozapine induced side effects. *J Pharm Technol* 2004, 20:155–64.

4. Stahl SM. *Stahl's Essential Psychopharmacology: The Prescriber's Guide*, 5th edn. New York, NY: Cambridge University Press, 2014.

The Case: The figment of a man who looked upon the lady

The Question: Are atypical antipsychotics anti-manic, antidepressant, anxiolytic, and hypnotic as well?

The Psychopharmacological Dilemma: How to improve insomnia that is caused by depression, anxiety, mood swings, and hallucinations

Pretest self-assessment question (answer at the end of the case)

Which of the following properties of certain atypical antipsychotics lend to their ability to promote and maintain sleep?

A. Histamine-1 receptor antagonism
B. Serotonin-2A receptor antagonism
C. Serotonin-7 receptor antagonism
D. A and B
E. All of the above

Patient evaluation on intake

- 42-year-old woman with a chief complaint of depression and interpersonal stress

Psychiatric history

- The patient states she was horribly abused as a child and had been addicted to alcohol and other substances for many years. Now has been sober for 10 years and attends AA and Narcotics Anonymous (NA) routinely with good results
- Admits moderate levels of PTSD symptoms with nightmares, flashbacks, and panic attacks
- Routinely experiences dysthymia (persistent depressive disorder) with intermittent full MDEs
- Psychiatric review of symptoms suggests symptoms of marked mood lability, affective dyscontrol, empty depression, dissociative events consistent with mild borderline personality disorder (BPDO)
- There is no history of inpatient psychiatric admissions, and rarely any suicidal gestures or self-injurious behaviors
- Denies hallucinations and delusions, but states she is paranoid that people might mean her harm and always needs to "be aware of her environment"
- She has been in legal trouble for reacting to social situations by striking out
  - This occurs usually when narcissistic injury occurs or if emotions are triggered by reminders of past abuse

- The patient has been tried on
  - One SSRI, paroxetine (Paxil) 40 mg/d
  - One TCA, nortriptyline (Pamelor) 75 mg/d
- Both monotherapies allowed for moderate improvements in her symptoms at best
- Has attended supportive psychotherapy weekly for many years
- Attends AA or NA daily and has a sponsor who is supportive

Social and personal history

- Single, never married, and has no children
- Has a General Education Diploma and attends college classes sporadically now
- Past alcohol and SUD, but has been in remission for 10 years
- No current legal issues but has some financial hardships

Medical History

- Patient is overweight
- Has CAD, DM2, chronic obstructive pulmonary disease (COPD), hyperlipidemia, GERD, HTN, glaucoma
- Compliant with her primary care clinician who collaborates well with her psychiatrist

Family History

- MDD in mother and aunts
- SUD throughout her extended family
- GAD in her mother
- Possible ADHD in siblings

Current psychiatric medications

- Paroxetine (Paxil) 40 mg/d (SSRI)

Current medical medications

- Exenatide (Byetta)
- Metformin (Glucophage)
- Glipizide (Glucotrol)
- Ramipril (Altace)
- Albuterol (Ventolin inhaler)
- Fluticasone/salmeterol (Advair Diskus)
- Latanoprost (Xalatan)
- Ezetimibe (Zetia)
- Pravastatin (Pravachol)
- Protonix (Pantoprazole)

Question

Based on this patient's history and the available evidence, what might you do next, given that she still has moderate, residual depression and PTSD symptoms?

- Try another SSRI
- Switch to an SNRI
- Augment with a mood stabilizer
- Augment with an NDRI, like bupropion-XL (Wellbutrin-XL)
- Augment with a 5-HT1A receptor partial agonist, like buspirone (BuSpar)
- Augment with an atypical antipsychotic

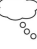

Attending physician's mental notes: initial evaluation

- Patient has worked hard on sobriety and even to control her personality disorder symptoms
- She is clearly depressed and agitated with PTSD
- At the time, the only other approved agent for PTSD was sertraline (Zoloft), an SSR
- Buspirone (BuSpar) and bupropion-XL (Wellbutrin-XL) are widely used, off-label depression augmentation options, which might help her
- Perhaps it is best to see what symptoms the patient deems most important to treat first, PTSD or depression
- As she is overweight with metabolic comorbidities, it may be worth choosing medications that limit risk of weight gain

Further investigation

Is there anything else you would especially like to know about this patient?
- What symptoms does the patient consider critical?
  - Insomnia – she does not sleep well in general and this may be caused either by depression, PTSD, or her current SSRI
  - Nightmares and flashbacks – these are very problematic as they trigger in the patient other symptoms such as mood lability and potential for violence and drug use
  - Depression – for her, this is secondary. Her depression is usually caused by PTSD flare-ups, their aftermath, and her interpersonal stressors
  - She feels that controlling her PTSD and sobriety will mitigate her depression

Question

Based on what you know about this patient's history, current symptoms, and medication, what would you do now?

- Try another SSRI
- Switch to an SNRI

- Augment with a mood stabilizer
- Augment with bupropion-XL (Wellbutrin-XL)
- Augment with buspirone (BuSpar)
- Augment with a sedating atypical antipsychotic
- Augment with prazosin (Minipress)
- Augment with a BZ sedative–hypnotic
- Augment with a melatonin receptor agonist hypnotic
- Augment with an antihistamine hypnotic

Attending physician's mental notes: initial evaluation (continued)

- Given the higher burden of PTSD and that she is failing an SSRI that is approved for PTSD and MDD, she will need to be tapered off and switched to another medication
- Will need to make a decision to try to treat all of her symptoms at once or treat single target symptoms in order of severity
- Formal CBT, such as exposure therapy for PTSD, is not available in the community and she has good rapport with her supportive therapist and her sponsors; therefore, these treatments should continue
- The other approved medication for PTSD is sertraline (Zoloft), which makes clinical, regulatory, and guideline-based sense
- Avoiding potentially addictive products is clearly warranted

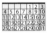

Case outcome: interim follow-ups through three months

- Next, she is cross-titrated off paroxetine (Paxil) and onto paroxetine-CR (Paxil-CR)
- The patient states she has been on paroxetine (Paxil) for some time now and is comfortable with it as it has helped partially
- As informed consent is given, steering her away from continued paroxetine use, her resistance increases
- States paroxetine at higher doses in past has been problematic for her
  - She is offered a newer option and she states she would like to try the slow-release CR preparation
  - It is titrated to 50 mg/d
  - There is no clear benefit
- Is offered a switch to another SSRI, sertraline (Zoloft), or to use a combination strategy bupropion-XL (Wellbutrin-XL)
- After weighing the options and giving informed consent, knowing that sertraline (Zoloft) is mechanistically similar to her paroxetine-XR (Paxil-CR), she opts for the NDRI bupropion-XL (Wellbutrin-XL) combination in the hope of a different outcome than with her SSRI, but also that it may curb her weight and improve her energy

- Titrated up to 450 mg/d as a combination with the SSRI, and the depression and vegetative symptoms do improve somewhat, but she continues with her usual partially treated PTSD symptoms and insomnia
  Considering her current medication regimen, do you have any concerns?
- Does she have a history of seizures or eating disorder, as bupropion products may induce seizures in these patients?
  - She does not
- The paroxetine-CR (Paxil-CR) is a robust inhibitor of the p450 2D6 enzyme system, for which bupropion products are a substrate
  - Is it possible that this drug interaction might elevate her bupropion plasma levels and induce a seizure?
- She is benefitting from this combination
  - Perhaps bupropion levels might be drawn, or
  - Perhaps augmenting her remaining PTSD symptoms with an antiepileptic medication might be a win–win situation, where symptoms and side effects are reduced simultaneously

Attending physician's mental notes: six months

- At the time of this treatment, the CYP450 interaction was a notable concern but this patient was significantly overweight, which likely accommodated this higher end of normal approved dosing
- Her depression appears well treated now but her PTSD residual symptoms continue to be problematic
- As she had modest gains from her first two medications, an SSRI and an NDRI, stopping them might cause relapse
- Adding another augmentation is likely warranted now, using a specific target symptom approach

Case outcome: interim follow-ups through nine months

- The patient agrees to augmentation with the antiepileptic selective GABA reuptake inhibitor (SGRI) tiagabine (Gabitril)
- This agent is not addictive, and in theory should elevate GABA availability, promote anxiolysis, and also protect against bupropion-induced seizures
- This augmentation was supported at this time by open-label trials but had no sanctioned approvals
  - Titrated to 16 mg/d
  - Sleep improves, but no other clear effects on the PTSD reliving events
  - It should be noted that this drug failed in controlled monotherapy trials in the treatment of PTSD some years later, and was also given a warning that despite being an approved epilepsy treating medication, it could actually cause seizures in non-epileptics
  - This patient suffered no such complications, however

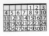

Case outcome: interim follow-ups through 12 months

- The patient gradually presents with more difficulty as random social events trigger PTSD reliving and some mood lability occurs
  - There are increased psychosocial stressors and a return of depressive symptoms
  - Sobriety continues
  - PTSD symptoms increase
  - Outside her usual insomnia and nightmares, she now has "a little man watching her"
    - Upon investigation, it is determined that she has a visual hallucination of a small man staring down at her when she is on the verge of falling asleep (hypnagogic hallucination)
    - This hallucination is not related to any PTSD themes, but she finds it very disturbing

Clinically, what types of patients typically suffer hypnagogic hallucinations?

- Narcolepsy patients
- Narcoleptics also may suffer sleep paralysis, cataplexy (drop attacks), as well as their usual REM-onset sleep attacks
- In this case, these hallucinations could also be related to a relapse into drug use or seizure activity (both of which were negative)

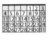

Case outcome: interim follow-ups through 12 months (continued)

- Evaluated for sleep disorder
  - Found to have OSA
  - Prescribed a continuous positive airway pressure (CPAP) machine and is compliant with its use
- The OSA appears to be unrelated to the hallucinations
- There is no relapse into drug use to explain the hallucinations
- She is not having seizures

Question

What would you do now?

- Escalate the tiagabine (Gabitril)
- Augment with a 5-HT1A receptor partial agonist
- Augment with an anxiolytic or hypnotic agent that is not addictive
- Add an atypical antipsychotic
- Taper off the now ineffective medications and start a new regimen

Attending physician's mental notes: 12 month follow-ups

- Despite increasing progress on her initial three medication regimen (SSRI, NDRI, SGRI), this was thwarted by social stress and exposure to PTSD-triggering stimuli

- Given her increased mood lability, irritability, potential for violence, flashbacks, and now limited hallucinations, an antipsychotic might be warranted
- At this time, it was becoming known that the atypical antipsychotics could drive an increase in weight but it was unclear if they would increase the metabolic syndrome
- This patient already has the metabolic syndrome, but it is very well controlled and followed very closely by her PCP

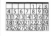

Case outcome: interim follow-up, 24 months

- This patient had fully relapsed
- The SSRI, paroxetine-CR (Paxil-CR), is discontinued due to its ineffectiveness
- The SGRI tiagabine (Gabitril) is tapered off as it was only partially effective, but mounting evidence suggests it may create seizures in non-epileptic patients
- Continues on bupropion (Wellbutrin-XL) as she recollects this being the most beneficial for her depressive symptoms. It also has halted her weight gain and curbed her appetite
- Next, she starts the more SERT-selective SSRI escitalopram (Lexapro) up to 20 mg/d to treat PTSD and residual depressive symptoms
- She is also given low-dose atypical antipsychotic quetiapine (Seroquel) 25–50 mg at bedtime to help induce sleep, possibly improve depression, PTSD, and mood lability
  - It is felt to be too risky to use a potentially addictive BZ sedative–hypnotic, given her SUD history and well-maintained sobriety
  - This low-dose quetiapine is not expected to cause metabolic complications
  - If she has persistent hallucinations, then the dose could be increased to full antipsychotic potential at doses greater than 400 mg/d
  - Warned of low but possible TD/EPS risks
  - Warned of metabolic risks and primary care clinician is consulted
- Does well on this combination and gradually has very good control of depression and PTSD symptoms
- The "little man" leaves
- A few weeks later, the "little man" hallucination comes back but without a full PTSD exacerbation
  - The quetiapine (Seroquel) is increased to 100 mg at bedtime with good effect once again
- A few weeks later, the patient has increased problems with lability and anger at her AA and NA meetings, which is putting her sobriety at risk

- Now offered a daytime 25–50 mg quetiapine (Seroquel) dose, which is utilized with good effect
  - In total, takes 150 mg daily along with the SSRI and NDRI combination therapy
- After several weeks of no hallucinations and good affect control, she opts to lower the atypical antipsychotic slowly to avoid prolonged exposure and side effects
- This goes well clinically and she continues on her baseline SSRI plus NDRI

Attending physician's mental notes: 36-month follow-ups

- Patient now is fairly stable and doing better
- The SSRI and NDRI work well together
  - Symptoms are much less problematic
  - They appear to cancel each other's side effects out in a win–win scenario
  - Denies side effects altogether
- There is no increase in metabolic issues with the short-term, low-dose quetiapine (Seroquel) use, and an eye examination for cataracts was negative
- Patient is compliant and we can extend her visits to quarterly, short appointments while we continue her supportive psychotherapy

Case outcome and multiple interim follow-ups to 60 months

- The patient, throughout this time, has sustained months of doing very well with regard to relationships, returning to school, and being active in the community
- She has occasional mild flare-ups of PTSD and BPDO symptoms but these are less frequent and less severe, likely as a result of ongoing sobriety, supportive psychotherapy, and a consistent set of well-tolerated medications
- Occasionally, increased PTSD nightmares and the "little man" return
  - The patient self-titrates as-needed quetiapine (Seroquel) 50–150 mg daily doses
    - This treats insomnia and restores her sleep cycle
    - This treats bedtime hallucinations
    - This improves affective lability during the daytime
- It is also determined that she has two types of insomnia
  - The spells mentioned here are usually PTSD related and fairly extreme in the patient's point of view
    - The rapid onset of sleep, maintenance of sleep, and possible antipsychotic effect of her atypical antipsychotic is warranted and works well here

- There is a second type of insomnia that is more insidious, where she has difficulty initiating sleep, increasing her fatigue and irritability with consequences next day
- Does not wish to take the atypical antipsychotic routinely as it was "quite strong" with morning fatigue and potentially more serious risks (TD/EPS/metabolic)
- For these transient bouts of insomnia that would last a few weeks at a time, she was offered the MT1/MT2 receptor agonist approved, non-addictive hypnotic (ramelteon [Rozerem] 8 mg at bedtime) with good results and no side effects
- Now reliably alternates the quetiapine (Seroquel), ramelteon (Rozerem), or no treatment, depending upon the type of sleep she is, or is not, having

Case debrief

- The patient has the common comorbidity of MDD, PTSD, and SUD
- She has personality traits that leave her vulnerable to relapses
- She had an uncommon hypnogogic hallucination presentation
- She has been fairly stable now for many years likely due to sobriety, sustained supportive psychotherapy, steady consistent medication management with fully dosed and rationally used polypharmacy (instead of many rapid medicine changes in reaction to new psychosocial, adjustment disorders)
- The treating team was very good about communicating about the patient's situations, symptoms, and likely etiology (adjustment based versus syndromal based) so that systems-based care was evident and very effective
- The medication regimen continues in this fashion with continual good results

Take-home points

- The patient had a balanced biopsychosocial approach by treating team members and great support through the AA and NA communities and her primary care team
  - This is a win–win, textbook collaboration situation that ideally should be emulated in these complex patient types, in that all providers were communicating and working together
- The patient had, in addition, win–win polypharmacy situations
  - Her SSRI and NDRI canceled out each other's side effects while providing additive clinical effectiveness regarding her many comorbidities
  - Her quetiapine (Seroquel) low dose was able to function as a multipurpose drug in that it: (a) induced and (b) maintained

her sleep, (c) alleviated her hallucination, and (d) provided agitation control and mood stability during the day AND it did not increase her metabolic disorder given its low dose and intermittent use

- The atypical antipsychotics likely should not be considered first-line drugs for insomnia, as they do carry risk for TD, EPS, and metabolic disorder that approved and other off-label hypnotics do not carry

Performance in practice: confessions of a psychopharmacologist

- *What could have been done better here?*
  - Hindsight is 20/20
  - It likely was a bit risky, in terms of potential drug interactions, having the patient on a full dose of paroxetine and bupropion simultaneously
    - If she happened to be a poor CYP450 2D6 enzyme metabolizer, then her seizure risk could increase as her bupropion levels could have elevated
    - Use of tiagabine (Gabitril) in addition to these two medications and the 2D6 interaction risk promoted an even greater seizure risk
  - Use of a more metabolically friendly atypical antipsychotic with a mild to moderate sedating profile might have been preferred to the quetiapine (Seroquel) used in this case (perhaps asenapine (Saphris))
- *Possible action items for improvement in practice*
  - Memorize drug interaction tables or use software or the internet to screen for interactions
  - If more risky combinations are used, consider a blood draw laboratory test for CYP450 isoenzyme quantification or drug levels
  - Be aware that atypical antipsychotics possess positive mechanisms for inducing and maintaining sleep that are not just side effects but reasonable positive clinical effects

Tips and pearls

- Two SSRI antidepressants are approved for treating PTSD: paroxetine (Paxil) and sertraline (Zoloft)
- In recent years, prazosin (Minipress) has acquired an evidence base to support its off-label use in alleviating PTSD nightmares specifically. This would have been a reasonable option in this case
- The beta-blockers have some limited evidence that, if utilized quickly after a trauma, they blunt hyperautonomic responses and that the risk for

developing full syndromal PTSD may be less. This would have been less helpful in this case as her trauma was not recent
- The atypical antipsychotics and antiepileptic medications also have a limited evidence base that supports their use in PTSD
- The sedatives are controversial as PTSD patients have high addiction rates

A pharmacodynamic moment

Why do some atypical antipsychotics make good hypnotic agents?
- First, using an atypical antipsychotic to treat insomnia has risks and benefits
  - Pros
    - Relatively fast onset
    - Non-addictive
    - May induce sleep onset and improve deep sleep propensity
  - Cons
    - Risk of serious side effects that other hypnotics do not have (TD, EPS, metabolics, cataracts [interestingly, follow-up long-term studies suggest little risk, but FDA language still suggests diligence in monitoring here for quetiapine], QTc prolongation, stroke in certain populations)
- Many atypical antipsychotics are antihistamines
  - H1 receptor antagonism causes sedation and somnolence as a result of lowering wakefulness center (tuberomammillary nucleus [TMN]) activity while promoting sleep center (ventrolateral preoptic [VLPO] area) activity
  - This enhances the brain's sleep–wake switch to favor sleep
  - The faster acting and reliably absorbed atypical antipsychotics, each with a shorter half-life, may be better suited as hypnotic agents as they may have more dependable sleep onset and less morning hangover effect
- Some atypical antipsychotics possess serotonin-2A (5-HT2A) receptor antagonism
  - This mechanism appears to help maintain patients in a sleeping state by promoting more efficient and deeper sleep
  - In this way, these antihistamine effects may initiate sleep and 5-HT2A blocking effects may maintain deeper or more efficient sleep
- At higher doses, atypical antipsychotics antagonize D2 receptors
  - This mechanism is known to calm agitated patients who are psychotic

- It is possible this calming effect lowers anxiety and cortical hyperarousal at bedtime, allowing better sleep onset
- This profile of H1, 5-HT2A, and D2 antagonism is unique to the atypical antipsychotics and is not found in any approved hypnotic agent
- If approved hypnotic agents fail to aid in sleep initiation or maintenance then atypical antipsychotics may be a reasonable choice

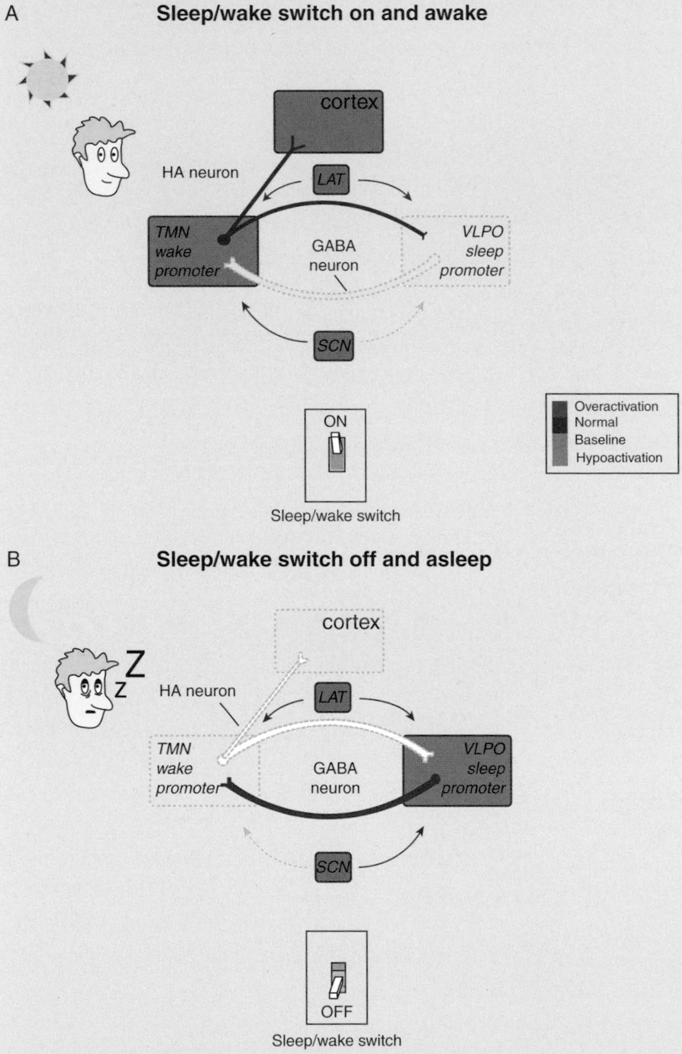

A **Sleep/wake switch on and awake**

B **Sleep/wake switch off and asleep**

Figure 11.1. A and B. Sleep/wake switch.

Antihistamine and the sleep–wake switch

- The hypothalamus is a key control center for sleep and wakefulness, and the specific circuitry that regulates sleep/wake is called the sleep/wake switch
- The "off" setting, or sleep promoter, is localized within the VLPO of the hypothalamus, while "on", wake promoter, is localized within the TMN of the hypothalamus
- Two key neurotransmitters regulate the sleep/wake switch: histamine from the TMN and GABA from the VLPO
  - When the TMN is active and histamine is released in the cortex and into the VLPO, the wake promoter is on and the sleep promoter is inhibited (Figure 11.1A)
    - ○ H1 receptor antagonists, antihistamines, block this wakefulness pathway whereby the released histamine transmitter cannot activate frontal lobe neurocircuitry, causing a loss of arousal and resultant fatigue
  - When the VLPO is active and GABA is released into the TMN, the sleep promoter is on and the wake promoter inhibited (Figure 11.1B)
  - The sleep/wake switch is also regulated by orexin/hypocretin neurons in the lateral hypothalamus (LAT), which stabilize wakefulness, and by the suprachiasmatic nucleus (SCN) of the hypothalamus, which is the body's internal clock and is activated by melatonin, light, and activity to promote either sleep or wakefulness

Serotonin receptor antagonism and sleep

- The 5-HT2 receptor subfamily is comprised of several types with the three most commonly studied subtypes: 5-HT2A, 5-HT1A, and 5-HT2C
- 5-HT7 and 5-HT1D receptors have also been evaluated more recently for their hypnotic, circadian, and antidepressant effects
- Evidence from both clinical and preclinical studies suggests that 5-HT2A receptors modulate and improve slow wave sleep (SWS) when blocked
  - This is considered deep and restorative
  - Is often lacking in depressed or fibromyalgia (FM) patients
- 5-HT2A receptor antagonists may not induce hypnosis, or sleep onset, but once sleep occurs, there is a shift toward more efficient and improved SWS
- 5-HT2A receptor blockade may promote better sleep by a complex mechanism
  - Serotonin typically diminishes cortical glutamatergic arousing neurons by agonizing 5-HT1A receptors and enhances glutamatergic excitatory arousal by stimulation of 5-HT2A receptors
  - In effect, antagonizing the 5-HT2A receptor dampens cortical activity to promote some somnolence and fatigue

- This may help maintain deeper sleep throughout the night as normal sleep cycle arousal is lowered (See Figure 11.2)
- Currently there are several compounds (volinanserin, esmirtazapine, pruvanserin, pimavanserin, APD125, AVE8488, HY-10275, ITI-722) in clinical development for the treatment of insomnia that utilize this 5-HT2A receptor antagonism, at least in part, as their hypnotic mechanism of action

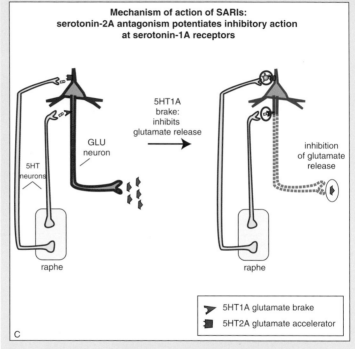

Mechanism of action of SARIs:
serotonin-2A antagonism potentiates inhibitory action
at serotonin-1A receptors

Figure 11.2. Mechanisms involved in the sleep/wake cycle.

In the image on the left, glutamate's excitatory influence arouses the cortex and promotes wakefulness, even at night. On the right, 5-HT2A receptor blockade is noted and glutamate activity lowers, and secondarily, cortical activity is dampened, resulting in deeper, more efficient sleep with less nocturnal awakenings

What about 5-HT1D receptor antagonism?

- This autoreceptor may be stimulated by use of triptans to treat migraine headaches
- However, as a presynaptic autoreceptor, it may be antagonized by some antipsychotics and result in:
  - Facilitated serotonin release
  - Facilitated NET as a postsynaptic heteroreceptor

PATIENT FILE

- Facilitated glutamate transmission as a heteroreceptor
- Rodent preclinical models suggest this mechanism may allow for antidepressant activity
- It is unclear if 5-HT1D promotes better sleep
- Combination 5-HT1D antagonist–SSRI antidepressants are being researched; vortioxetine is approved and an antidepressant now

What about 5-HT7 receptor antagonism?

- This case discusses some of the complex pharmacodynamics of quetiapine (Seroquel), but other atypical antipsychotics also have unique pharmacodynamic profiles that may contribute to their theoretical potential
- 5-HT7 receptor antagonism is not a property highly possessed by quetiapine (Seroquel), but is a potential novel mechanism by which other antipsychotics may allow for antidepressant and improved sleep effects
- The atypical antipsychotics asenapine (Saphris) and lurasidone (Latuda) possess a higher affinity for this receptor blockade, as does the classic atypical antipsychotic clozapine (Clozaril)
- The 5-HT7 receptor seems to be sensitive to light and circadian rhythms and may exert antidepressant potential through this complex mechanism
- Perhaps by improving sleep at night, energy and concentration during the daytime (depressive symptoms) may improve
- For example, rodent models show antidepressant properties when this receptor is blocked pharmacologically or removed genetically
- However, many of these effects will only occur at certain times of the day or the night
- It is also worth noting that the SSRI antidepressants boost synaptic serotonin levels, which ultimately causes the downregulation of these 5-HT7 receptors, and which is roughly equivalent to the blockade provided by the atypical antipsychotics noted earlier
  - The antidepressant vortioxetine has high affinity for 5-HT7 receptor antagonism
  - The atypical antipsychotic with high 5-HT7 receptor antagonism and approval to treat bipolar depression as a monotherapy is lurasidone (Latuda)

Posttest self-assessment question and answer

Which of the following properties of certain atypical antipsychotics lend to their ability to promote and maintain sleep?

A. Histamine-1 receptor antagonism
B. Serotonin-2A receptor antagonism
C. Serotonin-7 receptor antagonis
D. A and B
E. All of the above

161

Answer: E

The antihistamine property is common to the approved hypnotic doxepin (Silenor) and the over-the-counter sleep aid diphenhydramine (Benadryl), and is shared by some of the atypical antipsychotics. This property helps to initiate sleep while 5-HT2A receptor antagonism of the atypical antipsychotics tends to maintain and promote deeper sleep. 5-HT7 receptor antagonism appears to help circadian rhythms in order to promote appropriate timing and length of sleep duration.

References

1. American Psychiatric Association. *Treatment of Patients with Acute Stress Disorder and Posttraumatic Stress Disorder Guidelines*. Washington, DC: American Psychiatric Association, 2004.
2. Stahl SM. *Stahl's Essential Psychopharmacology*, 4th edn. New York, NY: Cambridge University Press, 2013.
3. Stahl SM. *Stahl's Essential Psychopharmacology: The Prescriber's Guide*, 5th edn. New York, NY: Cambridge University Press, 2014.
4. Ravindran LN, Stein MB. Pharmacotherapy of post-traumatic stress disorder. *Curr Top Behav Neurosci* 2010; 2:505–25.
5. Miller LJ. Prazosin for the treatment of posttraumatic stress disorder sleep disturbances. *Pharmacotherapy* 2008; 28:656–66.
6. Schwartz TL, Nihalani N. Tiagabine in anxiety disorders. *Expert Opin Pharmacother* 2006; 7:1977–87.
7. Berlin HA. Antiepileptic drugs for the treatment of post-traumatic stress disorder. *Curr Psychiatry Rep* 2007; 9:291–300.
8. Schwartz TL, Stahl SM. Treatment strategies for dosing the second generation antipsychotics. *CNS Neurosci Ther* 2011; 17:110–17.
9. Stahl SM. Multifunctional drugs: a novel concept for psychopharmacology. *CNS Spectr* 2009; 14:71–3.
10. Stahl SM. Selective histamine H1 antagonism: novel hypnotic and pharmacologic actions challenge classical notions of antihistamines. *CNS Spectr* 2008; 13:1027–38.
11. Sharpley AL, Solomon RA, Fernando AI, da Roza Davis JM, Cowen PJ. Dose-related effects of selective 5-HT2 receptor antagonists on slow wave sleep in humans. *Psychopharmacology (Berl)* 1990; 101:568–9.
12. Dugovic C, Wauquier A. 5-HT2 receptors could be primarily involved in the regulation of slow-wave sleep in rat. *Eur J Pharmacol* 1987; 137:145–6.
13. Teegarden BR, Al Shamma H, Xiong Y. 5-HT2A inverse-agonists for the treatment of insomnia. *Curr Top Med Chem* 2008; 8:969–76.
14. 5-HT2A inverse-agonists for the treatment of insomnia. http://www.intracellulartherapies.com/investor/2009_3_10.htm. Accessed August 6, 2010.

15. Abbas A, Roth B. Pimavanserin tartrate: a 5-HT2a inverse agonist with potential for treating various neuropsychiatric disorders. *Expert Opin Pharmacother* 2008; 9:3251–9.

16. Eplivanserin soothes insomnia without next morning effects. www. clinicalpsychiatrynews.com/article/S0270-6644(08)70780-X/ fulltext. Accessed August 6, 2010.

17. Ward SE, Watson JM. Recent advances in the discovery of selective and non-selective 5-HT1D receptor ligands. *Curr Top Med Chem* 2010; 10:479–92.

18. Davidson JR, Brady K, Mellman TA, Stein MB, Pollack MH. The efficacy and tolerability of tiagabine in adult patients with post-traumatic stress disorder. *J Clin Psychopharmacol* 2007; 27:85–8.

19. Wang Z, Kemp DE, Chan PK, et al. Comparisons of the tolerability and sensitivity of quetiapine-XR in the acute treatment of schizophrenia, bipolar mania, bipolar depression, major depressive disorder, and generalized anxiety disorder. *Int J Neuropsychopharmacol* 2011; 14:131–42.

20. Bauer M, El-Khalili N, Datto C, Szamosi J, Eriksson H. A pooled analysis of two randomised, placebo-controlled studies of extended release quetiapine fumarate adjunctive to antidepressant therapy in patients with major depressive disorder. *J Affect Disord* 2010; 127:19–30.

21. Guscott M, Bristow LJ, Hadingham K, et al. Genetic knockout and pharmacological blockade studies of the 5-HT7 receptor suggest therapeutic potential in depression. *Neuropharmacology* 2005; 48:492–502.

22. Kroeze WK, Roth BL. The molecular biology of serotonin receptors: therapeutic implications for the interface of mood and psychosis. *Biol Psychiatry* 1998; 44:1128–42.

The Case: The man who could not sell anymore

The Question: What to do when comorbid depression and social anxiety are resistant to treatment

The Dilemma: Rational subsequent polypharmacy trials may fail to achieve remission

Pretest self-assessment question (answer at the end of the case)

Why might certain atypical antipsychotics interact detrimentally with MAOI antidepressants?

A. Some atypical antipsychotics possess serotonin reuptake inhibitor (SRI) properties
B. Some atypical antipsychotics possess SNRI properties
C. Some atypical antipsychotics are partial agonists at 5-HT1A receptors
D. Some atypical antipsychotics are partial agonists at D3 receptors
E. A, B, and C
F. All of the above

Patient evaluation on intake

- 57-year-old man with a chief complaint of "horrible depression"
- Feels he "made a bad decision" late in his career and is now unemployed after many successful years in equipment sales
- Fearful and nervous that, at his age, he is too young to retire and too old to find a new job and be successful again

Psychiatric history

- He had been without major mental health issues until he left his gainful employment of 25 years as an equipment salesman
  - He left during poor corporate economic times assuming his company would fold
  - He left for a second company for a sales position in a different market, and performed poorly on commission and was let go
  - Psychiatric symptoms developed after this
- Has not been able to go back to work at all due to anxiety and fear about failing again
- He admits to full syndromal depressive symptoms
  - He has passive suicidal thoughts and ideational guilt that he is a bad spouse in that he has let his family down by being unsuccessful and unemployed
  - Additionally, he is amotivated, fatigued, and states he is hopeless and pessimistic about the future
- He now worries about everything, all the time, cannot focus, and is tense. He states he was never like this before

- Additionally, he can barely "look people in the eye" and talk to them
  - He is very concerned about doing and saying the right thing
  - After years of remembering many details in sales, he can barely keep any facts straight, and is convinced that he will fail
  - Panic attacks have occurred at recent job interviews, and since then is avoiding most situations where he has to speak to superiors
- He has relatively few friends as most were colleagues at his previous job
- While he is at home more, he is experiencing more conflict with his wife, although states she is supportive

Social and personal history

- He graduated high school and served successfully in the military without traumatic experience
- He was gainfully employed in sales for many years before changing jobs as noted
- His wife is employed now but they are having difficulties financially
- He does not use drugs or alcohol

Medical history

- He has experienced 10 lbs of weight loss while depressed over last several months and is slightly underweight
- He has no acute or chronic medical issues
- He has no liver or renal disease

Family history

- Denies any known psychiatric illness in any family member

Medication history

- One treatment so far while in the care of his PCP
  - He failed to respond to SSRI, paroxetine (Paxil) 40 mg/d
  - Currently, perhaps 10% improvement in intensity and duration of symptoms at most because he feels less sad and weepy, but is still socially not functioning well

Psychotherapy history

- Recently, started outpatient CBT with an adept clinician in the local area
- Little to no response to these psychotherapeutic interventions, but acknowledges it is early in the course of this intervention and feels comfortable conversing about his problems

PATIENT FILE

Patient evaluation on initial visit

- Acute onset of MDD symptoms with associated, or possibly comorbid anxiety disorder roughly six months ago
- Suffers immensely with guilt over his decision to leave his successful job for a new job this late in his career
- Very compliant with medication management and has started psychotherapy
- Good insight into his illness and wants to get better
- He has current, fleeting passive suicidal ideation
- There is possible guilt-based delusions (current ideation noted) but no other signs of psychosis
- Reports no current side effects

Current medications

- Duloxetine (Cymbalta) 90 mg/d (SNRI was started after his SSRI failure by PCP)
- Alprazolam (Xanax) 1 mg two times per day (BZ)

Question

In your clinical experience, would you expect a patient such as this to recover?

- Yes, his premorbid health and functioning were very good
- No, sometimes a devastating, late-life event causes chronic, unremitting depression

Attending physician's mental notes: initial evaluation

- This patient has his first MDE now. It is acute and triggered by a psychosocial stressor
- It seems more than an adjustment disorder as it is pervasive, lasting over time, and clearly disabling
- His initial failure on an SSRI is not alarming and he has recently been given a higher dose of an SNRI and started CBT, fostering a good prognosis
- However, his older age of onset, loss of income, status, and some mild marital strife are concerning

Question

Which of the following would be your next step?

- Increase the duloxetine (Cymbalta) to the full FDA dose of 120 mg
- Increase the alprazolam (Xanax) to a higher, more effective dose
- Augment the current medications with a third agent to accelerate response
- Do nothing additionally outside waiting for SNRI and CBT effectiveness to occur

Attending physician's mental notes: initial evaluation (continued)

- This patient seems to be on one of the gold standard approaches to treating depression
- First, an adequate trial dose/duration of an SSRI
- Now started on an adequate dose/duration of an SNRI
- Is starting bona fide CBT
- Things look good in that the current regimen is a reasonable one
- However, there is concern regarding his passive suicidal thoughts, which provoked a discussion about safety planning
- He also seems very guilt ridden and ruminative about his failure. Will need to continue to investigate if this is delusional
- He does meet criteria for MDD, SAD, and GAD
- It is unclear if these are truly comorbid or if his depression is fostering the anxiety symptoms
  - The latter seems appropriate as he had no premorbid anxiety prior to the onset of his depression
- If comorbid anxiety becomes more evident, his prognosis worsens

Further investigation

Is there anything else you would especially like to know about this patient?

- What about details concerning his past medication treatment and his current CBT?
  - Has taken paroxetine (Paxil) up to 40 mg/d
    - He tolerated it well and only had a minimal clinical response, which he states was not meaningful
  - CBT has just started
    - He has had three sessions so far
    - He likes his therapist and seems to have good rapport
    - This therapist is well known in the community and has a good reputation, where many CBT techniques are utilized although in an eclectic manner, over a longer time than the usual manualized 12–20 week duration

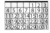

Case outcome: first interim follow-up visit four weeks later

- Patient now has more CBT and time on his SNRI
- He is no better and acknowledges the same symptoms as on his first appointment
- He states that he has no side effects, which he appreciates

PATIENT FILE

Question

Would you increase his current medications or change strategies?

- Yes, continue both duloxetine and alprazolam at even higher doses
- Continue duloxetine at higher doses but keep alprazolam as it is
- Continue alprazolam at higher doses but keep duloxetine as it is
- No, discontinue both agents as they have failed to allow for a clinical response and start new regimen

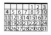

Case outcome: second interim follow-up visit at two months

- The patient had his duolextine (Cymbalta) increased to 120 mg/d and his alprazolam (Xanax) increased to 1 mg three times a day
- He has no side effects, is normotensive, and is reliably using his controlled substance
- This approach maximizes his antidepressant and the anxiolytic augmentation increase may help his secondary anxiety symptoms
- This approach leaves no doubt that a full trial was given and also allows more time for CBT to become clinically effective
- The patient shows moderately better affective ranges, less psychomotor symptoms, and states an absence of suicidal thoughts as a result
- He is felt to be 20%–30% better

Attending physician's mental notes: second interim follow-up visit at two months

- Despite being a little better, the patient is still not in remission after two months of treatment
- He is half-way through a clinical course of CBT
- He has a clinically meaningful response now in that he is not suicidal and has a better affective range
- He is a bit less anxious and ruminative but he is not a 50% responder yet
- As his primary illness is MDD, it is doubtful that escalating his BZ sedative–anxiolytic will help further
- He is side effect free, which is positive
- As this patient is now becoming possibly more treatment resistant with regard to his MDD, and he continues with comorbid anxiety features and has his first clinically meaningful response, switching away from his current SNRI may cause a loss of this initial clinical effect
- Waiting longer will likely not promote full remission
- His prognosis seems a bit worse compared to that assumed at the first visit
- Increasing his sedative–anxiolytic is unlikely to remit his depression
- Combination or augmentation strategies are discussed and considered by the patient

169

Question

What would you do next?

- As he is a partial responder with minimal response, discontinue his SNRI and try a new antidepressant
- As he is a partial responder with minimal response, has now failed two therapeutic trials, would combine with a second approved antidepressant
- As he is a partial responder with minimal response, has now failed two therapeutic trials, would combine with an evidence-based augmentation agent
- Continue to wait on the current regimen and CBT for full effectiveness to occur as he is side effect free

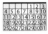

Case outcome: interim follow-up visits through seven months

- The patient agrees to start a NaSSA antidepressant combination by adding mirtazapine (Remeron) to the existing regimen (SNRI plus BZ)
- There is no initial change in status, patient is still depressed and anxious but not suicidal
- Mirtazapine (Remeron) is increased to 45 mg/d
  - At this dose, profuse night sweats develop and cannot be tolerated
  - Outside diaphoresis, he was normotensive with no other side effects
- Attempts are made to slowly lower both antidepressants (SNRI plus NaSSA) to mitigate side effects and to maintain his partial efficacy, but to no avail
- Patient chooses to discontinue both antidepressants
- Other strategies are considered and he agrees
  - To start bupropion-XL (Wellbutrin-XL), an NDRI, and is gradually titrated to 450 mg/d, and
  - To have the alprazolam converted to the slow-release preparation (Xanax-XR) for ease of use and once daily dosing
- He continues with same MDD symptoms. The night sweats resolve but he now develops insomnia and nightmares
- He has now failed to improve after 20 sessions of CBT

PATIENT FILE

Question

What would you do next?

- Discontinue the bupropion-XL as it has been dose maximized and is not being tolerated, and change to a more classic antidepressant in another class such as a TCA or an MAOI
- Change to another novel antidepressant in another class such as trazodone (Desyrel/Oleptro) or nefazodone (Serzone), vilazodone (Viibryd), vortioxetine (Brintellix)
- Lower the bupropion-XL to a dose where diaphoresis is alleviated and augment with an antiepileptic or mood stabilizer such as lamotrigine (Lamictal) or gabapentin (Neurontin)
- Augment with an atypical antipsychotic such as aripiprazole (Abilify), quetiapine-XR (Seroquel-XR), lurasidone (Latuda)
- Augment with lithium or thyroid hormone

Attending physician's mental notes: interim follow-up visits through seven months

- Patient has now failed SSRI, SNRI, NaSSA, NDRI antidepressant trials and CBT
- His prognosis for full depressive remission seems poorer
- Discussions around changing the class of medication to an MAOI, or augmenting with an atypical antipsychotic, or use of ECT are held

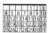

Case outcome: interim follow-up visits through 24 months

- MAOI is selected by the patient based on balance of efficacy and tolerability
  - Prefers less risk of movement disorder and metabolic syndrome
  - Feels he can be safe with diet and drug interactions
- Titrated on the selegiline transdermal patch (Emsam 6 mg/d initially and then to 9 mg/d), to which there is a 30% improvement at best
  - Unfortunately develops an allergic glue reaction (contact dermatitis) to the patch and it is discontinued, and the MAOI washed out over two weeks
- Changing to a new MAOI would require a two-week washout, and use of another MAOI might limit future augmentation strategies
- Other available MAOIs appear to have greater side-effect burden with regard to sedation, orthostasis, weight gain, and sexual dysfunction
  - Next choice is an atypical antipsychotic augmentation as he is afraid of the washout period again needed for a new MAOI

- He also requires a new approved antidepressant monotherapy
  - He is titrated onto venlafaxine-XR (Effexor-XR) SNRI therapy and also onto quetiapine (Seroquel) atypical antipsychotic as an augmentation therapy in a CIT strategy
    - Doses reach 300 mg/d and 400 mg/d, respectively
    - He tolerates these well without issue and finally gains a 50% response in his symptoms, which is his best to date
  - Able to lower alprazolam anxiolytic dose as he is calmer and sleeping better
  - He is still not in remission
- Next, there is failure to remit with
  - L-methylfolate (Deplin) augmentation
  - Modafinil (Provigil) augmentation
  - Intolerability to d-amphetamine (Dexedrine) augmentation
- Begins couples counseling and chooses to officially retire early, which lowers social stress
  - For the latter, he does not have to confront his performance anxiety and these symptoms are mitigated
  - He begins working out at a gym routinely, which restores some self-esteem
  - He is about 60% improved in MDD symptoms
  - His generalized anxiety-type symptoms resolve

Case debrief

- Two-thirds of patients have TRD
- Treatment resistance in this case appeared to be low initially as the patient had a clear stressor induce his first, and only, MDE
- However, his anxiety and fear of failure and performance seemed to increase his pharmacological treatment resistance, where he failed to respond to SSRI, SNRI, NDRI, NaSSA, and MAOI treatments, as well as several augmentations
- He was also resistant to a trial of CBT and marital therapy
- He finally achieved a sustained response, but not remission, on an SNRI plus an atypical antipsychotic and a BZ
- Dynamically, he lowered his stress by finally deciding to take a financial loss, by retiring early, which also contributed to symptom reduction
- This way, much of his anxiety about the future and guilt about his past was no longer relevant

Take-home points

- Many patients with depression and agitated features either do not respond to SSRIs or do not respond sufficiently to achieve functional independence, a return to vocation, or a social life. This patient had some symptom reduction but not a reduction in disability
- Many patients with depression also do not respond to CBT, if available
- Nevertheless, some patients can improve with pharmacologic approaches that have not been exhausted
- In this case, high-dose antidepressant monotherapies, combinations, and augmentations were utilized, allowing a response eventually
- In practice, this patient continues to try new combination and augmentation approaches in the hope of gaining remission

Performance in practice: confessions of a psychopharmacologist

What could have been done better here?

- Is eclectic CBT less effective than manualized, research-based CBT?
  - This patient could have been referred for the latter or even a change in psychotherapy technique toward a dynamic or interpersonal approach
  - Sometimes, psychotherapy needs to be "dosed" like a medication in that once a full dose and duration is tried, clinicians have to admit treatment failure and aggressively move toward a new treatment or psychotherapy option
- Should failure of the newer MAOI (selagiline patch) warrant a trial on an older "tried and true" MAOI such as phenelzine (Nardil) or tranylcypromine (Parnate)?
- Should more bona fide approved augmentation strategies (quetiapine-XR or aripiprazole) been initiated before the less evidence-based ones used here?

Possible action items for improvement in practice

- Research data for augmentation strategies that are not FDA approved
  - Determine if effect sizes are comparable, or not, to help guide future choices in TRD
- Research available United States and international guidelines regarding TRD
  - These often compile a summary list, that is easier to interpret, of evidence-based treatments and the stringency of the available data to support their use

- If this patient's guilt was actually delusional in nature, achieving a reasonable dose of antipsychotic may have alleviated this and his other depressive symptoms
  - In this case, using an atypical antipsychotic sooner may have been warranted

Tips and pearls

- The MAOI class of drugs is likely underutilized due to the overemphasized risk of hypertensive crisis and serotonin syndrome that surrounds their use
- In this case, only a moderate dose of one MAOI was tried. There likely was room for other MAOI trials
- Transdermal skin reactions in practice are difficult to treat and often fail to be relieved by oral/topical antihistamines or corticosteroids
- MAOIs are clearly approved for treating depression but also have a good evidence base for treating social anxiety and atypical presentations of MDD
- One negative to using MAOIs is the washout required between MAOI and other antidepressant trials
  - This often leaves patients unmedicated and prone to worsening of symptoms
  - Similar to switching among SSRI, SNRI, and TCAs, sometimes patients will respond to one MAOI better than another
- Occasionally, patients can be treated with BZ anxiolytics or mood stabilizers during a washout to help avoid insomnia and agitation, at least to make the transition easier
- However, certain typical and atypical antipsychotics have serotonergic and/or noreadrenergic potential, and despite not being officially contraindicated, probably should be avoided during washout or concurrent use of an MAOI (see following discussion)

Mechanism of action moment

Why might some antipsychotics interact with MAOI and create serotonin syndrome despite not being officially contraindicated?

- All atypical antipsychotics are 5-HT2A receptor antagonists and some are 5-HT2C antagonists
- Some atypical antipsychotics carry more MAOI interaction possibilities
  - Ziprasidone (Geodon) has functional SNRI pharmacodynamics

- SNRIs are fully contraindicated in MAOI use due to serotonin syndrome potential
- Ziprasidone (Geodon), aripiprazole (Abilify), brexpiprazole (Rexult), asenapine (Saphris), lurasidone (Latuda), and the active metabolite of quetiapine (Seroquel), norquetiapine, have functional 5-HT1A agonism properties
  - This pharmacodynamic property is utilized by the anxiolytic buspirone (BuSpar) and is also contraindicated in MAOI use
  - However, antipsychotic agents like this may be combined with MAOI by experienced clinicians, using much caution, in very treatment-resistant cases, as some of the serotonin drug interaction properties are weak or sometimes theoretical
    ◦ Risks and benefits need to be weighed on a case-by-case basis in these situations, not unlike when advanced clinicians therapeutically combine MAOI and TCA in TRD patients
- Clinically, knowing which atypical antipsychotics carry greater serotonergic activity also predicts those that may theoretically interact negatively with MAOI and should likely be avoided in combination

Two-minute tutorial

5-HT1A receptor agonism in treating depression

- How does 5-HT1A receptor agonism help treat depression or anxiety? This mechanism seems important in that
  - Buspirone (BuSpar) antidepressant augmentation is an evidence-based treatment
  - As noted here, many atypical antipsychotics employ this mechanism and are MDD augmentation strategies
  - Two of the latest antidepressants approved, vilazodone (Viibryd) and vortioxetine (Brintellix), utilize this mechanism

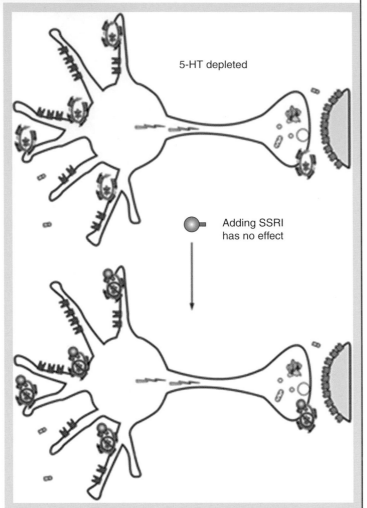

Figure 12.1. Mechanism of action of buspirone augmentation.

- SSRIs act indirectly by increasing synaptic levels of serotonin (5-HT)
- If 5-HT is depleted, there is no 5-HT release and SSRIs are ineffective
- This has been postulated to be the explanation for the lack of SSRI therapeutic actions or loss of therapeutic action of SSRI in some patients

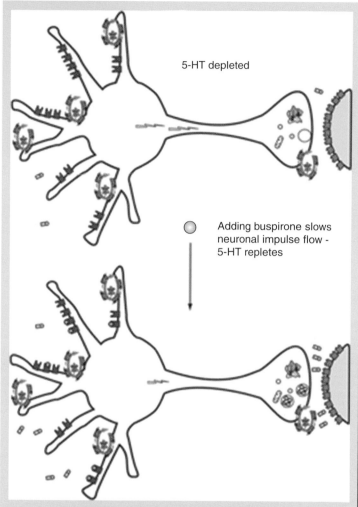

5-HT depleted

Adding buspirone slows
neuronal impulse flow -
5-HT repletes

Figure 12.2. Mechanism of action of buspirone augmentation.

- Shown here is how buspirone may augment the action of SSRIs both by repleting serotonin (5-HT) and directly desensitizing 5-HT1A receptors
- One theoretical mechanism of how 5-HT is allowed to reaccumulate in the 5-HT-depleted neuron is the shutdown of neuronal impulse flow
- If 5-HT release is essentially turned off for a while so that the neuron retains all the 5-HT it synthesizes; this may allow repletion of 5-HT stores
- A 5-HT partial agonist such as buspirone, or certain antidepressants or atypical antipsychotics, act directly on somatodendritic autoreceptors to inhibit neuronal impulse flow, possibly allowing repletion of 5-HT stores

- Additionally, these agents might boost actions directly at 5-HT1A receptors to help the small amount of 5-HT available in this scenario accomplish the targeted desensitization of 5-HT1A somatodendritic autoreceptors that is necessary for antidepressant actions

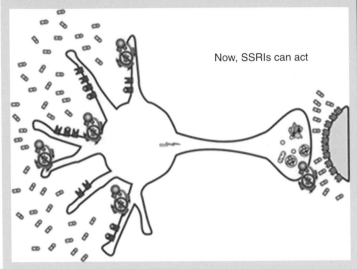

Now, SSRIs can act

Figure 12.3. Mechanism of action of buspirone augmentation.

- Shown here is how buspirone or other 5-HT1A agonists potentiate ineffective SSRI action at 5-HT1A somatodendritic autoreceptors, resulting in the desired disinhibition of the 5-HT neuron
- This combination of 5-HT1A agonists plus SSRIs may be more effective, not only in depression but also in other disorders treated by SSRIs, such as OCD and PD

Posttest self-assessment question and answer

Why might certain atypical antipsychotics interact detrimentally with MAOI antidepressants?

A. Some atypical antipsychotics possess SRI properties
B. Some atypical antipsychotics possess SNRI properties
C. Some atypical antipsychotics are partial agonists at 5-HT1A receptors
D. Some atypical antipsychotics are partial agonists at D3 receptors
E. A, B, and C
F. All of the above

Answer: E

As discussed in this chapter, some atypical antipsychotics utilize SSRI, SNRI, and partial 5-HT1A receptor agonism, which may contribute to their antidepressant potential but certainly may lead to hypertensive crisis or serotonin syndrome when combined with an MAOI. D3 receptor agonism is unlikely to affect MAOI use and is a mechanism solely possessed by aripiprazole (Abilify).

References

1. Nandagopal JJ, DelBello MP. Selegiline transdermal system: a novel treatment option for major depressive disorder. *Expert Opin Pharmacother* 2009; 10:1665–73.
2. Stahl SM. *Stahl's Essential Psychopharmacology*, 4th edn. New York, NY: Cambridge University Press, 2013.
3. Stahl SM. *Stahl's Essential Psychopharmacology: The Prescriber's Guide*, 5th edn. New York, NY: Cambridge University Press, 2014.
4. Schwartz TL, Nihalani N. Tiagabine in anxiety disorders. *Expert Opin Pharmacother* 2006; 7:1977–87.
5. Schwartz TL, Stahl SM. Optimizing antidepressant management of depression: current status and future perspectives. In: Cryan JF, Leonard BE, eds. *Depression: From Psychopathology to Pharmacotherapy*. Basel: Karger, 2010; pp. 254–67.
6. Schwartz TL, Petersen T, eds. Depression: Treatment Strategies and Management, 2nd edn. New York, NY: Informa, 2009.
7. Keller D. MAO inhibitors. *Cleve Clin J Med* 2011; 78:81.

The Case: The woman who thought she was ill, then was ill

The Question: What to do when medication is not absorbed, nor effective

The Dilemma: Treating anxiety and agitation in the severely medically ill

Pretest self-assessment question (answer at the end of the case)

What are some usual benefits of slow-release preparation medications?

A. Lower blood plasma levels often allow for less severe adverse effects

B. Extended half-life often allows for once-daily dosing and improved adherence

C. Cost is usually lowered as once-daily dosing is less costly to manufacture

D. Improved effectiveness over the parent immediate-release preparation

E. A and B

F. A, B, and C

G. All of the above

Patient evaluation on intake

- 44-year-old woman with a chief complaint of "being confused"
- Many clinicians have issued several diagnoses and she presents for a consultation
- Patient states that she has been "depressed and anxious as long as she can remember"

Psychiatric history

- The patient reports chronic and relapsing MDEs throughout her life
- At the initial visit, she feels minor to moderate amounts of depressive symptoms
  - She admits to poor sleep, mood, interest, energy, concentration, and appetite
  - She has increased guilt and worthlessness at times
  - She denies any active suicidal thinking
- There is no evidence of psychosis; however, she does seem to have dissociative spells during times of stress
- She may have had one episode of hypomania, but this was poorly defined, and she was smoking marijuana and drinking alcohol at the time
  - She has been completely sober for three years
- The patient does not meet full diagnostic criteria for GAD, but does worry excessively when depressed
- She has occasional panic attacks, but does not meet criteria for PD as these are often induced by interpersonal stressors
- Admits to suffering from AN in her teens and early adulthood but has had no weight-related symptomatology in last two decades

- Current body mass index (BMI) is 22, which is within normal range
- Denies having a distorted body image at this time
- Longitudinally, she admits to many dependent personality traits and borderline personality traits
  - She admits to having abandonment, dependency, and control issues, impulsive self-destructive behaviors, anger management problems, and she tends to see things in an "all-or-none" manner
  - The patient experiences idealization and devaluation in her relationships, and this pattern is also noted when she deals with medical professionals
- The patient had one suicide gesture by way of a minor overdose approximately a month and a half prior to consultation
- Denies any current suicidal symptoms
- She has had two psychiatric admissions, one as a teenager and the other after the recent overdose noted here

Social and personal history

- Graduated high school and college
- Gainfully employed at times but developed many medical problems, which prevents her working now
- She has relatively few friends and relies heavily on her significant other for support
- Does not use drugs or alcohol now
  - Sober for more than three years
  - In college, she misused barbiturates for a short time

Medical history

- This patient sees multiple medical providers and suffers from:
  - FM
  - Temporomandibular joint (TMJ) arthritis
  - Hypothyroidism
  - GERD
  - Osteoporosis
  - Migraine headaches
  - Myofacial dystonia
  - Pelvic floor dysfunction

Family history

- Bipolar disorder in one aunt
- MDD throughout her family
- GAD in one aunt

Medication history

- The patient reports that she has tried, with minimal sustained improvements
  - Three SSRIs: sertraline (Zoloft) 200 mg/d, citalopram (Celexa) 40 mg/d, escitalopram (Lexapro) 20 mg/d
  - An NDRI: bupropion-XL (WellbutrinXL) 450 mg/d
  - An SNRI venlafaxine-XR (Effexor-XR) 225 mg/d
  - Two antiepileptic medications used for anxiolysis: divalproex sodium (Depakote) 1500 mg/d, gabapentin (Neurontin) 1800 mg/d
- Has never had a trial of MAOIs, TCAs, NaSSAs, SARIs, lithium, stimulants, or atypical antipsychotics (serotonin–dopamine antagonists [SDAs])
  - Sometimes, the atypical antipsychotics are classified as SDAs as they simultaneously block 5-HT2A and D2 receptors
- She has not maintained a euthymic state for more than two months in many years

Psychotherapy history

- Many years of weekly, individual eclectic psychotherapy
- Most recently was seeing a psychiatrist for combined weekly supportive therapy and medication management
- There is no clear course of dedicated PDP, DBT, or CBT
- Little to no response to these psychotherapeutic interventions is noted, but acknowledges that she seems to function better when involved in psychotherapy

Patient evaluation on initial visit

- Patient has chronic depressive symptoms with comorbid personality disorder and many somatic symptoms, which she has experienced for many years
- Initially, she seems to be more debilitated by her medical complaints
- She has been compliant with medication management and psychotherapy
- She brings a case of medical records with her to her initial appointment to make sure everything is covered adequately
- She has good insight into her MDD and the need to treat her symptoms, but less so with regard to her personality traits and her somatic symptoms
- She denies current side effects on her psychiatric medications but states that she is often sensitive to side effects overall
- There is no evidence of misuse of her controlled medication
- She has no liver or renal disease, is normotensive, and has a normal body habitus

Current medications

- Psychiatrically, she takes
  - Duloxetine (Cymbalta) 60 mg/d (SNRI)
  - Alprazolam (Xanax) 6 mg/d (BZ)
  - Hydroxyzine (Vistaril) 125 mg/d (antihistamine)
- Medically, she takes
  - Fentanyl transdermal (Duragesic) 12 mcg/h
  - Levothyroxine (Synthroid) 125 mcg/d
  - Omeprazole (Prilosec) 40 mg/d
  - Ibandronate (Boniva) 150 mg/mo
  - Eletriptan (Relpax) 40 mg/d as needed for migraines
  - Odansetron (Zofran) 8 mg twice a day as needed for migraines
  - Naproxen sodium (Naprosyn) 500 mg twice a day
  - Onaboutulinumtoxin-A injection (Botox) 300 units as needed for muscle spasm

Question

In your clinical experience, would you suggest that this patient's symptoms were?

- Psychic and "all in her head"
- Depression and anxiety based with somatic features
- Personality based with much somatizing

Attending physician's mental notes: initial evaluation

- This patient has chronic MDD
- She has a lot of comorbidity
  - Anxiety
  - Maladaptive personality traits
  - Distant substance misuse
  - Many somatic and real medical issues
- Failure to remit on any of previous treatments
- These failures may not be alarming in that she is side-effect sensitive and some of these treatments were likely not for a full dose or adequate duration
- Her multiple comorbidities will increase treatment resistance and lower her likelihood of remission even in the face of excellent psychopharmacologic care
- She has not had a bona fide trial of PDP, dynamic deconstructive psychotherapy (DDP), or DBT
  - DDP is a psychodynamic therapy specifically geared to treat BPDO that is comorbid with AUD

- Prognosis is only fair unless better pharmacological therapy and psychotherapy occurs and is adhered to
- However, she is very compliant with office visits, is personable, and seems more motivated for care at this point

Question

Which of the following would be your next step?

- Increase the duloxetine (Cymbalta) to the full FDA dose of 120 mg
- Increase the alprazolam (Xanax) to a higher, more effective dose for anxiolysis
- Augment the current medications with another agent that has antidepressant properties
- Augment the current medications with another agent that has mood stabilizing properties
- Augment the current medications with another agent that has antipsychotic properties
- Augment the current medications with another agent that has pain dampening properties
- Change nothing and refer for more specific psychotherapy

Attending physician's mental notes: initial evaluation (continued)

- It is unclear whether this patient has had therapeutic trials on all medications, although some are well documented
- Will need to build rapport, increase trust, and try to enhance adherence
- Need to get to a good dose/duration for her current SNRI (duloxetine [Cymbalta]) as it has the ability to treat depression, anxiety, and neuropathic pain
- However, there is concern regarding her suicidal thoughts from one to two months ago, which will need further exploration and a discussion about safety planning
- She joined the practice already on higher doses of BZ use
  - There is no current indication of any misuse, but up until a few years ago, she had some substance misuse and was addicted to mechanistically similar barbiturate sedatives decades ago
  - Will need to continue to closely monitor and likely try to discontinue her controlled prescriptions over time
  - She states that her current treatment has helped her anxiety by at least 50%
- Meets many criteria for various personality disorders, but on the mild to moderate severity spectrum
  - Will have to keep these dynamics in mind, again to improve rapport and medication adherence

Further investigation

Is there anything else you would especially like to know about this patient?

- What about details concerning her dissociative spells or mood swings?
  - She reports that she will just "zone out" when stressed
    - She will lose track of time
    - These episodes may last minutes to a few hours
    - She does not "wake" up in new or different places and there is no evidence of personality change
    - She cannot remember what she was thinking about during these times
- She often has mood swings that go from euthymia to sadness, anger, or excessive happiness
  - These are never sustained more than one to two days, but often last only hours
  - These are often triggered by events in her environment
  - Her suicidal thoughts, intentions, and plans always occur after a stressful event with her significant other

Case outcome: first interim follow-up visit eight weeks later

- Patient has decided to leave her current provider and attend sessions for psychopharmacology medication management in this setting
- She has now additionally been placed on modafinil (Provigil) 200 mg/d and pregabalin (Lyrica) 150 mg/d by her rheumatologist to treat her fatigue and pain from FM
  - The other medications (duloxetine and alprazolam) remain unchanged
- She feels no better and acknowledges the same symptoms as upon the first visit
- She is experiencing a bit more fatigue on the alpha-2-delta calcium channel blocking neuropathic pain medication, pregabalin (Lyrica)
- She states that she has no major, compliance-limiting side effects thus far and there is no misuse of any of her current controlled medications

Question

Would you increase her current medications or change strategies?

- Yes, continue duloxetine, alprazolam, pregabalin, and modafinil at higher doses
- Continue duloxetine at higher doses but keep others as they are
- Continue modafinil at higher doses but keep others as they are

- Continue pregabalin at higher doses but keep others as they are
- No, discontinue these agents as they have failed to allow for a full clinical response, and start new regimen

Case outcome: second and third interim follow-up visits at three months

- Care was coordinated with her rheumatologist
  - Modafinil (Provigil) is increased to 300 mg/d to improve fatigue and increase wakefulness for her FM
  - Pregabalin (Lyrica) is lowered to 50 mg twice a day to lessen fatigue adverse effects
  - Other medications are left unchanged
- This approach begins to maximize the stimulant-like treatment while trying to minimize side effects
- Patient was counseled and supported regarding her ability to tolerate the side effects and efforts to balance these versus promoting greater effectiveness
- Despite these efforts, patient returns later stating she is too scared and had left her dose of modafinil (Provigil) at the previous 200 mg/d
  - The patient was supportively shown the approved package insert
  - She was also shown a well-renowned psychopharmacology guide
  - Both clearly delineated safe dosing strategies; she then was agreeable to dose escalation
- After this, unfortunately, the patient showed no symptom improvement as she did not make the suggested changes yet again

Attending physician's mental notes: second interim follow-up visit at three months

- This is going to be a difficult case given the patient's fear and ambivalence about medications and health issues, her hypochondriasis, and possible functional somatic syndromes
- On a positive note, she is relatively side-effect free for now

Question

What would you do next?

- Further escalate one medication at a time to balance efficacy and tolerability
- Begin removing ineffective medications to streamline her regimen and improve compliance
- Refer for more organized, specific psychotherapy

Attending physician's mental notes: second interim follow-up visit at three months (continued)

- As this patient is somewhat accepting of using her wakefulness medicine and sees it as bridging the gap between her mental and medical issues, it makes sense to work with this drug instead of adding anything else
- Increasing her sedative–anxiolytic or neuropathic pain medication are unlikely to remit her MDD and may promote more fatiguing side effects
- Combination or augmentation strategies can certainly be utilized in both depressive and pain disorders
  - Therefore, an increase in her SNRI (duloxetine [Cymbalta]) may also be called for to enhance noradrenergic functioning, but given her side-effect prone nature, changing one medication at a time is likely warranted
- Escalating the SNRI would have been a better monotherapy choice, but the intervention of multiple providers has increased her polypharmacy, and in her case, a likely risk of adverse effects and more non-adherence

Case outcome: interim follow-up visits through five months

- No change in status; patient is still depressed, anxious, in pain, but not suicidal
- Modafinil (Provigil) is increased to full 400 mg/d dose
- Patient calls one to two weeks later stating she has ankle edema
  - She insists on lowering and discontinuing the modafinil
  - A few days later the swelling continues
  - Conversation with primary care provider shows no other medical issue at hand
  - Usual side-effect profile suggests this might be her pregabalin (Lyrica), even though there was no recent dose change
  - Pregabalin was discontinued and the edema resolved

Question

What would you do next?

- Maximize the SNRI
- Maximize the BZ
- Augment with something else to better treat MDD

Attending physician's mental notes: interim follow-up visits through nine months

- Patient is still depressed and has mounting side effects and treatment ambivalence
- It would make sense to keep her regimen simple and to monitor her

Case outcome: interim follow-up visits through 12 months

- Elects to increase the SNRI, duloxetine (Cymbalta), but is nervous about increasing to 90 mg/d
- She does agree to adding a smaller 20 mg capsule making her dose 80 mg/d instead, which she more readily accepts
- The patient states later that she was more anxious on the higher SNRI dose and asked to taper it off
- Next, she was advised to consider a TCA given their ability to treat depression and reduce pain
  - She agreed to desipramine (Norpramin)
  - It tends to have less sedation and anticholinergic properties than other TCAs
  - It is largely NE facilitating
  - The TCAs tend to have double the dropout rate, or medication discontinuation rate, when compared to the SSRI
- After titration to the 50 mg/d low dose, she states that she again is too anxious, agitated, and insomnic on the TCA, and it is stopped
- She is willing to try another antidepressant medication, but not another TCA as she feels they are "too dangerous"
- Another SNRI, desvenlafaxine (Pristiq), is started, which she tolerated well and ultimately it was increased to 100 mg/d
- She starts outpatient DBT as an augmentation strategy
- She returns next with improved energy and concentration
- Her desvenlafaxine (Pristiq) is increased to 200 mg/d for better effectiveness, theoretically enhancing noradrenergic tone
- She continues on alprazolam (Xanax) 6 mg/d but begins to admit routine anxiety breakthrough symptoms between her doses
  - Assumption is made that this is tachyphylaxis with breakthrough anxiogenic withdrawal symptoms
  - She is converted to the slow-release preparation of alprazolam-ER (Xanax-XR) at 2 mg three times per day

Attending physician mental notes

- Finally have been able to work through and maximize a bona fide antidepressant treatment and troubleshoot her breakthrough anxiety spells
- The patient's depressive vegetative symptoms begin to respond and she is also less anxious
- Plan on every four to six weeks increasing her SNRI for better effect, and hopefully, remission
- DBT should also help navigate personality- and adjustment-based mood exacerbations

Case outcome: interim follow-up visits through 15 months

- The patient becomes critically ill, is hospitalized and undergoes major surgery for bowel infarction, which appears idiopathic and unrelated to any of her medications
- Delirium develops in the intensive care unit, likely due to
  - The pain medications that are administered
  - Serotonin discontinuation syndrome and sedative withdrawal while being off all of her psychotropics, as she was on bowel rest and unable to take oral medicines
- Upon consultation, she was given
  - Intravenous lorazepam (Ativan) to cover her sedative withdrawal
  - The typical antipsychotic perphenazine (Trilafon) for her medical delirium, with good resolution of her symptoms
- During surgery, she was given an ostomy and had a shortened gastrointestinal tract (GIT)
- Once she was able to eat and back in the outpatient setting
  - The usual alprazolam-ER (Xanax-XR) 2 mg three times a day is restarted
  - The antidepressant desvenlafaxine (Pristiq) was not restarted as she was denying depression symptoms
- She appeared to have better mood control on her low-dose typical antipsychotic perphenazine (Trilafon) and it was continued
- The patient later reported an acute increase in anxiety again a few days after the transition to her oral BZ anxiolytic
  - She transitioned from approximately 4 mg/d of intravenous lorazepam (Ativan)
    - This is equivalent to 8 mg of oral dosing
  - Regarding her current alprazolam-ER (Xanax-XR) 6 mg/d use, it is clearly a higher equivalent dose, hence withdrawal rebound anxiety was initially ruled out
- Patient next reported seeing medication tablets in her ostomy bag
  - These were identified as her slow-release preparation alprazolam-XR (Xanax-XR)
  - With her shortened GI tract, she was not absorbing these types of tablets
  - She appeared to be in mild BZ sedative withdrawal

Question

What would you do next?

- Request a home visiting nurse and restart intravenous or intramuscular lorazepam (Ativan), as these are parenteral routes and were effective in the hospital

- Convert this patient to a longer half-life BZ sedative, such as diazepam (Valium), assuming she can absorb some of this immediate-release drug and avoid withdrawal due to its extensively long half-life and metabolites
- Convert this patient back to the immediate-release alprazolam at an equivalent dose as it should be absorbed better without the slow-release mechanism in place

Case debrief

- This is a complex patient with many psychiatric comorbidities, psychosomatic conditions, and now a surgical emergency
- She was making consistent progress in rapport, trust, and an adequate and aggressively dosed antidepressant was administered
- However, she had to work through many ambivalences and anxieties regarding her medications to get to this point
- Her progress was thwarted by her bowel infarction and poor ability to absorb medications
  - Parenteral substitute medications were chosen and found to be effective acutely
  - Upon conversion back to oral tablets in the outpatient setting, it became clear she could not absorb some of her oral slow-release medications
  - She was placed back on immediate-release preparations with good anxiolysis, and continued on her perphenazine (Trilafon) longer term as a mood elevator and stabilizer as well as antipsychotic
    - At low doses, this typical antipsychotic possesses atypical properties of 5-HT2A receptor antagonism, and has been used to treat depression in an off-label manner. It had been FDA approved as a combination antidepressant, when it is commercially combined with the TCA amitriptyline
    - She should be monitored for TD and EPS
    - She could be switched to an atypical antipsychotic as an alternative
    - The patient opted to keep this medication as it is because it is helpful and well tolerated
- The patient remains on this combination (alprazolam plus perphenazine)
- She had to stop DBT while hospitalized but restarted psychotherapy with a dynamically oriented couples' therapist and is seeing gradual improvements in her personality traits
- She remains sober and shows no misuse of her controlled medications

Take-home points

- Treating this patient involved using many psychotherapeutic skills in order to maintain compliance and achieve therapeutic doses

- A 12-minute rapid medication management session approach likely would have backfired and allowed for a continuation of many subtherapeutic, side-effect riddled medication trials
- Spending more time with this patient, processing ambivalence about medications, increasing her ability to tolerate side effects, and gaining her trust by titrating slowly with one agent at a time appeared to be helpful in promoting symptom relief, until her surgical emergency warranted medication changes
- Steering away from the urge to treat patients with many symptoms of differing etiologies with a myriad of low-dose medications, given her personality traits, it made clinical sense to attempt solid monotherapy adjustments when possible
- This approach also allows more time for psychotherapeutic approaches to become effective
- This lowers the risk of excessive, unwarranted polypharmacy and the excessive collection of adverse effects

Performance in practice: confessions of a psychopharmacologist

- *What could have been done better here?*
  - Psychopharmacologists do not act in a vacuum
    - This patient's rheumatologist began the patient on two medications, which generally are warranted in the treatment of certain FM patients (approved pregabalin and off-label modafinil)
    - Outside treating her FM, these medications may actually have helped to dampen her anxiety, improve her cognition, and even depression
    - However, the use of these multiple medications ended with side-effect issues and delayed the psychiatrist's more aggressive monotherapy approach
    - Earlier discussion with the outside provider may have avoided this intervention
  - Inpatient providers should have been aware that her SNRI and her BZ would likely produce withdrawal syndromes when abruptly stopped
    - A parenteral BZ should have been started earlier
    - There is no easy way to provide parenteral antidepressants outside possible use of intravenous clomipramine
    - Certain opiate pain medications (tramadol, meperidine, fentanyl) possess SRI and NRI properties, and could be utilized for acute pain management and might avoid SNRI discontinuation syndrome
      - Recollect that this patient was taking fentanyl throughout her care in this case

- *Possible action items for improvement in practice*
  - Research guidelines and review articles regarding treating FM
    - Many rational polypharmacy approaches and techniques that are employed in the treatment of MDD may be applied similarly to treating FM
    - The SNRI class has two approvals (duloxetine and milnacipran) that may be able to help comorbid FM patients
  - Understand the complexity of drug delivery systems
    - Many psychotropics now come in immediate-, intermediate-, and slow-release preparations
    - Some agents are produced as prodrugs and as patches
    - Some drugs require to be taken with food, others without for optimal dosing and absorption
    - Understanding the mechanism of release, rate of absorption, and pharmacokinetics may mean the difference between having efficacy or not, side effects or not

Tips and pearls

- Generally, the slower the release mechanism or process that a drug preparation utilizes, the fewer side effects it will have
  - Lower initial blood plasma levels will be maintained and avoidance of initial rapid peak plasma levels allow for this
  - This is generally a good thing except for those patients who cannot absorb medications in the GI tract due to a shortened tract or malabsorption syndrome
- Slow-release products extend the natural half-life of most drugs and may sometimes lower inter-dosing withdrawal effects
- Generally, the slower the release mechanism is, the more likely the drug may be employed as a once-a-day drug, thus improving compliance

Pharmacoeconomic and regulatory moment

- Slower-release preparations are often more costly as the drug manufacturer has to pay for the development of the immediate-release drug itself and also pay for the development, or patent use, of the slow-release mechanism that surrounds the molecules of the immediate-release drug. This way, there are two costs for one drug
- The FDA allows for approximately 20% bioavailability differential between original brand name drugs and their generics
  - Generally, this is not a problem for most patients, but some will be more sensitive and gather more side effects if the generic is 15% more bioavailable
  - Some patients will relapse if the generic is 15% less bioavailable

- The slow-release technology between the brand name and generic drugs may also be different in bioavailability
  - Therefore, a generic slow-release drug may have two generic properties
    - The generic drug itself
    - The generic slow-release mechanism
  - If the generic slow-release mechanism allows faster release than the brand name, new side effects may appear when the brand is changed to generic, as peak plasma levels occur faster and to a higher concentration
  - The FDA has alerted prescribers that extended slow-release bupropion and slow-release methylphenidate (osmotically controlled-release oral delivery system [OROS]) generics are, in fact, different pharmacokinetically from the brand name version, as examples

Two-minute tutorial

How many ways can a drug be turned into a slow-release preparation?

- Adding a coating – e.g., bupropion-SR (Wellbutrin-SR)
  - A solid pill consisting of active drug is layered with a single, more inert coating that protects the drug from digestion and absorption early in the GIT. This allows absorption to occur more gradually further along the GIT
- Adding layers – e.g., zolpidem-ER (Ambien-CR)
  - In this instance, this drug has a tablet consisting of two layers. The initial layer of a more easily digestible coating is dissolved quickly in the GIT allowing onset of action quickly. The second, deeper layer also contains immediate-release drug but the layers are harder to break down and digest so drug release occurs later and further down the GI tract. These drugs actually give two separate releases instead of a longer, single, gradual release
- OROS – e.g., methylphenidate (Concerta) and paliperidone (Invega)
  - First, this technique uses a capsule that has a larger hole on one end, and a smaller hole on the other end. Second, inside the capsule is the immediate-release drug and a small sponge-like substance. As this complex capsule travels through the GIT, water from the GIT is drawn into the large hole, saturates the sponge, which expands, thus driving the active drug gradually out the small hole on the other side of the capsule via hydrostatic pressure
- Matrix – e.g., trazodone-ER (Oleptro)
  - An insoluble and difficult-to-digest web of material is created and the active drug is inserted throughout the matrix. As this slow-release

package is not easily digested, it takes the active drug time to percolate and leak out of the matrix gradually as it traverses the GIT

- Prodrugs – e.g., lisdexamfetamine (Vyvanse) and clorazepate (Tranxene)
  - A prodrug is a drug that is not clinically active in its natural state. A prodrug must be swallowed and digested in the GIT and then be passed to the liver. During hepatic metabolism, an enzyme, or series of enzymes, then alters the structure of the prodrug, which is released post-hepatically in this new form into the bloodstream. This digested new metabolite is the active therapeutic drug. The process of hepatic filtration and enzymatic metabolism is the slow-release mechanism. Essentially, the liver slows down production and release of the active drug
- SODAS microbeads (spheroidal oral drug absorption system) – e.g., methylphenidate (Ritalin-LA, Focalin-XR)
  - In this process, active drug molecules (beads) are suspended and then are coated with varying numbers of layers, or coats of inert materials, that must be slowly dissolved to release the active drug. The more layers, the slower the release in the GIT per individual bead. By placing spheres with a few layers, some layers, and many layers all in one capsule, the drug is released gradually throughout the day as they are degraded further and further along in the GIT in sequential fashion. Unlike the two-layered tablet, which allows two distinct releases, the SODAS technology allows many differently timed releases throughout the day, giving a picture that resembles a more gradual, or smooth, release process
- Transdermal delivery systems (patches) – e.g., methylphenidate (Daytrana) and selegiline (Emsam)
  - Essentially, the active drug is placed into a gel-like substance that is adhered to an impermeable backing. Next, adhesive glue is placed along the perimeter of the patch to adhere it to the patient's skin. Pressure and constant drug-to-skin contact is ensured and the active drug is gradually absorbed through the skin's capillaries, allowing for slow, constant absorption

Posttest self-assessment question and answer

What are some usual benefits of slow-release preparation medications?

A. Lower blood plasma levels often allow for less severe adverse effects
B. Extended half-life often allows for once-daily dosing and improved adherence
C. Cost is usually lowered as once-daily dosing is less costly to manufacture
D. Improved effectiveness over the parent immediate-release preparation

E. A and B
F. A, B, and C
G. All of the above
Answer: E
Lower plasma levels often offer less toxicity and thus fewer clinical side effects and make the drug easier to take, usually in once-daily fashion. Cost usually increases due to the technology involved in the slow-release drug mechanism, and in general, slow-release preparations are equally effective but engender less acute side effects, making C and D false.

References

1. Joshi HN. Recent advances in drug delivery systems: polymeric prodrugs. *Pharmaceut Technol* 1988; 118–30.
2. Roberts DM, Buckley NA. Pharmacokinetic considerations in clinical toxicology: clinical applications. *Clin Pharmacokinet* 2007; 46:897–939.
3. Dingemanse J, Appel-Dingemanse S. Integrated pharmacokinetics and pharmacodynamics in drug development. *Clin Pharmacokinet* 2007; 46:713–37.
4. Bateman DN, Eddleston M. Clinical pharmacology: the basics. *Medicine* 2008; 36:339–43.
5. Park K, ed. *Controlled Drug Delivery: Challenges and Strategies.* Washington, DC: American Chemical Society, 1997.
6. Soler J, Pascual JC, Campins J, et al. Double-blind, placebo-controlled study of dialectical behavior therapy plus olanzapine for borderline personality disorder. *Am J Psychiatry* 2005; 162:1221–4.
7. Leichsenring F, Leibing E.The effectiveness of psychodynamic therapy and cognitive behavior therapy in the treatment of personality disorders: a meta-analysis. *Am J Psychiatry* 2003; 160:1223–32.
8. Palmer RL. Dialectical behaviour therapy for borderline personality disorder. *Adv Psychiatr Treat* 2002; 8:10–16.
9. Gregory RJ, Chlebowski S, Kang D, et al. A controlled trial of psychodynamic psychotherapy for co-occurring borderline personality disorder and alcohol use disorder. *Psychotherapy* 2008; 45:28–41.
10. Goldman GA, Gregory RJ. Preliminary relationships between adherence and outcome in dynamic deconstructive psychotherapy. *Psychotherapy* 2009; 46:480–5.
11. Gregory RJ, Delucia-Deranja E, Mogle JA. Dynamic deconstructive psychotherapy versus optimized community care for borderline personality disorder co-occurring with alcohol use disorders: a 30-month follow-up. *J Nerv Ment Dis* 2010; 198:292–8.

12. Goldman GA, Gregory RJ. Relationships between techniques and outcomes in borderline personality disorder. *Am J Psychother* 2010; 64:359–71.
13. Stahl SM. *Stahl's Essential Psychopharmacology: The Prescriber's Guide*, 5th edn. New York, NY: Cambridge University Press, 2014.

The Case: Generically speaking, generics are adequate

The Question: What to do when using a generic is detrimental to a patient

The Dilemma: Navigating clinical care when generic medications are not always equal

Pretest self-assessment question (answer at the end of the case)

How much different can a generic drug be from its brand name counterpart, based upon individual regulatory tests of bioequivalence?

A. 0%
B. 5%
C. 15%
D. 25%

Patient evaluation on intake

- Patient #1
  - 60-year-old man with a chief complaint of "being angry and down"
- Patient #2
  - 15-year-old girl with a chief complaint of "everything sucks"
- Patient #1 states that he was involved in a fracas at work, was pushed down the stairs, and was in a coma for a week
- Patient #2 states that she has been having a difficult time at home and at school

Psychiatric history

- Patient #1 had been without any psychiatric issues until his head injury. He states his symptoms developed after this
- Patient #2 states that she has gradually become more emotionally labile, depressed, and anxious over the last one to two years
- Patient #1 has not been able to go back to work at all due to his depression, amotivation, and anger management problems
- Patient #2 has been absent from school due to her inability to get up and get ready for school
- Patient #1 admits to full syndrome MDD
  - He has passive suicidal thoughts that there is "not much to life" and he "wouldn't mind if he didn't wake up"
  - Admits to poor focus, concentration, and amotivation as chief complaints
- He states that little things make him angry quickly
  - Experiences road rage and followed fellow drivers after incidents
    - He states that he was never like this prior to his accident

- Denies PTSD-related avoidance, flashbacks, or nightmares as he does not remember the accident due to his head injury and coma
  - Is tense and hyperaroused most of the time
- He has relatively few friends as most were colleagues at his previous job. He is at home more and not motivated to leave his home
- Patient #2 admits to full MDD symptoms
  - Has suicidal thoughts that occur more when stressed
  - Admits to having an inability to focus, poor concentration, and lack of enjoyment as chief complaints
- She states that "little things make her angry quickly"
  - She is afraid that going to school puts her in situations where she may strike out and get into fights, even though this has never been her social pattern
  - She has friends but feels disenfranchised from them
  - She gets along with her grandmother but not her parents

Medication history

- Patient #1
  - Has had a few treatments so far while in the care of his PCP
  - He failed to respond to a low-dose SSRI
    - Fluoxetine (Prozac) 20 mg/d
    - Sertraline (Zoloft) 100 mg/d
    - Paroxetine (Paxil) 20 mg/d
  - SNRIs as well
    - Venlafaxine-XR (Effexor-XR) 75 mg/d
    - Duloxetine (Cymbalta) 60 mg/d
  - Additionally, an NDRI
    - bupropion-SR (Wellbutrin-SR) 300 mg/d
  - He stopped his medication several weeks ago due to lack of clinical improvement
- Patient #2
  - A few subtherapeutic treatments so far while in the care of her PCP
  - Failed to respond
    - To a low-dose SSRI (fluoxetine [Prozac]) 10 mg/d due to agitation side effects
    - To an SNRI (venlafaxine-XR [Effexor-XR]) 75 mg/d due to agitation side effects
    - Each of these treatments lasted less than one week

Psychotherapy history

- Patient #1 has never been involved in psychotherapy
- Patient #2 has just started supportive psychotherapy on a weekly basis

Social and personal history

- Patient #1
  - Graduated high school
  - Worked in law enforcement for many years and now is a disabled delivery driver since his accident
  - Does not use drugs or alcohol
- Patient #2
  - Attends high school, and despite her symptoms, is passing her classes for the most part
  - However, her grades have dropped from their usual levels
  - She only attends school 50% of the time
  - She does not use drugs or alcohol

Medical history

- Patient #1 has suffered a head injury, is overweight but otherwise in good health
- Patient #2 is healthy and has no history of eating disorder or epilepsy

Family history

- Patient #1 denies any known psychiatric illness in any family member
- Patient #2 has a family history of
  - MDD and GAD in her mother
  - AUD and questionable bipolar illness in her father

Patient evaluation on initial visit

- Patient #1
  - Acute onset of anxious and agitated MDD after head injury one to two years ago
  - Has not been compliant with medication and declines psychotherapy
  - Admits passive suicidal ideation
  - He has taken a few antidepressants at moderately therapeutic levels
- Patient #2
  - Gradual onset of symptoms as she entered her teenage years
  - There is no single stressor identified that predates her symptoms
  - She is gradually getting worse and is at risk of failing her classes and her grade level
  - She has been compliant with her medication but may have become more symptomatic with its use, and has only taken subtherapeutic doses as such

Current medications

- Patient #1
  - None

- Patient #2
  - Sertraline (Zoloft) 25 mg/d (was recently lowered from 50 mg/d), an SSRI

Question

In your clinical experience, which patient has a worse prognosis?

- Not sure, it is too early to tell
- Patient #1 is older, has failed more antidepressant trials, and has a worse prognosis
- Patient #1 has more comorbidity and has a worse prognosis
- Patient #2 is younger and cannot tolerate her medications and may be activated by them and has a worse prognosis
- Not sure as this is like comparing apples and oranges as they are both depressed, but for very different reasons, and both have different phenomenology for their depressive symptoms

Attending physician's mental notes: initial evaluation

- Patient #1
  - This patient has his first MDE now with associated anxiety features (subsyndromal PTSD likely)
  - It is acute and triggered by the psychosocial stressor but complicated by a traumatic brain injury (TBI)
  - It seems more than an adjustment disorder as it is pervasive, lasting over time, and clearly disabling at this point
  - His prognosis is likely fair but made worse by his medication resistance and non-adherence
- Patient #2
  - This patient is relatively untreated due to medication intolerance but psychotherapy and family interventions should be helpful
  - The reported activation and escalation is concerning on her current SSRI
    - Will need to work with the patient and family regarding safety planning, given FDA suicidal warnings associated with antidepressants in her age group
    - There is no clear family history of bipolarity, but "mood swings, alcoholism, and possible bipolar illness" have been noted in a first-degree relative
    - The SSRI activation may be a precursor of true bipolarity

Question

Which of the following would be your next step?

- Try a new SSRI for both of these patients
- Switch to an SNRI for both of these patients

- Switch to an NDRI for both of these patients
- Insist upon psychotherapy for both of these patients

Attending physician's mental notes: initial evaluation (continued)

- Both patients are currently undertreated and have not had a fair, therapeutic full dose and full duration SSRI trial
  - Patient #1 should be advised about the remaining SSRI medications
  - Patient #2 and her parents should be specifically advised about the two approved SSRIs for treatment of depression in adolescents (fluoxetine [Prozac] and escitalopram [Lexapro]) as her failing sertraline (Zoloft) is actually approved for pediatric OCD

Further investigation

Is there anything else you would especially like to know about these patients?

- What about details concerning Patient #1's brain injury?
  - He was injured one and a half years ago
  - He was in a coma for several days
  - His brain has likely healed to its fullest extent possible by now
  - His head was impacted on the right side, and according to the patient, he sustained bruising to his cortex in the right parietal area and also to a lesser degree on the left side (contrecoup injury)
  - He did not suffer any brain hemorrhage as a result
- What about details concerning Patient #2's previous antidepressant side effects?
  - The patient and family report that with low-dose SSRI and then an SNRI, she had to stop them due to acute behavioral changes
    - ○ She became more mood labile, angry, and irritable
    - ○ There was no evidence of insomnia, grandiosity, hyperactivity, or impulsivity
    - ○ Further questioning also suggests that the patient has these types of "mood swings" often and regardless of medication being used
    - ○ This activation was not accompanied with any increase in suicidal symptoms

Case outcome: first interim follow-up visit four to six weeks later

- Patient #1 was placed on an SSRI, citalopram (Celexa) 20 mg/d, to which he had never been exposed, and advised strongly to stick with a full-dosed trial
  - He returns no better

- He has mild fatigue as a side effect
- Patient #2 was placed on an SSRI, escitalopram (Lexapro), which was novel to her, but at a low 5 mg/d dose to avoid the acute side effect of agitation
  ○ Patient and family are fully educated about side effects and suicide monitoring
  ○ She returns with slightly improved affective range and energy, and is having no side effects

Question

Would you increase their current medications or change strategies?

- Yes, continue both patients at higher SSRI doses
- Continue Patient #1 at higher dose but keep Patient #2 at current dose
- Continue Patient #2 at higher dose but keep Patient #1 at current dose
- No, continue both patients at current dose and wait for full clinical effect to occur

Attending physician's mental notes: interim follow-up visits through three months

- Two rashes, two patients, two different drugs
- All drugs carry risk of rashes and allergies
- Patient #2 seems more severe, given the facial edema
- Likely have to stop both drugs in both patients despite some early clinical improvement

Case outcome: interim follow-up visits through three months

- Patient #1
  - Citalopram (Celexa) was increased to 40 mg/d for better effect
  - It caused minor increase in fatigue, but he had less dysphoria and mood lability
  - He developed a drug rash on his arms and legs
- Patient #2
  - Escitalopram (Lexapro) was increased to 10 mg/d with some initial improvement, but then a regression toward anhedonia, failure to thrive, and inability to attend school
  - She was hospitalized for the first time
    ○ She was placed on bupropion-IR (Wellbutrin-IR) 75 mg twice a day by her inpatient psychiatrist, and her SSRI discontinued
    ○ She showed initial improvement in her depressive symptoms globally
    ○ She developed a rash and facial swelling a few days after discharge

Question

What would you do next?

- Taper off both drugs in both patients
- Taper off both drugs in both patients while treating with antihistamines
- Taper off both drugs in both patients, treat with antihistamines, and start new SSRI monotherapies once rash clears
- Taper off both drugs in both patients, treat with antihistamines until rash clears, then rechallenge with different preparation of same antidepressant, if available given their initial improvements

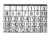

Attending physician's mental notes: interim follow-up visits through three months (continued)

- The patients were both improving on their respective medications
- If possible, and safe, would like them to be on the same, or closest similar medication next, to perpetuate their initial responses to their last medication
- Sometimes changing preparation of a drug may alleviate allergies
  - Certain tablets or capsules may have dyes or sugars that create the allergic response
    - The allergy is not caused by the antidepressant molecule itself, but rather by the dyes or fillers
    - However, if the allergy is to the specific drug molecule, the allergic response will happen again when the drug is restarted

Case outcome: interim follow-up visits through six months

- Patient #1
  - Is tapered off his generic citalopram, and given antihistamines until his rash clears
  - He agrees to try the brand name citalopram (Celexa) as it will have the same drug molecule but different fillers
  - He is titrated to 40 mg/d
  - This allows for gradual improvement in some of his MDD symptoms again
  - No rash develops
  - He was likely allergic to the dye or fillers in the previous generic preparation
- Patient #2
  - Is tapered off her purple dye-colored bupropion-IR tablets
  - Is given antihistamines until her rash and swelling clears
  - Pharmacy is called and asked to locate an all-white, non-colored preparation of bupropion-SR
    - This assumes that the patient was allergic to only the dye of bupropion-IR, not the drug molecule

- Patient is placed on low-dose, white 100 mg tablet, SR preparation
  - ○ Rash and facial swelling returns
  - ○ Her antidepressant is discontinued
  - ○ She is presumed allergic to the bupropion molecule itself
  - ○ No further rechallenges with any preparation are warranted

Attending physician's mental notes: interim follow-up visits through six months

- Sometimes allergies are due to the medication's molecule itself, such as in Patient #2, and the medication should be avoided in the future, regardless of preparation (immediate versus slow release, brand name versus generic)
  - This allergy to the medication should be listed in the patient's chart
- Sometimes allergies are due to the fillers (excipients, dyes, sugars, slow-release polymers) inside a tablet or capsule, not the drug molecule, as seen in Patient #1
  - In these situations, rechallenging is worthwhile, if the patient was improving on the initial antidepressant and tolerating it well
  - If the type of dye causing the reaction can be determined or triangulated, it should be listed specifically as the allergen in the patient's chart
- Some drugs that are more prone to skin rashes and disruptions, however, are likely not worth a rechallenge, such as lamotrigine (Lamictal), topiramate (Topamax), modafinil (Provigil), etc., as the risk of serious or even life-threatening rashes is higher

Case debrief

- Allergic reactions happen and can be managed like any other side effects
- In both of these cases, side effects were controlled by tapering off the medication and prescribing antihistamines
- As both patients were doing a little better, the prescriber next tried to maintain the patients on the rash-prone, but initially effective medications (albeit different preparations), with one patient continuing to improve and the other patient doing worse again with rash-based side effects
- Patient #2 was eventually placed on sertraline (Zoloft), which previously made her agitated prior to admission to the practice
  - However, this was started at the low dose of 12.5 mg/d and titrated much more slowly to avoid activating side effects
  - This approach was effective and she eventually was titrated up to 150 mg/d (a more therapeutic trial to the previous one), and has started a gradual response

Take-home points

- All drugs may cause rashes
- Providers should be aware that certain drugs carry greater risks
- Providers have options on how to manage these
- Often, maintaining a good clinical response is worth an attempt at trying the offending agent again
  - Treating and mitigating its side effects, such as rashes in these cases
    ○ Rash side-effect mitigation might be considered similar to treating extrapyramidal symptoms in psychotic patients with anticholinergics
- Treating side effects often builds patient rapport and trust in that one is actively trying to improve their outcome and tolerability
- Attempts to maintain patients on their initially effective medication may actually be of great importance as treatment resistance increases, as patients are tried on many short-term medication trials and then begin to run out of treatment options

Performance in practice: confessions of a psychopharmacologist

- *What could have been done better here?*
  - Rashes can be serious
  - Rechallenging patients who are rash sensitive should be done with a high degree of patient education and support
  - During a rechallenge, patients should be warned that any throat tightening, facial swelling, shortness of breath should trigger a call to the office or trip to the emergency room
- *Possible action items for improvement in practice*
  - Try to minimize risk to the patient
  - There are many antidepressants available. It may have been easier (in Patient #2) to switch to an unrelated, chemically distinct, new antidepressant

Tips and pearls

- Clinicians should be aware of drugs that have a higher tendency toward rashes. These drugs often contain dyes
- Clinicians should be aware of all of the different preparations that a certain drug has, so that changing among them can be done if clinically warranted
- Generics and brand name drugs may be pharmacokinetically "bioequivalent" within FDA-approved ranges, but may have different side-effect profiles
  - Depending on differing absorption rates
  - Depending upon the different dyes and fillers used
  - They may not be equal from a tolerability standpoint

Two-minute tutorial

What are the rules for being a generic drug?

- A generic drug is comparable to the initial brand name drug product in dosage form, strength, route of administration, quality, and intended use
- A generic must be bioequivalent to the original manufactured brand name drug
  - This is often measured by evaluating the time it takes the generic drug to reach the bloodstream as compared to the brand name drug
  - The generic drug's absorption must deliver roughly the same amount (within 25% - see later) of active brand name drug product
  - The FDA requires the bioequivalence of the generic product to be between 80% and 125% of that of the parent branded product
  - Studies suggest that the average difference is often 3.5%
  - The *Drug Price Competition and Patent Term Restoration Act of 1984*, also known as the Waxman–Hatch Act (now Public Law No: 98–417) set this standard into place
    - This Act allows generic drug makers to create their version of the product but without repeating similar human patient trials
    - It is assumed that a bioequivalent drug will be equally safe and effective as the brand name
    - The FDA does not demand a brand name versus generic trial to prove this, nor does it insist that the generic drug be studied against a placebo
    - This saves the generic manufacturer certain costs and they can place the generic product on the market for less as a result
    - When generic products become available, the market competition often leads to substantially lower prices for both the original brand name product and the generic forms
    - Often, multiple generic manufacturers will make their own version of the brand name product in question
    - This way, there are multiple versions of generics available for pharmacies to purchase and stock at any given time
    - This competition often lowers the generic drug's price even further
- The time it takes a generic drug to appear on the market varies
  - In the United States, drug patents give 20 years of protection
  - This patent is often filed when the drug molecule is discovered
  - It is tested in the bench-top laboratory, then preclinically in animal models, and finally in human trials of increasing complexity and size
  - By the time a brand name drug is available for patients to take, its remaining brand name life and patent protection is often between seven and 12 years

Diagnosing and treating rashes in clinical practice

Overview

- Drug hypersensitivity results from interactions between a pharmacologic agent and the immune system
- Allergic reactions to medications represent a specific class of drug-hypersensitivity reactions mediated by the immunoglobulin IgE
- However, some reactions involve additional, poorly understood mechanisms that are not easily classified
- Drug-induced reactions are likely the most common iatrogenic illness
  - Complicating 5%–15% of therapeutic drug trials
  - Causing more than 100,000 deaths due to serious adverse drug-allergic reactions
- Epidemiologic data support the existence of specific factors that increase the risk of general adverse drug reactions, such as female gender, history of asthma, systemic lupus erythematosus, or use of beta-blockers. Although atopic patients do not have a higher rate of sensitization to drugs, they are at increased risk for serious allergic reactions
- Identifiable risk factors for drug-hypersensitivity reactions include age, female gender, concurrent illnesses, and previous hypersensitivity to related drugs
- Larger molecular drugs with greater structural complexity are more likely to be immunogenic, although some drugs may have a smaller molecular weight but may become immunogenic by being coupled with carrier proteins
- Another factor increasing the frequency of hypersensitivity drug reactions is the route of drug administration
  - Topical, intramuscular, and intravenous administrations are more likely to cause hypersensitivity reactions
  - These effects are caused by the efficiency and higher amount of allergic antigen being presented to the skin
  - Oral medications are less likely to result in drug hypersensitivity

Classification

- Drug hypersensitivity is a clinical diagnosis based on available data at hand
- Drug reactions can be classified into immunologic and nonimmunologic
- The majority of adverse drug reactions are caused by predictable, nonimmunologic effects
- The remaining minority of adverse drug events are caused by unpredictable effects that may or may not be immune mediated
- Immune-mediated reactions account for 5%–10% of all drug reactions and constitute true drug-allergic hypersensitivity, with IgE-mediated drug allergies falling into this category

- The more common, yet unpredictable, nonimmune drug reactions seen often in practice can be classified in three ways
  - Pseudoallergic reactions are the result of direct mast cell activating, histamine releasing by exposure to drugs such as opiates, vancomycin (Vancocin), and radiocontrast media
  - These reactions may be clinically indistinguishable from true immune-related drug reactions, but do not involve drug-specific IgE
- Idiosyncratic reactions are qualitatively aberrant reactions that cannot be explained by the known pharmacologic action of the drug and occur only in a small percent of the population
  - A classic example of an idiosyncratic reaction is drug-induced hemolysis in persons with glucose-6-phosphate dehydrogenase (G6PD) deficiency
- Drug intolerance occurs when a patient has a lower threshold toward experiencing the normal pharmacologic action of a drug
  - An example might include developing tinnitus after a single average dose of aspirin instead of the usual experience after chronic high-dose utilization
  - These are likely not true allergies and are often erroneously reported on hospital charts and electronic medical records (EMRs) as true allergies instead of side effect intolerances

Clinical manifestations

- True hypersensitivity adverse drug reactions are great imitators of disease and may present with involvement of any organ system, including systemic reactions such as anaphylaxis
- Drug reactions commonly manifest with dermatologic symptoms caused by the metabolic and immunologic activity of the skin
  - The most common dermatologic manifestation of drug reaction is morbilliform rashes
    ○ Typically, an erythematous (red), maculopapular (flat to bumpy) rash that appears within one to three weeks after drug exposure, originates on the trunk, and eventually spreads to the limbs
    ○ Urticaria (hives) and swelling may be a typical manifestation of a truly allergic reaction, but it may appear with pseudoallergic reactions as well
  - Rarer severe nonallergic, hypersensitivity cutaneous reactions may also occur
    ○ For example, erythema multiforme, Stevens–Johnson syndrome (SJS), and toxic epidermal necrolysis (TEN), are severe and life-threatening reactions
    ○ These represent bullous skin diseases that require prompt recognition because of their association with significant morbidity and mortality

- These conditions are associated often with development of a fever, blistering lesions, and mucous membrane involvement

Therapy and management

- The most important and effective therapeutic measure in managing drug-hypersensitivity reactions is the discontinuation of the offending medication, when possible
- Alternative medications with unrelated chemical structures should be substituted where possible
- The clinical consequences of medication cessation or substitution should be closely monitored (precipitation of an SSRI or BZ withdrawal)
- In the majority of patients, rash symptoms will resolve within two weeks if the diagnosis of drug hypersensitivity is correct
- Additional therapy for drug-hypersensitivity reactions is largely supportive and symptomatic (antihistamine)
    - Systemic corticosteroids may speed recovery in severe cases of drug hypersensitivity
    - Topical corticosteroids and oral antihistamines may improve dermatologic symptoms
- The severe drug reactions of SJS or TEN require additional intensive therapy where patients should be evaluated and admitted to the hospital
- Anaphylactic responses, which include rashes, facial swelling, stridor, or difficulty breathing require prompt and urgent care
    - In an emergency room setting, epinephrine may be injected and systemic steroids administered while airway and vital sign support are ongoing

Posttest self-assessment question and answer

How much different can a generic drug be from its brand name counterpart, based upon individual regulatory tests of bioequivalence?

A. 0%

B. 5%

C. 15%

D. 25%

Answer: D

A generic drug may differ by 21% from the parent brand name product. When switching from a brand name to a generic, some patients may develop new side effects if the generic is actually more bioavailable. Other patients may have a return of psychiatric symptoms if the generic is less bioavailable. In another scenario, a patient may be changed from one generic to another as pharmacies try to purchase the most economical generic available. Take an example where a patient is actually on a generic antidepressant that is 20% more bioavailable than the brand name drug, but a year later is switched by the pharmacy to a new generic that is 10% less bioavailable than the parent brand name drug. This is actually a 30% lessening of antidepressant dose and tempts fate for a psychiatric relapse, even more than the initial brand name-to-generic scenario noted initially. Thankfully, this is often the exception and not the rule. However, clinicians must be astute regarding this relationship in certain acutely relapsing patients.

References

1. Orange Book Annual Preface, Statistical Criteria for Bioequivalence. *Approved Drug Products with Therapeutic Equivalence Evaluations*, 29th edn. U.S. Food and Drug Administration Center for Drug Evaluation and Research, 2009. http://www.fda.gov/Drugs/DevelopmentApprovalProcess/ucm079068.htm. Accessed August 10, 2009.
2. http://www.fda.gov/Drugs/ResourcesForYou/Consumers/BuyingUsingMedicineSafely/UnderstandingGenericDrugs/ucm167991.htm. Accessed May 9, 2011.
3. Davit BM, Nwakama PE, Buehler GJ, et al. Comparing generic and innovator drugs: a review of 12 years of bioequivalence data from the United States Food and Drug Administration. *Ann Pharmacother* 2009; 43:1583–97.
4. Riedl MA, Casillas AM. Adverse drug reactions: types and treatment option. *Am Fam Phys* 2003; 68:1781–91.

The Case: The woman who would not leave her car

The Question: What to do when obsessive compulsive disorder with poor insight is resistant to treatment

The Dilemma: Rational subsequent polypharmacy trials may help, but fail to achieve remission

Pretest self-assessment question (answer at the end of the case)

While OCD may develop postpartum in some cases, which is not true *of postpartum OCD?*

A. It is less common than postpartum blues
B. It is less common than postpartum depression
C. It occurs in up to 5% of postpartum women
D. Obsessions are most frequently related to contamination fears

Patient evaluation on intake

- 56-year-old woman with a chief complaint of "not doing well for many years"
- Has suffered anxiety and depression for over 30 years

Psychiatric history

- Was without major psychiatric symptoms until her late twenties
- Lost a child in utero and a few weeks after this there was an outbreak of pinworms in her household
- Since this time she has never recovered
- Has been depressed, and has obsessive thoughts about contamination
- Is essentially dependent on husband and family, does not drive, cannot work as a result
- Admits to MDD symptoms
  - Reasonable sleep but only with medication
  - Low interest
  - Low energy
  - Poor concentration and worsening short-term memory
  - Ideational guilt but not to a psychotic level
  - Poor appetite
  - Denies suicidal thinking
- Does not meet criteria for PTSD, PD (although she has frequent acute episodes of agitation), or GAD
  - She does meet criteria for SAD and the patient and husband describe her as being shy and avoidant her whole life
    - ○ Given the longevity of rejection sensitivity, avoidant personality disorder might be considered

- Meets criterion for OCD
  - Obsessions of excessive contamination are frequently encountered
  - Compulsively, she used to wash hands hundreds of times a day
    - A course of exposure and response prevention (ERP) therapy helped to decrease this many years ago
    - Interestingly, this compulsion was largely replaced by her actions of living in her car in her garage for extended periods of time
      - She often will leave the house in the morning and spend the whole day in her car in the garage reading books as the car is not contaminated nearly as much as the rest of the house
    - Denies other OCD symptoms
    - It is clear that much of daily routine and life revolves around the symptoms of OCD, which are deemed more disabling
- While screening for mania, she and her husband do acknowledge bipolar-like symptoms with sustained hypomania and possible mania in the distant past
  - These are ill defined and without any clear consequences
  - There is subtle mood elevation at times
  - More often, these appear to be sustained agitation episodes
- There is no evidence of eating disorder or substance abuse

Social and personal history

- Graduated high school and was gainfully employed as a clerk/secretary thereafter, but stopped work after she was married and started a family
- Now is married with grown children
- Drinks coffee in the morning, does not smoke or take drugs

Medical history

- Hyperlipidemia
- HTN
- No drug allergies, no vision problems, no skin problems

Family history

- SAD, avoidant personality, MDD in the patient's mother

Medication history

- Has tried a myriad of TCA, SSRI, SNRI, and BZ throughout the years
- Augmented with low-dose atypical antipsychotics in the past

Psychotherapy history

- Eclectic, supportive psychotherapy intermittently attended over last 30 years

- Some behavioral therapy but unclear if a full ERP behavioral therapy protocol was completed
- Little to no sustained response to these psychotherapeutic interventions, as she continues with fluctuating symptoms that never fully remit

Patient evaluation on initial visit

- Acute onset of apparent MDD symptoms associated with trauma of loss of an unborn child
  - Will need to consider postpartum MDD, or even postpartum OCD
- Symptoms of MDD have remitted at times
- OCD has not ever fully remitted
- Has fair insight, at best, into the OCD symptoms and better insight into the distress caused by the depressive symptoms
- Possible history of hypomania
- Despite symptoms, she has no suicidal ideation and no recent history of psychiatric inpatient admissions
  - 30 years ago, admitted twice for inpatient hospitalizations for suicidal thoughts, which in retrospect may have been postpartum induced
- Reports no current side effects but does have pre-existing metabolic illness

Current medications

- Fluoxetine (Prozac) 40 mg/d (SSRI)
- Quetiapine (Seroquel) 300 mg/d (atypical antipsychotic)

Question

In your clinical experience, would you consider her current medication regimen a therapeutically dosed one?

- Yes
- No

Attending physician's mental notes: initial evaluation

- This patient seems to have recovered from her index episode of postpartum MDD, but often relapses
- There is some corroborative evidence to suggest hypomania episodes
- Has comorbid OCD that has never fully remitted
- Seems content to be at home and not working but clearly is distressed by some symptoms
- Presents with a supportive spouse, which will help prognosis and treatment adherence
- Has been on many psychotropics over the last 30 years
  - It is unclear if these have been therapeutically dosed, but regardless, is likely fairly treatment resistant

- Current regimen's SSRI is too low a dose to be effective in treating OCD
- The combination of the SSRI and this particular atypical antipsychotic would be considered adequate for treating MDD

Question

Which of the following would be your next step?

- Increase the fluoxetine (Prozac) to the full FDA dose toward 80 mg/d for OCD
- Increase the quetiapine (Seroquel) to a higher, possibly more effective dose, toward 600 mg/d
- Increase both agents simultaneously
- Augment the current two medications with a third agent to improve response

Attending physician's mental notes: initial evaluation (continued)

- This patient seems to be on a standard approach for treating MDD
  - Good dose/duration of therapeutic SSRI
  - A therapeutic dose of her quetiapine (Seroquel) is being utilized now
    - The original quetiapine (Seroquel) immediate release is not approved as adjunctive treatment for unipolar MDD
      - Its longer-acting preparation, quetiapine-XR (Seroquel-XR), is at doses of 150–300 mg/d
    - The immediate-release preparation is approved for treating bipolar depression as a monotherapy at doses 300–600 mg/d
    - Suspect either preparation could be helpful in her case
- The atypical antipsychotics are often used clinically to treat resistant OCD, but the current SSRI is likely at too low a dose to be helpful
  - SSRIs typically need much higher doses in place for longer durations than those usually needed for treating other types of anxiety disorder
- Care may be complicated in that she has elevated cholesterol and blood pressure and the atypical antipsychotics are associated with escalation of metabolic disorder
- Quetiapine (Seroquel) seems to have a dose-related escalation in metabolic disorder
  - These adverse effects may increase remarkably at doses greater than 150 mg/d, according to MDD studies utilizing the XR preparation
- Developing better insight into her contamination fears and a referral for a bona fide CBT/ERP course may be warranted

216

Further investigation

Is there anything else you would especially like to know about this patient?

- What about details concerning her current HTN and hyperlipidemia?
  - Takes verapamil (Calan) 120 mg/d for HTN and is stable and routinely normotensive
  - Takes simvastatin (Zocor) 40 mg/d for hyperlipidemia and is well controlled
    - Cholesterol is 221 mg/dL, but HDL is 78 mg/dL, and triglycerides 75 mg/dL
    - Blood glucose is 86 mg/dL
- What about details regarding her longitudinal disability and family support?
  - Her illness struck while she decided to be a homemaker and raise children
  - Did not leave work due to her psychiatric symptoms
  - Was able to raise children without difficulty
  - Spouse is currently very supportive but reports that the patient only really functions well within the immediate family
  - Over time they have not challenged her idiosyncratic OCD symptoms, but do feel she suffers more when concomitantly depressed and agitated

Case outcome: first interim follow-up visit six weeks later

- Patient was given the choice to escalate the SSRI or the atypical antipsychotic, as both were felt to still have room to therapeutically increase dosing
- Patient suggested that the atypical had allowed better sleep and more calming effects
  - Quetiapine was raised to 400 mg at bedtime
  - This escalation was also warranted in that there is a potential history for bipolar II symptoms, and as she has fair insight at best into the OCD
  - Was converted to the once-daily quetiapine-XR in case symptoms were more representative of a bipolar disorder and would require even higher dosing in the future to prevent onset of mania, while treating the OCD with higher-dose SSRI therapy
  - This preparation is approved officially for depression adjunctive treatment as well, but at the lower doses already used. Up to 600 mg/d is approved for bipolar depression

- After this, husband reported that this is the "best she has done in years" and asks how long the effect will last?
  - Patient agrees in that the MDD and agitation are completely gone
  - Is spending less time in her car and seems less concerned with regard to contamination fears
- No side effects reported

Question

How would you answer the husband's question about longevity of response?

- She will stay in remission for many years
- She will likely relapse within the year
- She will likely do well, but requires ongoing minor medication changes to maintain her response

Attending physician's mental notes: interim follow-up visits through six months

- Despite being a little better clinically, now the patient is resistant to higher dose (fluoxetine 60 mg/d) and atypical antipsychotic (quetiapine-XR 500 mg/d) trials
- She has a clinically meaningful response in that she is less agitated, sleeping well, but she is not even a 50% responder
- She is side effect free, which is positive

Case outcome: interim follow-up visits through six months

- Patient calls between appointments stating that she and her spouse feel she is more depressed and agitated again despite there being no clear stress-related events
- Quetiapine-XR (Seroquel-XR) is increased to 500 mg/d without improvement
- At an office visit with apparent clinical decline noted, agrees to increase the SSRI, fluoxetine (Prozac), to 60 mg/d
  - This approach begins to maximize both medications toward a full-dosing strategy
- Mild improvement is noted but not to the same degree as the first medication adjustment
  - Compared to baseline, she is perhaps
    - 30% better with regards to MDD symptoms
    - 15% better with regard to OCD

Question

Do you consider her to be on optimal medication doses?

- Yes, both agents are dosed above the moderate approved range and should be considered therapeutic failures
- No, neither agent is dosed high enough to be considered a full trial, especially if her differential diagnosis includes OCD with potential bipolar or psychotic illness

Attending physician's mental notes: interim follow-up visit through six months (continued)

- Symptoms continue to fluctuate despite increasing medications
- There is an element of patient and family pessimism as she was robustly better, perhaps at her baseline best ever, only to decline again
- From a unipolar MDD point of view, quetiapine-XR (500 mg) and fluoxetine (60 mg) are maximized
- If there is a psychotic element to the depression, then the quetiapine-XR could be increased further
- From an OCD point of view, the fluoxetine or quetiapine-XR could be escalated for better effectiveness
- If the atypical antipsychotic is continued, laboratory values likely need to be obtained from the PCP to make sure there is no metabolic worsening

Case outcome: interim follow-up visits through nine months

- Fluoxetine (Prozac) and quetiapine-XR (Seroquel-XR) were both escalated to 80 mg/d and 700 mg/d, respectively
- Patient returns depression free with only minor bouts of agitation
- No longer stays in her car, but spends more time in her house
  - Still cleans a lot and assumes things are contaminated, but is more tolerant of these feelings
  - OCD symptoms are 50% better
- Currently has no medication side effects
- Collaboration with PCP shows
  - No metabolic worsening
  - Eye examinations are negative for cataracts
- Patient declines further medication alterations as she feels better and also sees gradual improvement

Question

What would you do next?

- Leave all medications as they are because the patient is in MDD remission and has a solid OCD response

- Strongly encourage patient to escalate her medications further to attempt gaining OCD remission
- Encourage patient to augment her current regimen with a third medication to attempt gaining OCD remission
- Refer for a new course of CBT/ERP to attempt to gain OCD remission

Attending physician's mental notes: interim follow-up visits through nine months

- The goal is always to achieve remission where safe and possible
- The patient is tolerating her medications very well with almost no adverse effects
- It makes clinical sense to escalate her medication doses further
- She has also been somewhat avoidant to going through a new course of psychotherapy as she has avoidant traits on top of her OCD symptoms
- Another option would be to motivate her to attempt a new course of CBT/ERP to alleviate her remaining OCD symptoms
  - The short-term, time-limited approach might be more acceptable to her

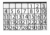

Case outcome: interim follow-up visits through 15 months

- Declines other medication options, feeling comfortable with her improvement thus far and relative absence of side effects
- Agrees to undergo a 20-week CBT/ERP response prevention protocol to help her better address and cope with her contamination fears to specific areas of her house
- She created a hierarchy of challenges to her OCD and currently attends CBT sessions regularly

Case debrief

- Patients with OCD often develop depression as OCD frequently interferes immensely with psychosocial functioning
- OCD patients often avoid treatment as they are aware that the OCD symptoms are abnormal and are embarrassed or ashamed to present their symptoms to clinicians as well
- However, in this case, the patient was actually more comfortable with her OCD symptoms and less so with her depression and agitation
  - This poor insight into her contamination fear may have been poor insight-specified OCD or a depressive psychosis or delusion
  - This patient also began her MDD and OCD in a postpartum state

- ○ It Is possible that she has had a smoldering psychosis since then that finally began to resolve when a higher-dose antipsychotic regimen was established
- This patient is not currently depressed but still suffers mild to moderate fluctuating OCD
- CBT/ERP was helpful to a certain degree in that she is more comfortable in certain areas of her house and seems to cope better when her OCD symptoms fluctuate higher

Take-home points

- Patients with poor insight into their OCD might display more psychotic or delusional features
- These symptoms may respond to atypical antipsychotics as long as the antipsychotic is also dosed therapeutically
- Special attention should be given to each drug's approval status and guidelines for effective dosing, based upon each clinical indication
- Psychotherapy may be used as an augmentation strategy for residual symptoms

Performance in practice: confessions of a psychopharmacologist

- *What could have been done better here?*
  - Is one atypical antipsychotic better than another?
    - ○ In this case, the quetiapine-XR (Seroquel-XR) certainly is supported, given its approved status, clinical data evidence base, and indication for treating unipolar MDD adjunctively
    - ○ However, its higher dose is out of the approved range for unipolar or bipolar depression (not for psychosis), but in this case was helpful
    - ○ Aripiprazole (Abilify), brexpiprazole (Rexulti), or lurasidone (Latuda) has similar approvals and could have been used instead
      - As this patient came into treatment with certain metabolic illness problems, choosing a more metabolically friendly atypical antipsychotic like these may have been warranted initially
    - ○ However, in her case she did not develop any metabolic worsening
  - No atypical antipsychotic has approval for treating OCD, but treatment guidelines support their adjunctive use in resistant cases
- *Possible action items for improvement in practice*
  - Research clinical trials, off-label data for augmentation strategies for treatment-resistant OCD
  - Research-available US and international guidelines for OCD treatment, as these offer a summary list that is often easier to

interpret, and provide a discussion regarding evidence-based treatments and the stringency of the available data
- Review postpartum OCD as it is often under-recognized and undertreated
  - ○ It is estimated that anywhere from 60% to 80% of new mothers will experience the "baby blues"
  - ○ Postpartum depression is more severe and affects approximately 10%–20% of new mothers
  - ○ Postpartum OCD affects approximately 3%–5% of new mothers
    - ▪ The focus of the obsessions is often on the fear of purposely harming the newborn, or somehow being responsible for accidental harm
- If this patient's contamination fear were actually paranoid and delusional in nature, finally achieving a reasonable dose of antipsychotic may have alleviated this and her other depressive symptoms
  - ○ In this case, using a higher-dose atypical antipsychotic sooner may have been warranted

Tips and pearls

- Treating OCD often requires very high doses of SSRI antidepressant agents
- High doses often have to be maintained for several weeks to a few months to achieve clinical effectiveness
- Failure of OCD to respond to high-dose SSRI may be augmented with atypical antipsychotics to gain further response or remission

Neurocircuitry moment

Why are OCD brains OCD?
- Dysfunction in the orbitofrontosubcortical circuitry, composed of direct and indirect pathways from the frontal cortex and projecting into the striatum, are hypothetically implicated
- The direct pathway
  - Projects from the striatum to the globus pallidus interna/substantia nigra, pars reticulate complex (the primary output location of the basal ganglia)
  - Back to the cortex, which activates the thalamic system
  - This generates, promotes, and coordinates complex motor activities
- The indirect pathway

- Follows a longer route starting from the striatum and continuing through the globus pallidus externa, subthalamic nucleus, globus pallidus–substantia nigra pars reticula, thalamus
- Ultimately returning to the cortex
  - This is an inhibitory pathway that attempts to dampen complex motor activities
- A mentally well-functioning brain would have a balance between these two pathways, allowing the correct amount of motor activity
- OCD patients may show more activation of the *direct* pathway, thereby increasing activity in the OFC, ventromedial caudate, and medial dorsal thalamus, which could result in compulsive, repetitive behavior activity.
  - The indirect pathway appears unable to inhibit the more aggressive direct pathway's activity, allowing compulsive behaviors to continue
- The neurocircuitry of OCD and non-OCD anxiety disorders differs
  - OCD brains demonstrate dysfunction in the frontostriatal circuitry as noted here
  - Other anxiety disorders often involve the amygdala and a fear response component
  - This may explain why OCD tends to require higher doses and longer durations of treatment compared to other anxiety disorders as the neurocircuitry involved is dependent upon the disorder being treated

Two-minute tutorial

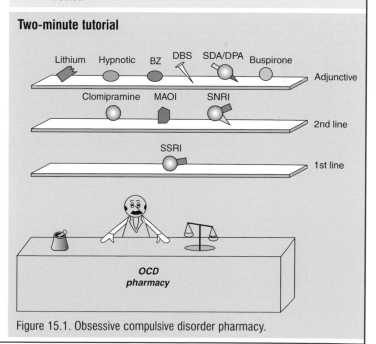

Figure 15.1. Obsessive compulsive disorder pharmacy.

Treatments for OCD

- SSRIs are the first-line recommendation for patients with OCD
    - Approved agents include fluoxetine (Prozac), sertraline (Zoloft), and paroxetine (Paxil)
- Second-line agents are considered off-label but have at least a minimum evidence base to support their use
    - SNRI agents (venlafaxine-XR [EffexorXR], duloxetine [Cymbalta], and desvenlafaxine [Pristiq]) all have potent serotonin reuptake inhibitor (SRI) activity, which may account for their anti-obsessive properties
    - MAOI agents cannot be added to SSRI or SNRI treatments safely, but may be used as monotherapy trials in more resistant OCD cases
        ○ The risk of serotonin syndrome or tyramine-induced hypertensive crises limits the safety and tolerability of this class, hence a second-tier rating
    - The TCA clomipramine (Anafranil) was actually the first approved agent
        ○ Its side-effect profile includes more sedation, weight gain, and anticholinergic effects than that of the SSRIs
        ○ Its cardiotoxicity in overdose limits it to second-tier use
        ○ This agent is considered the gold standard from outcomes-based trials
- Several medications may be used as adjuncts for residual symptoms or treatment-resistant OCD
    - Buspirone (BuSpar) and the atypical antipsychotics are often mentioned in treatment guidelines
    - The BZ anxiolytics and hypnotics are noted in some studies to lower agitation associated with obsessive thinking, but often do little to limit compulsive behaviors
    - Deep Brain Stimulation (DBS) is approved for compassionate use for treatment-resistant OCD patients
        ○ DBS is less surgically invasive than traditional or gamma knife anterior capsulotomy psychosurgery for truly refractory cases of OCD

Posttest-self assessment question and answer

Obsessive compulsive disorder (OCD) may develop postpartum in some cases, which is not true *of postpartum OCD*

A. It is less common than postpartum blues

B. It is less common than postpartum depression

C. It occurs in up to 5% of postpartum women

D. Obsessions are most frequently related to contamination fears

Answer: D
Obsessions most frequently noted are images or impulses about causing harm to the newborn or being unable to intervene and stop harm from involving the infant. Contamination was predominant in this case, but is not the most typical presentation postpartum.

References

1. Saxena S, Rauch SL. Functional neuroimaging and the neuroanatomy of obsessive-compulsive disorder. *Psychiatr Clin North Am* 2000; 23:563–86.
2. Hollander E, Kim S, Khanna S, Pallanti S. Obsessive-compulsive disorder and obsessive-compulsive spectrum disorders: diagnostic and dimensional issues. *CNS Spectr* 2007; 12:5–13.
3. Stahl SM. *Stahl's Essential Psychopharmacology: The Prescriber's Guide*, 5th edn. New York, NY: Cambridge University Press, 2014.
4. American Psychiatric Association Work Group on Obsessive-Compulsive Disorder. Practice guideline for the treatment of patients with obsessive-compulsive disorder. *Am J Psychiatry* 2007; 164:1–56.
5. Greenberg BD, Malone DA, Friehs GM, et al. Three-year outcomes in deep brain stimulation for highly resistant obsessive-compulsive disorder. *Neuropsychopharmacology* 2006; 31:2384–93.
6. Greist JH, Jefferson JW, Kobak KA, Katzelnick DJ, Serlin RC. Efficacy and tolerability of serotonin transport inhibitors in obsessive-compulsive disorder. A meta-analysis. *Arch Gen Psychiatry* 1995; 52:53–60.
7. Kobak KA, Greist JH, Jefferson JW, Katzelnick DJ, Henk HJ. Behavioral versus pharmacological treatments of obsessive compulsive disorder: a meta-analysis. *Psychopharmacology (Berl)* 1998; 136:205–16.
8. Bloch MH, Landeros-Weisenberger A, Kelmendi B, et al. A systematic review: antipsychotic augmentation with treatment refractory obsessive-compulsive disorder. *Mol Psychiatry* 2006; 11:622–32.
9. Bauer M, Pretorius HW, Constant EL, et al. Extended-release quetiapine as adjunct to an antidepressant in patients with major depressive disorder: results of a randomized, placebo-controlled, double-blind study. *J Clin Psychiatry* 2009; 70:540–9.

The Case: The woman who liked late-night TV

The Question: What to do when comorbid depression and sleep disorders are resistant to treatment

The Dilemma: Continuous positive airway pressure (CPAP) may not be a reasonable option for treating apnea; polypharmacy is needed but complicated by adverse effects

Pretest self-assessment question (answer at the end of the case)

Which of the following hypnotic agents is less likely to be addictive, impair psychomotor function, or cause respiratory suppression?

A. Ramelteon (Rozerem)
B. Zolpidem (Ambien)
C. Doxepin (Silenor)
D. Temazepam (Restoril)
E. A and C
F. B and D
G. None of the above

Patient evaluation on intake

- 70-year-old female with a chief complaint of "being sad"
- Feels she had been doing well until her hearing began to diminish in both ears
  - Candidate for cochlear implants in the future, but this is a long way off
  - Despite the promise of improved hearing, she often has crying spells for no clear reason

Psychiatric history

- The patient has been without psychiatric disorder throughout her life
- Has felt increasingly sad over the last year and these feelings were not triggered by an acute stressor
- Lives alone with the help of a home aide
  - Her spouse died many years ago due to CAD
  - Despite her aide and her son who visits often, she is having a harder time coping with both instrumental and basic activities of daily living
- She admits to full MDD symptoms
  - She is sad, has lost interest in things she used to enjoy, and is fatigued with poor focus and concentration
  - Denies feelings of guilt, worthlessness, or any suicidal thoughts
  - Appears mildly psychomotor slowed
  - Additionally states that sleep is "awful"
    ◦ Does not fall asleep easily as her legs "ache and jump"

  - ○ Takes frequent naps during the day as a result
  - ○ She admits to snoring frequently
- There is no evidence of cognitive decline or memory problems
- She has a supportive son who accompanies her to all appointments and helps provide her care

Social and personal history

- Graduated high school, was married, and raised her children
- Denied any academic issues, learning disability, or ADHD symptoms growing up
- Having and maintaining friendships has been easy and successful over the years
- At times, she is lonely at home
- Her mobility has declined somewhat, which limits her going out
- Participates in activities at a local elders' center
- No history of drug or alcohol problems

Medical history

- HTN
- Hypothyroidism
- CAD
- Anemia
- Environmental allergies
- Obesity

Family history

- Reports AUD throughout her extended family
- MDD reportedly suffered by her mother

Medication history

- Never taken psychotropic medications

Psychotherapy history

- Recently, has gone to a few sessions of outpatient supportive psychotherapy, but her hearing loss makes this modality almost impossible
  - – Hearing aids have failed to help
  - – May be a candidate for cochlear implants
- She has a fax machine at home and states that she and her therapist often fax notes back and forth, which she finds helpful as receiving them brightens her mood
  - – Perhaps this is "supportive facsimile therapy"

Patient evaluation on initial visit

- Gradual onset of geriatric, first-episode MDD symptoms likely as a result of hearing loss and mobility loss
- This caused interpersonal disconnectedness, loneliness, and onset of MDD
- Suffers from daily crying spells and seems very tired
- Has good insight into her illness and wants to get better
- There appears to be no suicidal or safety concerns clinically
- The fatigue and possible infirmities of strength and balance may be problematic if side effects compound these symptoms

Current medications

- Furosemide (Lasix) 40 mg/d
- Lisinopril (Zestril) 40 mg/d
- Levothyroxine (Synthroid) 100 mcg/d
- Enteric-coated aspirin 325 mg/d
- Fexofenadine (Allegra) 180 mg/d
- Ferrous sulfate 1000 mg/d

Question

Interpersonal approaches to psychotherapy would suggest that social disconnection and loss of role function causes depression, and treating this patient by changing the way she thinks, feels, and acts in problematic relationships may help. Does this make sense for this particular patient?

- Yes, this approach is evidence based in terms of providing IPT
- Yes, this approach clinically fits this patient's precipitating events prior to developing MDD
- Yes, for the reasons noted. However, her inability to hear well might render IPT difficult to apply and outcomes difficult to achieve

Attending physician's mental notes: initial evaluation

- Patient has her first MDE now
- It appears chronic in nature, but essentially, has been untreated
- It seems more than an adjustment disorder as it is pervasive, lasting over time, and clearly disabling at this point
- As this is an initial MDE and an initial foray into treatment with good family support, her prognosis is good
- However, her older age of onset, loss of hearing, mobility, and marked medical comorbidity are concerning
- Psychotherapy, especially IPT-based, would be clearly indicated but difficult to deliver adequately

Question

Which of the following would be your next step?

- Start an SSRI such as citalopram (Celexa)
- Start an SNRI such as duloxetine (Cymbalta)
- Start an NDRI such as buporpion-XL (Wellbutrin-XL)
- Start an NaSSA such as mirtazapine (Remeron)
- Start a SPARI such as vilazodone (Viibryd)
- Start a SARI such as trazodone-ER (Oleptro)
- Start a multimodal serotonin receptor modulating antidepressant with geriatric depression/cognition data, such as vortioxetine (Brintellix)

Attending physician's mental notes: initial evaluation (continued)

- This case seems easy in that she is untreated up to this point; therefore, any antidepressant has a chance of working
- However, there is concern regarding her obesity and lethargy; thus, avoiding medications with high weight-gain side-effect burden is warranted
- Sleep is also very disrupted
  - By initial insomnia, which may be caused by her depression
  - Perhaps by restless legs syndrome (RLS)
  - It is unclear if she snores and has OSA
- Hearing loss and inability to communicate well is also problematic in providing her with good psychotherapy
  - Even delineating symptoms in the medication management session is a difficult task
  - Likely need to pressure and advocate for the cochlear implants acting as an antidepressant in order to advance this process

Further investigation

Is there anything else you would especially like to know about this patient?

- She has marked fatigue; have medical causes been ruled out?
  - She is euthyroid and her anemia is stable with a normal hematocrit
  - Her cardiac function is stable and without compromise
  - If she has RLS, this could account for her fatigue and should be investigated
  - If she has OSA, this could account for her fatigue and should be investigated

Case outcome: first interim follow-up visit four weeks later

- Citalopram (Celexa), an SSRI, was started at 10 mg/d and titrated to 20 mg/d
- She appears less weepy and is in a partial response
- Still is not sleeping well
- Denies any typical side effects

Question

Would you increase her current SSRI medication?

- Yes
- Yes, only if it appears that she is partially better and her response has reached a plateau in this partial response range
- No, she is a partial responder with only four weeks of treatment. Longer treatment may allow for remission
- No, addition of a sleeping pill may treat insomnia and result in improved energy and concentration, thus facilitating a better overall response via polypharmacy
- No, citalopram carries cardiac warnings, especially in geriatric MDD patients

Attending physician's mental notes: second interim follow-up visit at two months

- Despite being a little better, the patient is still suffering
- She is crying less but there is now more of a need to improve her sleep and daytime fatigue issues
- She has clinical risks for OSA (HTN, obesity, large neck size), and if this is a positive finding, CPAP treatment may be an excellent choice for her apnea and her depression residual symptoms
- Her access to a sleep laboratory is limited and it may take months to have the study completed

Case outcome: second interim follow-up visit at two months

- Citalopram (Celexa) is increased gradually, given her age, to 30 mg/d
  - Historically, the QTc prolongation warning did not exist when this patient was prescribed this medication
  - Currently, use above 20 mg/d is discouraged in the elderly
    - If a higher dose is needed clinically, it would make sense to obtain plasma levels and an EKG in the current era
- Sleep electrophysiology is ordered to rule out OSA, RLS
- She is placed on off-label tiagabine (Gabitril) as a hypnotic in order to avoid more respiratory suppressing, psychomotor impairing, sedative-hypnotic BZ or BZRA agents

- This agent has human sleep laboratory data suggesting it increases slow wave, restorative deep sleep
- Its theoretical mechanism of action is GABA reuptake inhibition, selectively at the GAT1 transporter, making it an SGRI
- She is allowed to titrate to 6 mg/d at bedtime
- This agent, interestingly, is approved to treat epilepsy but came out with a warning, well after this patient utilized this "drug" therapy that tiagabine might actually induce seizures in non-epileptic patients

- The patient subsequently shows moderate improvement in her affect
- Experiences slightly less RLS
- Is not initiating sleep any better
- She is felt to be 20%–30% better globally, but is plagued by daytime fatigue as a chief complaint
  - This may actually be occurring due to the adverse effect profile of tiagabine (Gabitril)

Question

What would you do next?

- Continue escalating her SSRI to a higher dose
- Switch or augment with a more stimulating antidepressant
- Augment with a formal stimulant
- Add a formal hypnotic agent to better improve sleep

Attending physician's mental notes: second interim follow-up visit at two months (continued)

- Cannot wait months for a sleep study
- Her SSRI is at a reasonable, moderate dose, and has effectively treated the target symptom of sadness and dysphoria
  - Switching from this may cause a relapse
- Adding a noradrenergic or dopaminergic agent may target her fatigue symptoms a little better
- Adding a hypnotic may improve her sleep, and secondarily, her next day wakefulness, but need to watch for respiratory suppression and psychomotor impairment, especially if she has severe undiagnosed OSA

Case outcome: interim follow-up visits through four months

- The NDRI bupropion-XL (Wellbutrin-XL) is added to her SSRI and titrated to 300 mg/d
  - There is moderate improvement in her vegetative MDD symptoms and her drive and motivation improves slightly
- Zaleplon (Sonata) 5 mg at bedtime is started in place of tiagabine (Gabitril) with improved sleep onset overall, but she still reports RLS

– Zaleplon is chosen as the shortest half-life (1 h) BZRA, and in theory, should have least impact on psychomotor impairment or respiratory suppression in this class of sleep-inducing agents
• Further workup suggests she meets criteria for RLS. Sleep study is still pending
• Cochlear implants are approved and surgery scheduled

Question

What would you do next?

• Increase the bupropion-XL (Wellbutrin-XL) to the approved maximum 450 mg/d
• Increase the citalopram (Celexa) further above the geriatric approved maximum dose
• Increase zaleplon (Sonata) toward the approved maximum of 20 mg/d (10 mg/d in the elderly)
• As she is a partial responder, make no changes until her cochlear implants are in place and her sleep study is performed

Attending physician's mental notes: interim follow-up visits through four months

• Fairly good resolution of dysphoria is reported but insomnia and fatigue are still a major problem
• It will still be a while for her to obtain a sleep study and she likely has OSA clinically, thus markedly increasing a sedative at night is worrisome
• RLS is now more concerning to the patient, and she admits she likes to stay up watching late-night TV
  – The initial insomnia may be more of a circadian rhythm sleep disorder (CRSD) in that she is choosing to stay up late and then has to get up early when her home health aide arrives
  – She is inappropriately awake in the early morning hours and inappropriately tired during the daytime. A circadian delayed phase shift has occurred
• Perhaps a "win–win" situation exists where her RLS and initial insomnia could be treated with one medication
  – This was attempted with tiagabine (Gabitril)
    ○ This helped the RLS
    ○ Did not improve her sleep onset
    ○ Left her more fatigued in the morning
    ○ Could consider using another off-label antiepileptic medication, given her partial RLS response to tiagabine and hope for less daytime fatigue

- A literature search suggests that gabapentin (Neurontin) does have a limited evidence base showing effectiveness in RLS
  - Otherwise, an option would be to choose a formal RLS-approved dopaminergic medication such as pramipexole (Mirapex) or ropinirole (Requip)
  - These D2 receptor agonists have some data suggesting they may provide antidepressant response but fatigue is a key side effect
  - It might help fatigue at night, but the daytime fatigue may be a problem

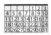

Case outcome: interim follow-up visits through nine months

- Gabapentin (Neurontin) is titrated to 300 mg twice a day as patient also has RLS symptoms intermittently through the day as well
- Zaleplon (Sonata) 5 mg at bedtime is still allowed, but only as needed for severe insomnia
- SSRI (citalopram [Celexa]) and NDRI (bupropion-XL [Wellbutrin-XL]) are continued at the same doses, 30 mg/d and 300 mg/d, respectively
- There is remission of MDD symptoms
- RLS resolves and she sleeps better with minimal morning fatigue
- However, she still seems to go to bed after midnight due to watching TV
  - Patient and family educated about sleep hygiene and behavioral management of sleep initiation
  - It is not possible to ask the home health aide to arrive later due to her schedule, so the patient cannot sleep late to allow for an adequate number of hours of sleep
- Her sleep study shows moderate OSA
  - She is fitted for a CPAP mask, which causes discomfort and claustrophobia and she declines to wear it
- Medications with known sedation side effects are moved to afternoon or dinner-time to avoid iatrogenic sedation in the morning

Attending physician's mental notes: interim follow-up visits through 12 months

- Patient has been doing very well on moderate dose of two antidepressants and a hypnotic agent used as needed
- RLS is well treated with a low-dose antiepileptic
- Cochlear implants are implanted and work very well. She is able to hear and converse, which has helped lower her social isolation and likely has helped her depression
- There are minimal to no side effects and she agrees to maintain these medications
- Compliance and family support are excellent

Case outcome: interim follow-up visits through 18 months

- There is a resurgence of insomnia and daytime fatigue
- Zaleplon (Sonata) is increased to a 10 mg dose at bedtime, which is used more routinely, but is ineffective
  - This is discontinued and she is allowed to take the next longest half-life BZRA hypnotic, zolpidem (Ambien) up to 10 mg at bedtime
- Sleep improves some, but sometimes she still chooses to watch TV and go to bed late
  - One morning she falls asleep at the breakfast table in front of her home health aide
  - She later falls and fractures her arm and requires inpatient physical rehabilitation
  - While there, develops panic attacks and is treated by the inpatient physician successfully with the BZ anxiolytic, alprazolam (Xanax), in low doses (0.25 mg as needed)
- Upon returning home, she discontinues the alprazolam anxiolytic
  - Is not depressed but her insomnia and fatigue continue
  - Still refuses CPAP treatment and behavioral modification measures fail to help
  - It becomes clear that at night, her sleep patterns and use of her zolpidem (Ambien) are erratic
- Instead of trying to induce sleep to improve daytime fatigue, which is likely due to OSA, the patient and son agree to approach her case with regard to providing more daytime wakefulness with a stimulant medication
  - Starts modafinil (Provigil) as it is approved for OSA fatigue and likely has fewer cardiac and blood pressure adverse effects than true stimulant-class medications
- Given her fall on full-dose zolpidem (Ambien) and her OSA, it is agreed to remove sedative-type medications
- However, providing better sleep initiation is still needed
  - Ramelteon (Rozerem), an MT1/MT2 receptor agonist hypnotic agent, is started
    ○ This should provide for better sleep onset without the risk of much respiratory suppression or falls
    ○ This combination should allow better daytime alertness with a relative absence of morning fatigue side effects and likely less risk for developing ataxia, psychomotor impairment, and fall potential

Case debrief

- Over the next several months, the patient ultimately is maintained in an MDD-free state, RLS-free state, and the OSA fatigue is reduced by at least 50% by use of modafinil (Provigil), which clearly improves her quality of life
- Her current regimen includes:
  - Citalopram (Celexa) 20 mg/d
  - Bupropion-XL (Wellbutrin-XL) 300 mg/d
  - Gabapentin (Neurontin) 600 mg/d
  - Modafinil (Provigil) 400 mg/d
  - Ramelteon (Rozerem) 16 mg/d
- Modafinil had to be escalated to its full dose to allow for its sustained response (400 mg/d)
- Ramelteon had to be doubled over the approved 8 mg dose for better effectiveness (16 mg at bedtime)
- Citalopram was reduced to 20 mg/d as it was felt to be contributing to fatigue
- Finally, after a physical rehabilitation stay, her need or desire to stay up late for TV watching diminished and her home health aide adjusted her schedule to arrive a bit later in the morning
  - These behavioral modifications seemed to improve her CRSD symptoms and improved her quality of life because her delayed phase shift was allowed to continue instead of being resisted
    - Essentially, as her health aide could come later, the patient was allowed to sleep in and obtain more consecutive hours of sleep

Take-home points

- Geriatric depression is complicated given the psychosocial issues that must be navigated, medical comorbidities that are present, and the possibility of more pronounced side-effect burden in this age group
- Sometimes treating the depression is simple, but treating the comorbidities require more effort or collaboration with other providers to optimize treatment
  - In this case, collaboration with otolaryngology, pulmonology–sleep medicine, primary care, physical medicine and rehabilitation, home healthcare, and the family often occurred

Performance in practice: confessions of a psychopharmacologist

- *What could have been done better here?*
  - Unlike other cases in this book, this patient was not escalated to the maximum higher dose monotherapy before combination therapy was started

- ○ Polypharmacy ultimately helped this patient and worked to lower her symptoms
- ○ It is possible that her medications could have been further streamlined by removing her SSRI and leaving her NDRI in place
- – Given her OSA and tendency toward falls, BZ and BZRA sleep-inducing agents likely should have been avoided
- – Interestingly, well after this patient was treated with citalopram and tiagabine, FDA warnings were given about QTc prolongation and seizure induction, respectively
    - ○ As such, these may be poor treatment options currently
- • *Possible action items for improvement in practice*
    - – Research information on CPAP equipment. It is possible that newer generations of equipment might be less cumbersome and claustrophobia inducing
        - ○ This information could be used in a motivational format to improve CPAP compliance and avoid excess medication use to treat residual fatigue
        - ○ Dental appliances that fit like mouth guards may be utilized instead of CPAP to keep her airways open more at night
    - – Become aware of available hypnotic agents that are not addictive and for those that have less psychomotor impairment and respiratory suppression, e.g., ramelteon (Rozerem), doxepin (Silenor), doxylamine (Unisom), suvorexant (Belsomra)
    - – These agents are Non-BZ and Non-BZRA

Tips and pearls

- • Shorter half-life hypnotic agents have a shorter span of clinical effectiveness and often provide somnolence for four to six hours, e.g., zaleplon (Sonata) and zolpidem (Ambien Intermezzo)
- • Shorter half-life hypnotic agents often are fully metabolized after four to eight hours of sleep and should have less impact with regard to causing morning sedation or impairment
    - – Despite this, the FDA recently suggested that lower doses of the BZRA agents be utilized to avoid psychomotor daytime impairment
- • Intermediate and longer-acting hypnotic agents provide for longer durations of sleep maintenance but may also allow for more side effects upon awakening, e.g., zolpidem-CR (Ambien-CR) and eszopiclone (Lunesta)

Mechanism of action moment

Does melatonin facilitation induce sleep or remove wakefulness?

- Endogenous melatonin is secreted by the pineal gland during darkness and acts mainly in the SCN to regulate circadian rhythms
- There are three types of receptors for melatonin: MT1 and MT2, which are both involved in sleep, and MT3, which is the enzyme NRH: quinone oxidoreductase-2, and not thought to be involved in sleep physiology
  - Specifically, MT1 receptor agonism, by way of endogenous melatonin at nighttime or by direct agonism through ramelteon use, may allow for inhibition of neurons in the SCN that are responsible for promoting wakefulness
    - With this mechanism, MT1 receptor activation removes wakefulness at the level of the circadian "clock" or "pacemaker"
    - The SCN's alerting signals, dampened by melatonin, likely do not stimulate the reticular activating system (RAS)
    - Monoamine transmission (DA, NE) from the brainstem is attenuated secondarily
    - This mechanism removes the brain's ability to create an aroused, wakeful state, thus allowing sleepiness to occur
  - Phase shifting (being routinely awake or somnolent at the wrong hours of the day/night) and circadian rhythm effects of the normal sleep/wake cycle are thought to be primarily mediated by MT2 receptors, which entrain these signals in the SCN
  - This is important for the following reasons
    - Worsening sleep, by way of phase-delayed circadian rhythms (similar to this patient), tends to worsen MDD symptoms
    - Brain neurogenesis, learning, and memory may also be impacted negatively
    - Deep sleep may increase neurotrophic factors and growth factors
    - Interestingly, SSRIs, TCAs, ECT, and possibly psychotherapy may also increase neurotropic factors in the CNS
- There are several different agents that act at melatonin receptors, as shown in Figure 16.1

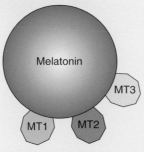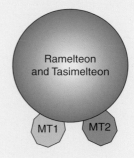

Figure 16.1. Melatonergic agents.

- Endogenous melatonin, or over-the-counter preparations, act at MT1 and MT2 receptors as well as at the MT3 site
- Ramelteon (Rozerem) is an MT1 and MT2 receptor agonist hypnotic agent available by prescription for sleep initiation
- Tasimelteon (Hetlioz) is also an MT1 and MT2 receptor agonist specifically approved for "non-24" patients. These patients are blind, do not respond to typical day/night cues, and develop persistent CRSD
  - By increasing brain derived neurotrophic factor (BDNF) and improving neurogenesis
  - By antagonizing 5-HT2C receptors, which facilitates NE and DA neurotransmission to the frontal cortex

Two-minute tutorial

Restless legs syndrome: what should psychiatrists know?

Diagnosis

- Patients develop an urge to move their legs, often accompanied by or felt to be caused by uncomfortable and unpleasant sensations in the legs
- The urge to move and unpleasant sensations begin, or worsen, during periods of rest or inactivity, such as lying down or sitting
- These sensations are often relieved by movement, such as walking or stretching, at least as long as the activity continues
- These symptoms occur or are worse in the evening or night compared to the day

Etiology

- 60% of RLS patients report a positive family history for RLS
- Genetic association studies have now identified five genes and 10 different risk alleles for RLS

- One of the allelic variations associated with increased risk of RLS is also associated with decreased serum ferritin, indicating relative reduction in body iron stores
- Theoretically, brain iron deficiency may produce dopaminergic pathology producing RLS symptoms. This iron–DA hypothesis may best explain the pathology of RLS
- Initial cerebrospinal fluid (CSF), autopsy, and brain imaging studies showed expected brain iron deficiency particularly affecting the DA-producing cells in the substantia nigra
- Animal and cellular iron deficiency studies have suggested that tyrosine hydroxylase activity in the substantia nigra, decreased D2 receptors in the striatum, decreased DAT functioning, and increased extracellular DA, with larger increases in the amplitude of the circadian variation of extracellular DA exist in RLS models
- These same findings have largely been replicated in RLS patients, revealing the iron–DA link
- Specifically, brain iron deficiency affects dopaminergic function
- First, by increasing tyrosine hydroxylase, which then increases extracellular DA
- This results in a decrease in DAT (reuptake pumps) on the cell surface (DAT downregulation)
- In extreme cases, it also causes a decrease in the number of D2 receptors on neuronal surfaces (receptor downregulation)
- In these cases, RLS is a hyperdopaminergic condition with an apparent postsynaptic dopaminergic desensitization that overcompensates during the circadian low point of dopaminergic activity in the evening and night
- Counterintuitively, this leads to the RLS symptoms that can be easily corrected by adding D2 receptor agonist medications at night
- Essentially, more DA activity is added to overcome the desensitization
- This D2 receptor agonist prescription-induced excess activity is very effective at calming RLS symptoms
- However, this sometimes leads to RLS augmentation where RLS may actually worsen in a select few patients over longer-term treatment because this creates a further imbalance of greater DA activity in the face of even more downregulation of receptors
- RLS may also be related to cortical sensorimotor dysfunction
- This would be consistent with the disruptions in the adenosine and dopaminergic systems regulating sensorimotor responses that have been reported for iron deficiencies noted here
- RLS often is comorbid with MDD, which is also known to have DLPFC hypoactivity

- In this manner, MDD and RLS may share overlapping dysfunctional frontocortical DA neurocircuits

RLS and comorbidity

- Health-related quality of life is substantially reduced in RLS patients and is comparable to other chronic neurological disorders such as Parkinson's disease and stroke
- Severity of RLS plus MDD symptoms have the most significant negative impact on quality of life
- RLS is also common in those who are pregnant, suffer from renal disease, or rheumatoid arthritis

RLS treatment

- Dopaminergic drugs are the first-line treatment and have been shown to relieve symptoms in 70%–90% of patients
- Ropinirole (Requip) and pramipexole (Mirapex) are approved agents that are D2 receptor agonists
- Adverse effects include induction of compulsive behaviors, nausea, asthenia, sedation, somnolence, syncope, hallucinations, or dyskinesias
- Oral iron treatment may significantly reduce RLS severity
- Opioids may be considered for patients presenting with neuropathy or painful dysthesias
- Alpha-2-delta calcium channel blocking anticonvulsants (gabapentin [Neurontin] or pregabalin [Lyrica]) have also been studied, showing RLS symptom reduction

Posttest self-assessment question and answer

Which of the following hypnotic agents is less likely to be addictive, impair psychomotor function, or cause respiratory suppression?

A. Ramelteon (Rozerem)
B. Zolpidem (Ambien)
C. Doxepin (Silenor)
D. Temazepam (Restoril)
E. A and C
F. B and D
G. None of the above

Answer: E

Ramelteon and doxepin are not GABA-A receptor positive allosteric modulators (PAMs), are therefore not related to the true BZ or BZRA class of hypnotics, are not associated with addiction, and appear to have little to no respiratory suppression or psychomotor impairment, comparatively speaking.

References

1. Salas RE, Gamaldo CE, Allen RP. Update in restless legs syndrome. *Curr Opin Neurol* 2010; 23:401–6.
2. Klerman GL, Weissman M, Rounsville BJ, Chevron ES. *Interpersonal Psychotherapy of Depression*. New York, NY: Basic Books Inc., 1984; pp. 14–16.
3. Stahl SM. *Stahl's Essential Psychopharmacology*, 4th edn. New York, NY: Cambridge University Press, 2013.
4. Stahl SM. *Stahl's Essential Psychopharmacology: The Prescriber's Guide*, 5th edn. New York, NY: Cambridge University Press, 2014.
5. Zarate CA Jr., Payne JL, Singh J, et al. Pramipexole for bipolar II depression: a placebo-controlled proof of concept study. *Biol Psychiatry* 2004; 56:54–60.
6. Walsh JK, Zammit G, Schweitzer PK, Ondrasik J, Roth T. Tiagabine enhances slow wave sleep and sleep maintenance in primary insomnia. *Sleep Med* 2006; 7:155–61.
7. Emens J, Lewy A, Kinzie JM, Arntz D, Rough J. Circadian misalignment in major depressive disorder. *Psychiatry Res* 2009; 168:259–61.
8. Lewy AJ. The dim light melatonin onset, melatonin assays and biological rhythm research in humans. *Biol Signals Recept* 1999; 8:79–83.
9. Aimone JB, Deng W, Gage FH. Adult neurogenesis: integrating theories and separating functions. *Trends Cogn Sci* 2010; 14:325–37.
10. Holmes MM, Galea LA, Mistlberger RE, Kempermann G. Adult hippocampal neurogenesis and voluntary running activity: circadian and dose-dependent effects. *J Neurosci Res* 2004; 76:216–22.
11. Molteni R, Calabrese F, Pisoni S, et al. Synergistic mechanisms in the modulation of the neurotrophin BDNF in the rat prefrontal cortex following acute agomelatine administration. *World J Biol Psychiatry* 2010; 11:148–53.
12. Armstrong SM, McNulty OM, Guardiola-Lemaitre B, Redman JR. Successful use of S20098 and melatonin in an animal model of delayed sleep-phase syndrome (DSPS). *Pharmacol Biochem Behav* 1993; 46:45–9.
13. Millan MJ, Gobert A, Lejeune F, et al. The novel melatonin agonist agomelatine (S20098) is an antagonist at 5-hydroxytryptamine2C receptors, blockade of which enhances the activity of frontocortical dopaminergic and adrenergic pathways. *J Pharmacol Exp Ther* 2003; 306:954–64.

14. Katona C, Hansen T, Olsen CK. A randomized, double-blind, placebo-controlled, duloxetine-referenced, fixed-dose study comparing the efficacy and safety of Lu AA21004 in elderly patients with major depressive disorder. *Intern Clin Psychopharmacol* 2012; 27:215–23.

The Case: The patient who interacted with everything

The Question: What to do when treating depression is thwarted by pharmacokinetic problems and side effects

The Dilemma: CYP450 enzyme genetic alterations may cause subtherapeutic, side effect-prone treatment

Pretest self-assessment question (answer at the end of the case)

Which of the following medications is often used in regulatory trials to determine if a CYP450 inhibition interaction exists with an experimental drug?

A. Temazepam (Restoril)
B. Desipramine (Norpramin)
C. Desvenlafaxine (Pristiq)
D. Paliperidone (Invega)

Patient evaluation on intake

- 54-year-old woman with a chief complaint of "being depressed"
- Patient started interferon treatment for hepatitis C and became alarmingly depressed

Psychiatric history

- The patient had been psychiatrically healthy until she was treated with interferon
- While on treatment she developed marked insomnia initially, which was then followed by more fulminant depression and anxiety symptoms
- Now experiencing full MDD symptoms
  - Except that she denies suicidal thoughts but has ideational guilt that she is a bad spouse and mother and that she has let her family down by being incapacitated and unable to do much of anything around the home
  - Experiencing marked agitation and restlessness routinely during the day and has insomnia at night
  - Is very tired, fatigued, unfocused, and unmotivated
- Does meet criteria for GAD prior to the onset of this MDE
  - Worries excessively
  - Is tense, keyed up, on edge
  - Has insomnia
  - Additionally admits to panic or agitation attacks that are sustained for hours
    - She did not experience these when euthymic, or prior to her interferon treatment
- There is no evidence of psychosis, mania, substance misuse
- Spouse and family are supportive

- She has traveled to specific inpatient depression treatment programs for advice and brings her extensive workup to her initial session

Social and personal history

- Graduated from college with a bachelor's degree
- Married and has a grown daughter
- A school teacher by trade, but has been unable to teach
- Does not misuse alcohol, caffeine, nicotine, or other drugs

Medical history

- Chronic severe head, neck, and shoulder pain, which is now exacerbated by MDD
- A report showing she is CYP450 hepatic enzyme deficient is reviewed
  - 2D6 is markedly deficient (a poor metabolizer)
  - 2C19 is moderately deficient
- Did not complete interferon treatment for hepatitis C, but is considered stable hepatically nonetheless

Family history

- Denies any known psychiatric disorder in any family member

Medication history

- Initial SSRI (escitalopram [Lexapro] 10 mg/d) and SNRI (desvenlafaxine [Pristiq] 50 mg/d) left her fraught with agitation and activation-based side effects

Psychotherapy history

- No previous experience with psychotherapy and has relied only on PCPs for outpatient pharmacotherapy and inpatient psychiatrists as well
- Somewhat receptive to the idea of attending psychotherapy as a treatment option

Patient evaluation on initial visit

- Acute onset of MDD symptoms with marked agitation and insomnia roughly six months ago
- She seems to be suffering immensely with guilt over her incapacity
  - This does not appear to be delusional at this time
- She has been noncompliant with medication management thus far as she has developed side effects even to small doses of antidepressants and has declined psychotherapy as an option
- She has apparent insight into her acute illness and wants to get better

- She has current distrust of medications, and given her workup for liver metabolism enzymes, is convinced that she will get side effects on all medications

Current medications

- Zolpidem-CR (Ambien-CR) 12.5mg/d (BZRA)
- Zolpidem (Ambien) 5 mg/d as needed for severe breakthrough insomnia (BZRA)
- Alprazolam (Xanax) 0.25 mg/d as needed for panic attacks (BZ)
- Mirtazapine (Remeron) 15 mg/d (NaSSA)
- Ibuprofen (Motrin) 1200 mg/d
- Tramadol (Ultram) 50 mg/d as needed for severe pain

Question

Should interferon-induced depression respond to antidepressant monotherapy?

- Yes
- No

Attending physician's mental notes: initial evaluation

- This patient has her first MDE now
- This seems superimposed upon GAD, which was likely pre-existing
- She is remarkably agitated and looks horribly withdrawn and fatigued
- It is acute and precipitated by a medication (Interferon) known to induce MDD in patients being treated for hepatitis
- There is some evidence that SSRI and TCA treat interferon-induced depression
  - Sometimes SSRIs are used prophylactically as a pretreatment
  - She could respond to initial monotherapies
- Her initial failure to a subtherapeutic SSRI and SNRI is possibly alarming, but her issue has been intolerance, not inefficacy
- She was recently started on a minimally therapeutic dose of a third antidepressant in a novel class
  - Mirtazapine (Remeron) is an NaSSA antidepressant
  - It is unlikely to be problematic
    - She has known CYP450 2D6 and 2C19 genetic enzyme deficiencies
    - Mirtazapine pharmacokinetics include
      - Approximately 100% of the orally administered dose is excreted via urine and feces within four days
      - Biotransformation is mainly mediated by the CYP2D6 *and* CYP3A4 isoenzymes

- Inhibitors of these isoenzymes (or those with genetic enzyme deficiencies) cause modest increases in mirtazapine plasma concentrations (17% and 32%, respectively) usually without leading to clinically relevant consequences as mirtazapine has multiple routes of metabolism and clearance
  - ○ Mirtazapine has little inhibitory effects on CYP isoenzymes and, therefore, the pharmacokinetics of co-administered drugs are usually unaffected
- However, her documented CYP450 2D6 liver enzyme deficiency will predispose her to side effects of many drugs and many psychotropics will need to be dose-modified during her care
  - – Her first two reactions (to an SSRI and SNRI) and side effects clearly worsened her agitation and her trust of psychotropics
    - ○ Escitalopram (Lexapro) requires CYP450 2C19 and 3A4 enzymes
      - Her 3A4 system should have been able to metabolize the escitalopram
      - However, 2C19-deficient patients can show a 1.8-fold increase in escitalopram, making her initial SSRI side effects possibly related to her 2C19 enzyme deficiency
    - ○ Desvenlafaxine (Pristiq) requires no CYP450 metabolism and is renally excreted; it should not have caused side effects based upon her CYP450 genetic deficiencies
      - Her side effects appear to be either usual activating side effects or hypochondriacal responses
  - – She seems convinced and determined that she will be hurt by all interventions
- Her clear isoenzyme deficiencies, anxiety, and hypochondriacal thought processes make her prognosis difficult to determine

Question

Which of the following would be your next step?

- Increase the mirtazapine (Remeron) to the full FDA dose of 45 mg/d
- Increase the alprazolam (Xanax) to a higher, more effective dose to treat her agitation
- Change to a more effective hypnotic agent to better treat her insomnia
- Review her current medications further to see if any are CYP450 2D6 or 2C19 substrates that are likely to be poorly metabolized and induce immense side effects
- Continue to motivationally suggest she consider psychotherapy as a side-effect-free treatment

Attending physician's mental notes: initial evaluation (continued)

- This patient seems to be undertreated due to
  - Clear medical reasons (CYP450 2D6 and 2C19 deficiencies)
  - Phobic reactions given her initial experience with interferon and her antidepressants
  - Good doses/duration of antidepressant treatment have not been utilized
  - Much rapport/trust building and very slow titrations will likely be needed to treat her effectively
- All prescribing will need to be cross-checked for CYP450 2D6 and 2C19 interactions as she is vulnerable to toxicity and side effects if agents are metabolized through these isoenzyme systems
- It is possible that her liver is more affected by her hepatitis C than we suspect, causing her to process medications even more poorly. Could she be a candidate for sofosbuvir (Sovaldi) as an alternate to interferon treatment?
- She seems very guilt-ridden and ruminative about her decline. Will need to continue to investigate if this is delusional
- She does meet criteria for MDD
- It is unclear if her anxiety is truly comorbid or if her MDD is fostering the anxiety symptoms
- If psychosis and comorbid anxiety become more evident, then her prognosis worsens further

Further investigation

Is there anything else you would especially like to know about this patient?

What about details concerning her CYP450 deficiencies? How poor of a metabolizer is she?

- Cytochrome CYP450 genotype revealed that she is a poor to intermediate 2D6 metabolizer, and an intermediate 2C19 metabolizer
- Therefore, drugs that are metabolized and broken down by these enzymes will not be processed efficiently hepatically, causing increased plasma drug levels and likely greater side effects
- In patients like this, each prescribed drug should have its metabolic pathways evaluated before prescribing
- Drugs known to interact could be used, but dosing must be adjusted to lower doses to avoid toxicity and side effects
- Her current medications may have some interactions

- Zolpidem (Ambien) is largely metabolized through 3A4 enzymes and should not present any interaction as she has no genetic enzyme deficiencies for this isoenzyme
- Alprazolam (Xanax) is metabolized by the 3A4 enzyme system as well
- Mirtazapine (Remeron) 15 mg/d is metabolized, as noted earlier, through 3A4 and 2C19. She should have minimal problems as her mild to moderately deficient 2C19 enzyme system can be adequately supported, again by 3A4 enzymes for which she has no deficiency

What about details regarding her liver functioning in face of her untreated hepatitis C?

- This patient has AST and ALT hepatic enzyme levels that fluctuate between 200 U/L and 300 U/L, which are considered three to four times greater than normal values
- She is considered to be stable by her gastroenterology physicians, but her liver is at risk for ongoing damage as a result of her hepatitis

Case outcome: first interim follow-up visit four weeks later

- Patient was tolerating the low-dose mirtazapine (Remeron) except for carbohydrate-craving side effects
  - It was increased to 30 mg/d
- Next, she is placed on chromium picolinate 200 mcg/d as an antidote to her carbohydrate cravings
  - Evidence base suggests that use of this agent up to 1000 mcg/d may reduce carbohydrate cravings in MDD patients
  - Anecdotal reports suggest it may reduce AAWG
  - A larger evidence base suggests it improves insulin sensitivity and may be mildly effective in treating some diabetes patients
- Between sessions insomnia escalates and she calls reporting that she had to take extra zolpidem (Ambien) to compensate
  - She panics more when she cannot sleep and her depressive symptoms worsen as a result
  - She does not seem to be abusing the hypnotic agent but the pattern is worrisome
- Upon return, there is slightly less dysphoria and agitation
- Affect is moderately brighter
- Carbohydrate craving is moderately diminished
- Insomnia is evaluated and appears partially driven by the MDD symptoms, but also has a phobic, fear-like quality more consistent with insomnia as if it were a clear comorbidity in itself
  - *DSM-5* allows insomnia to be a comorbid diagnosis if it is a focus of clinical attention even if, in part, the insomnia is felt to be secondary to MDD

- Admits now to mixing her zolpidem and zolpidem-CR and overusing them as she wakes up in the middle of the night sometimes

Question

What would you do next?

- Increase the mirtazapine (Remeron) as she seems to be responding better with each dose escalation
- Change her hypnotic agent to another with a longer half-life to allow better sleep maintenance
- Change her hypnotic agent from her current, sleep center-selective BZRA zolpidem to a true BZ hypnotic that is less selective and possibly able to allow for hypnosis, anxiolysis, and muscle relaxation
- Change her hypnotic to one that is not a controlled substance due to fear of pending addiction
- Leave medications the same as she is appearing to respond to moderate-dose mirtazapine

Attending physician's mental notes: second interim follow-up visit at two months

- Despite being a little better, she is not a full responder to full-dose mirtazapine (Remeron)
- This drug is involved in the CYP450 system, but its metabolism is divided among different enzymatic pathways
  - The patient is not deficient on all pathways and has tolerated this medication well, except for her reported hair loss
  - She does not seem to be having any major systemic side effects but is growing wary of the medication
  - It is possible that she is having side effects from her CYP450 enzymatic 2C19 deficiency regarding mirtazapine metabolism, but more likely at this point, is highly somatic and suffers anxiety-induced side effects
    - These are erroneously attributed to the medicine
    - These are often called "nocebo" effects as they are placebo-induced
- She is particularly fixed on the hair loss (approved package insert suggests 1/10,000 chance), refuses augmentation with zinc or selenium, and refuses to accept that it might be related to her stress, that in turn requires more aggressive treatment
- She states that she is "fed up" with antidepressants and just needs her sleep and wants to focus on treating her insomnia
- She believes that her insomnia drives her MDD symptoms and that her MDD will resolve if she sleeps better

Case outcome: second interim follow-up visit at two months

- Mirtazapine (Remeron) dose is maximized to 45 mg/d
- Now taken off all zolpidem preparations and instructed against using sleeping pills in an as-needed measure as these may be a prelude to addiction and misuse
- Is given eszopiclone (Lunesta) 2 mg at bedtime as it has a longer half-life for better sleep maintenance, and it is less selective for the BZ1 subreceptor and may have more anxiolytic effects
  - Her pill count and potential for overuse will be closely monitored
  - This hypnotic is metabolized via CYP3A4 and CYP2E1 enzymes and she should not develop marked side effects
- This approach maximizes her antidepressant while trying to treat her insomnia and agitation better
- The patient calls between sessions to state she is having marked hair loss since the mirtazapine was increased, has mild fatigue, and she wishes to consider stopping it
- There is no change in insomnia
- There is mild sustained improvement in affective range and activity level
- She is felt to be 10%–20% better at most but is hyper-focused on insomnia and side effects

Question

What would you do next?

- As she is a minimal responder, remove mirtazapine and try another antidepressant that does not utilize CYP450 2D6 or 2C19 metabolism
- As she is a minimal responder and is on a somewhat tolerated antidepressant agent that has less impact, try to convince patient to stay on the mirtazapine and consider an augmentation/combination approach
- As patient has 2D6 genetic liver enzyme deficiencies, is somewhat phobic of medications, is preoccupied with insomnia, next prioritize treatment of the insomnia and return to treating the depression once this chief complaint symptom is resolved
- Consider TMS or ECT, as these device-based treatments require no CYP450 system metabolism
- Consider a nutraceutical such as l-methylfolate (Deplin) at 15 mg/d or S-adenosyl methionine (SAMe) at 400–800 mg twice daily, as they may be useful adjunctive antidepressant agents and may have minimal if any side effects
  - This patient might be accepting and less side-effect prone by understanding that these complementary alternative medicine (CAM) treatments are "not real prescription antidepressants"

– They may be considered less risky, more holistic, and her comfort level with medication management may increase

Attending physician's mental notes: second interim follow-up visit at two months (continued)

- This patient has "put her foot down" regarding *not* using formal antidepressants
- Increasing her sedative–hypnotic dose or changing to one with faster absorption, longer half-life, or affinity for the GABA-A receptor is unlikely to remit her depression, but building rapport with the patient may improve her anxiety about medications
- If her sleep is improved and her symptoms do lessen, she may be more amenable to antidepressant treatment later

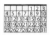

Case outcome: interim follow-up visits at three months

- The patient declines antidepressants but agrees to a trial of a bona fide BZ sedative–hypnotic (temazepam [Restoril])
  - As-needed use is not allowed, informed consent and pill counts are strict, and her spouse is now involved in dispensing
  - All BZRA products are discontinued
  - She has been taken off mirtazapine
  - Begins temazepam 7.5 mg at bedtime
  - This drug is chosen as it does not require extensive hepatic enzyme metabolism and is considered one of the safer sedatives to use in liver-impaired patients
    - It is glucuronidized in the liver and does not require p450 enzyme activity
    - It is excreted extensively in the urine
  - Lorazepam (Ativan) and oxazepam (Serax) are similar but approved for anxiolysis, not hypnosis
- No change in status, patient did not sleep well on temazepam and felt sedated the next day
  - Insists on stopping it and be returned to the zolpidem-CR (Ambien-CR) as she felt it was the best balance between efficacy and tolerability
- Depression, agitation, and insomnia continue
- Enters into a discussion regarding possibly restarting an antidepressant but wants absolute proof that one chosen will not bother her CYP450 issues
  - Bibliotherapy using *The Black Book of Psychotropic Dosing and Monitoring*, 10th edition, or *The Top 100 Drug Interactions: A Guide to Patient Management* is resourced [perhaps the *Epocrates Interaction Check* can be used electronically]

- It is shown to, and reviewed with, the patient present, as are internet resources and her records showing her p450 enzyme deficiencies
- This seems to improve her affect and lower her apprehension, as p450 medications that would likely render her toxic with side effects are dismissed and safer ones that she can metabolize easily are discussed as treatment possibilities
- She is given choices that fit her needs
- Many antidepressants are reviewed and sertraline (Zoloft) is seen as a low-affinity substrate for CYP450 isoenzymes with CYP2B6 contributing the greatest extent of metabolism, and lesser contributions from CYP2C19, CYP2C9, CYP3A4, and CYP2D6
- Similar to mirtazapine use in this patient; she is satisfied to try this drug as it is clearly metabolized through many enzymatic pathways for which she is not deficient
- Sertraline (Zoloft) also comes in small tablet (25 mg) and liquid preparations so that her dose may be started at extremely low levels

Question

Are you comfortable resourcing materials with the patient present in session?

- Yes, this type of informed consent is medicolegally protective
- Yes, this approach often increases patient's comfort level as it is felt to be a thorough process
- No, this takes too much time in session
- No, this likely makes the patient feel that the clinician does not know enough in that he/she needs to look it up

Case outcome: interim follow-up visit at four months

- The patient was started on low sertraline (Zoloft) 12.5 mg/d
  - Even though there is little CYP450 enzyme risk, given that it is metabolized by many pathways she is proficient in, she has had reactions to SSRI and SNRI in the past
  - Starting on a very low dose makes clinical sense to reduce potential side effects and nocebo effects
- She calls stating there is now marked anxiety and worsening depression
  - This is attributed to the sertraline
  - As a result, she is placed temporarily on alprazolam (Xanax-XR) 0.5 mg/d with some relief
  - This might be typical activating side effects due to excess serotonin that she experienced on previous SSRI and SNRI therapy
  - This might be anxiety and a nocebo effect (hysterical side effects)
  - It is unlikely that this is a CYP450 deficiency-induced toxicity because sertraline is metabolized through several CYP450 pathways

Attending physician's mental notes: interim follow-up visits through four months

- Patient has now failed two SSRIs and one SNRI due to side effects, and failed an NaSSA (mirtazapine) antidepressant
- Zolpidem-CR allows some improved sleep and she agreed to escalate alprazolam for daytime agitation control, but has gone back to adamantly refusing all potentially anxiogenic antidepressants
- As we seem to be restricted to treating patient's surface symptoms of insomnia and anxiety, she is reoriented and advised about proper sleep hygiene and motivated to start psychotherapy, which she agrees to do

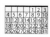

Case outcome: interim follow-up visits through six months

- Medications have reverted back to a combination of zolpidem and zolpidem-CR for sleep and alprazolam for daytime agitation, which again are manipulated with advice between visits
- She is a bit better in these areas but continues to have full MDD symptoms and to be incapacitated most of the time
- Psychotherapy has started but has not helped much as yet
- She asks about medication options that are not "full-blown" antidepressants, use different non-SSRI/SNRI mechanisms, and do not interfere with her CYP450 metabolic deficiencies
- She ultimately agrees that mirtazapine (Remeron) was helpful and asks to be retitrated, only to call back later stating it had to be stopped, again due to fatigue (which was not a significant problem when used previously at even higher doses)
- She asks again about medication options that are not full-blown antidepressants, use different mechanisms, and do not jeopardize her deficient CYP450 metabolic pathways
  - Offered lithium, which is 100% renally excreted and not CYP450 metabolized
  - Offered paliperidone (Invega), which is mostly renally excreted and requires no hepatic metabolism
    ○ It is an atypical antipsychotic that may help control agitation and possibly depressive symptoms in an off-label manner
  - Offered the selegiline transdermal patch (Emsam) MAOI antidepressant, which tends to avoid first-pass liver metabolism
  - Offered alpha-2-delta calcium channel blocking epilepsy medications such as gabapentin (Neurontin)
    ○ It is also renally excreted and may have off-label anxiolytic potential
- She accepts lithium now as a montherapy for MDD
  - Declines the patch as she feels that there was no way for her to "control her dose"

> ○ Further exploration of this reveals that she would often halve or quarter her doses of previous medications

Case debrief

- Interferon is well known to induce depression. This patient seems to have developed her first MDE after interferon
- She was highly anxious and agitated as well
- Throughout sessions it became clear that her anxiety was interfering with her ability to tolerate her medications more so than her well-known CYP450 vulnerabilities
- However, both of these needed to be taken into consideration routinely during her treatment
- The primary focus turned toward providing relief from her insomnia and anxiety target symptoms, only to be thwarted in that sedative–hypnotics were mildly effective but caused sedation, preventing her from being dose-escalated but better treated
- Finally, after being advised to take lithium, the patient terminated care as she was unwilling to be put on other medications
- She was essentially left on the zolpidem BZRA preparations, which was similar to her situation when she came to her first office visit
- Interestingly, during one session, device-based MDD treatments (ECT, VNS, TMS) were discussed
  - The patient later remembered the TMS discussion and inquired about this with an outside provider
  - She had a modest antidepressant response but not remission after she proceeded with a course of TMS therapy
    - ○ Daily right DLPFC stimulation for three to four weeks
  - TMS became a good choice as it has no drug interactions, is not a "medication," thus allowing for fewer side effects in her mind, and it matched her idea of what a better tolerated treatment would be
- This case shows that a patient's fear about taking medication can thwart his/her compliance, leaving him/her undertreated and remaining symptomatic
- Despite best efforts in psychoeducation, bibliotherapy, allowing patient freedom of choice and control of medication in a partnership fashion, micro-titrating at very subtherapeutic doses, using medications that would not interfere greatly with her CYP450 enzymatic deficiencies, enlisting help of a psychotherapist for psychotherapy, and use of much patience and countertransference containment, she continued with poor compliance and almost no sustained partial response at all
- TMS allowed for a good MDD response (nearly 70% symptom improvement)

Take-home points

- Anxious patients often do not respond well to medication management and often develop amplified side effects or even nocebo effects, where just the thought of being on a medication increases placebo-based side effects
- Many supportive techniques are often needed to help compliance and thus improve outcome
- Sometimes treating a chief complaint or prioritized symptom, instead of the syndrome or disorder, may be helpful at first

Performance in practice: confessions of a psychopharmacologist

- *What could have been done better here?*
  - Despite a change in strategy to treat her insomnia and agitation symptomatically, this approach did not work
    - This patient likely required higher doses of sedative
    - Even though she tolerated sedatives better than antidepressants, she was still left with fatigue, which was disheartening
    - Perhaps trying a myriad of different sedatives with differing absorption and half-lives may have worked better for her and the dose may have been escalated for better clinical effectiveness
- *Should TMS or device-based treatment been suggested sooner?*
  - ECT actually could have been utilized effectively, but the patient was fairly rigid that ECT was too frightening and too severe a treatment
  - VNS could be helpful but she really did not meet regulatory criteria of four failed, full antidepressant trials, and VNS could take months to work
  - TMS fits fairly well in this case in that she had one full antidepressant failure and a few very subtherapeutic trials
- *Possible action items for improvement in practice*
  - Research data for device-based treatments, specifically TMS, as it is the latest approved modality and contains regulatory wording for patients who have found antidepressants intolerable
  - Research the CYP450 enzyme systems or become more aware of available resources to use in patients with laboratory-based or clinically based diagnoses of CYP450 deficiencies
  - A simple technique is to internet search the drug's name plus the word "metabolism." Notice the many references at the end of this case
  - CYP450 drug interaction tables may also be searched and utilized, but sometimes these are more complicating and confusing

Tips and pearls

- Using micro-titration techniques may improve patient compliance and confidence in the prescriber and the drug prescribed
- Most approved antidepressants have an approved starting dose where it has been shown to outperform placebo
- Often, clinicians choose to start an off-label, lower dose knowing that it will probably not be therapeutic at all, but the lower dose will likely not have many side effects
- As such, patients will be more willing to escalate the dose later after initial success at lower dose and improved initial tolerability
- This also dynamically conveys that the prescriber is kind, worried about adverse effects, and wants to minimize suffering
- Micro-titrating takes this one step further
  - For example, in this case the patient was started on half of a 25 mg tablet, or 12.5 mg/d of sertraline
  - The usual starting dose is 50 mg/d
  - Sertraline actually comes in a liquid 20 mg/ml concentration
  - Using a 1 cc syringe, a clinician could actually dose this at 2 mg/d initially, if desired, to make a point of really starting at the lowest dose available – a micro-dose (0.1 cc)
  - Literally, her dose could be eye-dropper increased every few days to reach a therapeutic dose

Pharmacokinetic moment

What psychotropic drugs should you know about that inhibit CYP450 2D6?

- This patient had a genetic abnormality that rendered her poor and inefficient in processing drugs that require CYP450 2D6 enzyme activity
- Sometimes, psychopharmacologists prescribe drugs that iatrogenically create 2D6 deficiencies by inhibiting CYP450 with the same net result as this patient's genetic deficiencies, i.e., drug intolerability
  - Fluoxetine and paroxetine inhibit CYP450 2D6 maximally
  - Bupropion, duloxetine, haloperidol, perphenazine, thioridazine inhibit CYP450 2D6 moderately
  - Fluvoxamine, sertraline, citalopram, venlafaxine inhibit CYP450 2D6 weakly

Note: Inhibition means that other drugs (substrates) that require 2D6 for metabolism will therefore increase in blood plasma concentrations, likely increasing toxicity side effects.

What drugs should you know that require CYP450 2D6 to be properly metabolized (called substrates)?

- Patients who are deficient in CYP450 2D6 or who are inhibited iatrogenically may require lower dosing than normal
- Most TCAs are 2D6 substrates and require lower doses
  - In fact, desipramine is often used in testing newly approved drugs to see if they are 2D6 inhibitors
  - If a new drug, when combined with desipramine, elevates desipramine levels, the new drug is considered a 2D6 inhibitor
  - Dextromethorphan, a cough suppressant, may also be used in similar fashion
    - Interestingly, dextromethorphan may have antidepressant qualities when used in neurologically based affective disorders (pseudobulbar affect)
    - Mechanistically, it may dampen glutamate activity to improve crying spells
    - Pharmacokinetically, it is combined in one pill with quinidine
      - Quinidine inhibits CYP450 2D6 allowing for longer sustained plasma levels of the dextromethorphan
      - Here, a drug–drug interaction is used to create a slow-release mechanism for the therapeutic dextromethorphan
      - This combination product is called Nuedexta
- The following also may require dose-lowering strategies
  - Bupropion, duloxetine, paroxetine, trazodone, venlafaxine
  - Amphetamine products
  - Atomoxetine
  - Fluphenazine, perphenazine, thioridazine
  - Aripiprazole, risperidone, iloperidone, vortioxetine

What drug–drug interaction combinations are most likely to be seen in psychopharmacological practice?
- Notice that some of the previously listed products are both substrates *and* inhibitors
  - In this way, giving a monotherapy of one of these agents causes 2D6 inhibition, which also increases blood levels of the same drug
  - This is often accounted for when drug dosing is studied through regulatory processes
  - This may explain why certain 2D6-deficient patients might be exquisitely sensitive to even low-dose monotherapy approaches
- One of the most common and dangerous 2D6 interactions in practice often involves psychiatric care when there is overlap with primary care
  - This may occur when the psychiatrist is treating depression and the PCP is treating neuropathic pain
  - For example, the psychiatrist may prescribe paroxetine or fluoxetine (SSRIs), both of which are major 2D6 inhibitors

- The primary clinician may simultaneously prescribe anitriptyline (TCA) for pain or insomnia at seemingly low doses to treat these symptoms off-label
- However, the SSRI prescribed is likely tripling the plasma level of the TCA in this case
  - If the amitriptyline is 10 mg/d this might be acceptable, but if the TCA is dosed at 50 mg/d, it may be equivalent now to 150 mg/d
  - In this case, especially in those older than 50 years, an EKG and blood levels should be obtained and monitored
  - The likelihood of serotonin syndrome increases as both the TCA and the SSRI are at full doses and both markedly inhibit the SERT
- Another similar interaction occurs when primary care utilizes the muscle relaxant cyclobenzaprine (Flexeril), as this drug is essentially a TCA
- Carbamazepine (Equetro) is also a TCA-structured drug
- A common combination strategy for resistant depression includes the mixture of bupropion and an SSRI
  - As noted, bupropion may inhibit its own degradation, thus elevating its own levels
  - It has been shown to be safe at doses of 400–450 mg/d depending on the preparation used
  - Clearly doses higher than this elevate risks of seizure activity
  - If maximally dosed, bupropion is combined with an SSRI with known 2D6 inhibition, bupropion levels will elevate up to concentrations above safety levels, thus increasing seizure risk
  - Again, fluoxetine/paroxetine use will raise bupropion levels the most, citalopram moderately, sertraline and escitalopram the least
  - One should consider antidepressants that involve the least inhibition interference with 2D6 when combining with bupropion, such as desvenlafaxine or mirtazapine
- Finally, over-the-counter cough suppressants that contain dextromethorphan can also have their levels tripled by major 2D6 inhibitors
  - Similar to the TCA drug–drug CYP450 2D6 interactions discussed earlier, levels may increase that ultimately produce QTc prolongation and possible ventricular arrhythmias

Posttest self-assessment question and answer

Which of the following medications is often used in regulatory trials to determine if a CYP450 inhibition interaction exists with an experimental drug?

A. Temazepam (Restoril)
B. Desipramine (Norpramin)
C. Desvenlafaxine (Pristiq)
D. Paliperidone (Invega)

Answer: B
Desipramine is a TCA that has very easy-to-determine blood levels and may be tracked effortlessly in clinical trials. When an experimental new drug is going through federal regulatory processes, it is often tested in combination with desipramine to determine if this TCA's level will increase above the norm, thus signaling a CYP450 2D6 inhibition interaction by the experimental drug. The other three agents undergo hepatic glucuronidation and do not require CYP450 isoenzyme involvement, and would not be good tests for CYP450 interactions as such.

References

1. Estabrook R. A passion for P450s (remembrances of the early history of research on cytochrome P450). *Drug Metab Dispos* 2003; 31:1461–73.
2. Degtyarenko K. Directory of P450-containing systems. International Centre for Genetic Engineering and Biotechnology, 2009. http://www.icgeb.org/~p450srv/. Accessed July 12, 2011.
3. Flockhart DA. Cytochrome P450 drug interaction table. Indiana University-Purdue University Indianapolis, 2007. http://medicine.iupui.edu/flockhart/. Accessed July 12, 2011.
4. Kraus MR, Schäfer A, Schöttker K,et al. Therapy of interferon-induced depression in chronic hepatitis C with citalopram: a randomised, double-blind, placebo-controlled study. *Gut* 2008; 57:531–6.
5. Renault PF, Hoofnagle JH, Park Y, et al. Psychiatric complications of long-term interferon alfa therapy. *Arch Intern Med* 1987; 147:1577–80.
6. Valentine AD, Meyers CA, Kling MA, Richelson E, Hauser P. Mood and cognitive side effects of interferon alpha therapy. *Semin Oncol* 1998; 25:39–47.
7. Vollmer KO, von Hodenberg A, Kölle EU. Pharmacokinetics and metabolism of gabapentin in rat, dog and man. *Arzneimittelforschung* 1986; 36:830–9.
8. Levenson JL, Fallon HJ. Fluoxetine treatment of depression caused by interferon-alpha. *Am J Gastroenterol* 1993; 88:760–1.
9. Goldman LS. Successful treatment of interferon alpha-induced mood disorder with nortriptyline. *Psychosomatics* 1994; 35:412–13.
10. Timmer CJ, Sitsen JM, Delbressine LP. Clinical pharmacokinetics of mirtazapine. *Clin Pharmacokinet* 2000; 38:461–74.
11. Noehr-Jensen L, Zwisler ST, Larsen F, et al. Impact of CYP2C19 phenotypes on escitalopram metabolism and an evaluation of pupillometry as a serotonergic biomarker. *Eur J Clin Pharmacol* 2009; 65:887–94.

12. Von Moltke LL, Greenblatt DJ, Granda BW, et al. Zolpidem metabolism *in vitro*: responsible cytochromes, chemical inhibitors, and *in vivo* correlations. *Br J Clin Pharmacol* 1999; 48:89–97.
13. von Moltke LL, Greenblatt DJ, Cotreau-Bibbo MM, Harmatz JS, Shader RI. Inhibitors of alprazolam metabolism in vitro: effect of serotonin-reuptake-inhibitor antidepressants, ketoconazole and quinidine. *Br J Clin Pharmacol* 1994; 38:23–31.
14. Docherty JP, Sack DA, Roffman M, Finch M, Komorowski JR. A double-blind, placebo-controlled, exploratory trial of chromium picolinate in atypical depression: effect on carbohydrate craving. *J Psychiatr Pract* 2005; 11:302–14.
15. Broadhurst CL, Domenico P. Clinical studies on chromium picolinate supplementation in diabetes mellitus–a review. *Diabetes Technol Ther* 2006; 8:677–87.
16. Barsky AJ, Saintfort R, Rogers MP, Borus JF. Nonspecific medication side effects and the nocebo phenomenon. *JAMA* 2002; 287:655–6.
17. Obach RS, Cox LM, Tremaine LM. Sertraline is metabolized by multiple cytochrome P450 enzymes, monoamine oxidases, and glucuronyl transferases in human: an in vitro study. *Drug Metab Dispos* 2005; 33:262–70.
18. Schwarz HJ. Pharmacokinetics and metabolism of temazepam in man and several animal species. *Br J Clin Pharmacol* 1979; 8:23S–29S.
19. DeBattista C, Schatzberg AF. *The Black Book of Psychotropic Dosing and Monitoring*, 10th edn. New York, NY: MBL Communication, 2006.
20. Hansten PD, Horn JR. *The Top 100 Drug Interactions: A Guide to Patient Management*. Freeland, WA: H&H Publications, LLP, 2007; pp. 235–6.

The Case: The angry twins

The Question: Is pharmacologic treatment of personality traits effective?

The Dilemma: There are no approved medications for personality disordered patients

Pretest self-assessment question (answer at the end of the case)

Which of the following are approved for treating mood swings?

A. Fluoxetine (Prozac)
B. Lamotrigine (Lamictal)
C. Asenapine (Saphris)
D. Alprazolam (Xanax)
E. All of the above
F. None of the above

Patient evaluation on intake

- 30-year-old identical twins are referred separately for depression and anger problems
- Both state that external stressors, e.g., work, family, etc. have driven them to depression and "mood swings"

Psychiatric history

- Patient #1 states that he has a long history of mood swings, especially toward anger attacks, but over the last few years has been more "down and out" stressed, and suffering from insomnia
- Patient #2 is identical
- Patient #1 further admits to full MDD symptoms
  - Occasionally experiences passive suicidal thoughts, agitation and restlessness, fatigue, poor concentration, and amotivation
  - Does not have evidence of guilt or worthlessness symptoms
- Patient #2 is identical
- Patient #1 has no history of psychosis, mania, substance misuse, anxiety disorder
- Patient #2 is identical
- Patient #1 admits to a history of volatile and irritable temperament, difficulty in delaying gratification, poor frustration tolerance, and learning from an early age that aggression is often beneficial
- Patient #2 is identical

Social and personal history

- Patients #1 and #2 both graduated from high school

- Both have been gainfully employed in service industry jobs, but have had difficulty dealing with their supervisors
- Both are married with children
- Their relationships are generally supportive but with occasional bouts of conflict
- Both have a legal history of violent and assaultive behavior
- Neither have alcohol or drug addiction histories

Medical history

- Patient #1 has HTN, hypercholesterolemia, pre-diabetes, and an atrial cardiac arrhythmia
- Patient #2 is identical except for the arrhythmia

Family history

- Patient #1 admits distant family members have schizophrenia or bipolar disorder
- Patient #2 is identical

Medication history

- Patient #1 was started on the SNRI, venlafaxine-XR (Effexor-XR) 75 mg/d, by his PCP over a year ago
  - Self-discontinued it two weeks ago due to ineffectiveness. Continues to take the BZ, alprazolam 0.5 mg/d, as needed for agitation
  - There is no evidence of misuse
- Patient #2 is *not* identical here and had been placed on a stimulant, an NDRI, an SSRI, a BZRA, and an epilepsy medication, topiramate (Topamax), by his previous psychiatrist
  - Feels the latter medication was not helping, caused GI distress; he stopped it two weeks ago
- Therefore, they are identical at some level of medication non-compliance, but they are very different in that their previous provider engaged in either a slow, limited series of monotherapies *or* in aggressive polypharmacy

Psychotherapy history

- Patients #1 and #2 have been undergoing eclectic, supportive, individual psychotherapy over the last few months
- Neither has received formal CBT, IPT, DBT, or PDP

Patient evaluation on initial visit

- There is evidence of a gradual onset of MDD symptoms associated with multiple social stressors

- Premorbid, Cluster B personality traits are observed as well
  - *DSM-5* lists several personality disorders, and Cluster B disorders traditionally involve patients who suffer from marked mood swings, inability to control their affect, and are often considered to be dramatic and erratic
  - These include histrionic, narcissistic, antisocial, and borderline personality disorders
- Both seem to be moderately depressed and suffering
- Both seem motivated for medication management

Current medications

- Patient #1
  - Alprazolam (Xanax) 0.5 mg/d as needed for agitation (BZ)
- Patient #2
  - Methylphenidate-ER (Concerta) 18 mg/d (stimulant)
  - Bupropion-XL(Wellbutrin-XL) 300 mg/d (NDRI)
  - Sertraline (Zoloft) 100 mg/d (SSRI)
  - Zolpidem (Ambien) 10 mg at bedtime (BZRA)

Question

Do patients suffering from unstable, affectively labile, insatiable, frustration-inducing, volatile Cluster B moods respond to psychopharmacology?

- Yes
- No
- Maybe

Attending physician's mental notes: initial evaluation

- Both patients are motivated for treatment and have very similar presentations
- Both have initial failures with psychotropics
- Patient #1 was subtherapeutic on an antidepressant and he discontinued as it was not helping
  - He has been undertreated
- Patient #2 is the opposite and appears to be on many medications
  - Most of which are therapeutic
  - He may have been overtreated
- Both stopped some of their medications without consulting their individual prescribers, which is troubling
- The MDD symptoms should be easy to treat as they are relatively new
- The personality disorder symptoms will increase treatment resistance and likely predispose both patients to frequent depressive relapses

- Will need to better delineate adjustment disorders (that are numerous) versus state-dependent, full MDEs as well
- There will likely be clear interplay between stress adjustments, personality coping styles, and frank MDD

Question

Which of the following would be your next step for both patients?

- Use psychotherapy alone as there are no approved drugs for treating personality traits
- Use SSRI/SNRI as they are approved for MDD
- Use a mood stabilizing antiepileptic medication as some are approved for bipolar mood stabilization and have some data showing effectiveness in personality disorders where mood lability is problematic
- Use an atypical antipsychotic as some are approved for bipolar mood stabilization, depression, agitation, and have some nonregulatory data showing effectiveness in personality disorders, especially for cognitive, perceptual, and aggressivity symptoms
- Use buspirone or a beta-blocker as they have some off-label data showing effectiveness in treating anger and irritability

Attending physician's mental notes: initial evaluation (continued)

- Further discussion with the treating psychotherapists is needed to better delineate diagnoses
  - Their depressive spells seem legitimate and sustained for both patients
  - This is felt to be superimposed on top of long-standing Cluster B personality traits
- These traits are felt to be further exacerbated by stress and depression
- Likely, ongoing psychotherapy will be needed in order to maximize psychopharmacological response and prevent relapses
- Using an approved antidepressant makes on-label sense, but the level of mood lability may warrant a mood stabilizing antipsychotic or mood stabilizer, which is not unlike treating a bipolar patient

Further investigation

Is there anything else you would especially like to know about these patients?

- What about details concerning the patients' potential for metabolic disorder?
  - Both patients are overweight with centralized abdominal obesity
  - Both patients share HTN and elevated lipids

- Discussions with their PCPs suggest these are relatively well controlled with statins and antihypertensives
- Both patients have slightly elevated blood glucose levels suggesting pre-diabetes
- Both patients have family members who developed full metabolic disorder with age

Case outcome: first interim follow-up visit four weeks later

- Patient #1 agrees at initial evaluation to continue the BZ alprazolam (Xanax) and agrees to restart the SNRI, venlafaxine-ER(Effexor-XR), at 75 mg/d, knowing that it will need to be dosed higher to become more effective and maximized
  - Returns later minimally better but now refuses to escalate the SNRI as it may be associated with worsening blood pressure at higher doses
  - Reports that his PCP had to add another antihypertensive and that radio-ablation for his cardiac arrhythmia has failed
- Patient #2, at initial evaluation, stated that he liked his current medications and that each one added had some specific benefit
  - States he was partially better and is not comfortable making changes
  - However, does admit that the BZRA zolpidem is failing to maintain his sleep, thus a switch is made to zolpidem-ER (Ambien-CR) 12.5 mg at bedtime for better sleep maintenance
  - He returns later and states that he developed profuse diarrhea
  - He discontinued all of his psychotropics
  - The diarrhea resolved and he did not restart them

Question

What would you do next?

- For both patients, choosing a new monotherapy antidepressant is warranted
- For both patients, choosing a mood stabilizing atypical antipsychotic is warranted
- For both patients, choosing a mood stabilizer is warranted

Attending physician's mental notes: second interim follow-up visit at three months

- Both patients are not responding fully to SSRI treatment with anxiolytic and hypnotic augmentations

- Both now at least have full therapeutic SSRI trials, which they have tolerated well
- Both patients clearly state they are unwilling to titrate any higher as they have lost faith that these current SSRIs "will work"

Case outcome: second interim follow-up visit at three months

- Patient #1 starts the SSRI fluoxetine (Prozac) at 20 mg/d while the alprazolam is continued
  - Calls between visits feeling no effect and fluoxetine is increased to 40 mg/d
  - Returns stating that the MDD is a bit better, but during the session it is clear that the personality traits are still present and without change
- Patient #2 starts the SSRI paroxetine (Paxil) 20 mg/d
  - Reports that his mother was on this with good results
  - This patient also had a chief complaint of insomnia and was simultaneously started on an SARI, trazodone (Desyrel) 50 mg at bedtime
  - Between sessions he requests more paroxetine and it is titrated to 40 mg/d
  - Returns stating he is not better on any account

Question

What would you do next?

- For both patients, try another SSRI
- For both patients, try an SNRI
- For both patients, try an atypical antipsychotic
- For both patients, try a mood stabilizer

Attending physician's mental notes: second interim follow-up visit at three months (continued)

- Both patients like the fact that they have been relatively side-effect free on SSRI and are agreeable to trying another
  - Patient #1 is titrated to sertraline (Zoloft) 100 mg/d
  - Patient #2 is titrated to fluoxetine (Prozac) 40 mg/d
- This approach allows at least some more SSRI activity to be in place longer for each patient, and ongoing psychotherapy has more time to become effective
- This approach also allows further avoidance of side effects and helps to avoid the pattern of overmedicating using irrational polypharmacy, while trying to treat ongoing personality/Cluster B symptoms

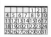

Case outcome: interim follow-up visits through 12 months

- Patient #1 now reports gradual improvements in many of his symptoms with consistent sertraline (Zoloft) plus alprazolam (Xanax) use but had an altercation with his boss and another healthcare provider and called for help containing his anger and violence propensity
  - Psychotherapeutic interventions failed and he was offered low-dose, as-needed haloperidol (Haldol) 1–2 mg/d
    - ○ This typical antipsychotic was chosen as the patient was at imminent risk of harming others and needed agitation control, not dissimilar to that required on some inpatient units where "as-needed" haloperidol is utilized with rapid effect
    - ○ Interestingly, the CATIE trial had just come out as well, spurring the need to evaluate the use of typical versus atypical antipsychotics
    - ○ At the time, the atypical agents were new, more expensive, and there was a push to really determine a cost–benefit analysis
    - ○ This typical antipsychotic was taken for a few days with the patient finding it to be very helpful
  - The following weekend, patient calls at night with "lockjaw" and a broken tooth
  - He is prescribed the anticholinergic EPS antidote benztropine (Cogentin) 2 mg/d with resolution of his trismus-based EPS and is taken off the typical antipsychotic
    - ○ In retrospect, the CATIE trial or a single study should not be evaluated and translationally used in a vacuum
- Patient #2 also reports gradual improvements in many symptoms with consistent fluoxetine (Prozac), zolpidem-CR (Ambien-CR), and trazodone (Desyrel) use
  - However, he begins having difficulty with his teenage son and reports a gradual return of mood lability and affective dyscontrol symptoms
  - Chief complaint still is marked insomnia, and the trazodone (Desyrel) is increased to 200 mg at bedtime with good effectiveness

Question

Are you comfortable prescribing psychotropics for personality disorder symptoms?

- Yes, they are clearly helpful in treating patients with pure personality disorder symptoms
- Yes, they are clearly helpful in treating patients who have personality disorder symptoms underlying true affective disorder illness

- Yes, there are no approved psychotropics here, but off-label use often may lower personality traits so that psychotherapy may proceed more efficiently
- No, the evidence base is too weak to support this practice
- No, personality disorders should be treated with an evidence-based psychotherapy such as DBT or DDP
  - DBT is an empirically supported, manualized treatment composed of both individual and group psychotherapy modalities
    - It is designed specifically for individuals who engage in self-destructive behaviors
    - It has also been found to be effective in treating eating disorders, SUD, and MDD in elderly patients
    - Considered a modification of CBT, DBT places equal emphasis on change-oriented and acceptance-based interventions
    - DBT skills groups are educational therapeutic classes aimed at reducing maladaptive behaviors by offering alternative ways to respond to stressful situations and intense emotions by teaching coping skills in mindfulness, interpersonal effectiveness, emotion regulation, and distress tolerance
  - DDP is a manual-based, PDP-based treatment developed for complex behavioral problems, including addiction, self-harm, eating disorder, and recurrent suicide attempts
    - In research studies, individuals with complex behavioral problems have demonstrated abnormalities in the way the brain processes negative emotions and interpersonal stresses
    - There is a relative deactivation of prefrontal brain regions and hyperactivation of other regions, including the amygdala and ventral striatum
    - These changes in brain functioning also account for the depression, anxiety, impulsivity, mood swings, and poor interpersonal functioning that so often accompany complex behavioral problems
    - DDP theoretically remediates and restores normal brain functioning by facilitating elaboration and integration of affect-laden interpersonal experiences and related attributions of self and other, as well as providing novel experiences in the patient–therapist relationship that promote self–other differentiation and a positive therapeutic alliance
    - Treatment involves weekly individual sessions for a 12-month period and follows sequential stages

Attending physician's mental notes: interim follow-up visits through 24 months

- After Patient #1's dystonia resolved, there was a return of his mood lability and dyscontrol while off the typical antipsychotic
  - He is given an atypical antipsychotic with less significant EPS risk and is titrated to 10 mg/d of aripiprazole (Abilify)
  - Experiences a gradual return of his better controlled affective state
  - Develops mild akathisia but tolerates this until it remits a few days later
  - This atypical antipsychotic did not escalate any metabolic symptoms
  - His cardiac condition is treated
  - MDD lifts and his ability to tolerate interpersonal stress improves
  - Returns to gainful employment
- Patient #2 experiences increases in interpersonal stressors, and develops full MDD, plus his mood lability markedly increases
  - Offered aripiprazole (Abilify) augmentation as this had benefitted his twin brother (Patient #1)
  - Given the use of fluoxetine (unlike his twin) with its ability to markedly inhibit the CYP450 2D6 enzyme, and thus elevate his aripiprazole levels abruptly; he is titrated much more slowly
  - Ultimately he is titrated to 8 mg/d (given his fluoxetine use, his blood levels could be double or triple his oral intake), but receives no benefit
- Patient #2 next is switched from the SSRI fluoxetine (Prozac) to the SNRI venlafaxine-XR (Effexor-XR) up to 150 mg/d in the hope that its noradrenergic potential would help alleviate his mounting MDD symptoms
- He continues the aripiprazole, trazodone, and zolpidem-CR
  - There is mild metabolic worsening (blood pressure increases with the addition of the SNRI)
  - Unfortunately, the aripiprazole was not as effective as in his brother's experience
- Asks to stop this medication
- SNRI could not be escalated due to HTN fears per the PCP
- Elects to start another atypical antipsychotic, risperidone (Risperdal), and it is titrated to 2 mg/d while closely watching for metabolic symptom worsening
  - Returns several weeks later feeling that he is moderately improved globally with regard to all symptoms
  - However, weight increased 10 lbs and blood glucose passes 100 mg/dL
- After informed consent, given only his partial risperidone plus venlafaxine-ER regimen response, and an acute increase in

metabolic symptoms, he is offered a trial of another atypical antipsychotic associated with less weight gain and metabolic syndrome risk
- Ziprasidone (Geodon) is now titrated to 120 mg/d
  - Insomnia is marked and a third sleep-inducing agent, ramelteon (Rozerem) is added up to 16 mg at bedtime
- The patient now takes zolpidem-CR (Ambien-CR), trazodone (Desyrel), ramelteon (Rozerem), venlafaxine-ER (Effexor-XR), and ziprasidone (Geodon)
  - The patient returns finally sleeping well, with gradual remission of the MDD symptoms
  - Experiences much less anger and tendency toward aggression. Seems to be able to better control his behaviors
  - Metabolic symptoms return to usual baseline

Case debrief

- Patients #1 and #2 are identical twins who both present with essentially the same type of MDD with clear comorbid personality disorder
- Both are involved in long-term supportive, eclectic psychotherapy
- Both were compliant with medication management once they noted some symptom reduction
- Both showed improvement with a combination of serotonergic agents plus atypical antipsychotics
- Both showed a remission of depression and better ability to cope with interpersonal stress with improved affective control
- Both received supportive, problem-oriented psychotherapy but no formalized CBT, IPT, DBT, or DDP approaches

Take-home points

- Patients with a mixture of MDD and personality disorder symptoms should have psychotherapy, ideally as maladaptive personality traits and defenses likely lead to increased stress and interpersonal difficulty; all of which are known to trigger recurrent MDEs
- When possible, this should consist of evidence-based psychotherapies
- Patients' personality traits are often reciprocally exacerbated by MDD, and adequate treatment of the depression may lower the impact of their personality traits on their psychosocial functioning and improve functional outcomes, social wellbeing, and support
- Rational polypharmacy techniques may be applied to treating psychiatric disorders such as MDD, but may also be applied to individual psychiatric symptoms, such as insomnia, as seen in Patient #2

- In this case, hypnotic agents of differing mechanisms were added to ultimately achieve better sleep
  - GABAergic, antihistaminergic, and melatonergic agents were combined safely and successfully in a stepwise manner

Performance in practice: confessions of a psychopharmacologist

- *What could have been done better here?*
  - The evidence base for the effectiveness of both medication management and for eclectic, supportive psychotherapy in the treatment of personality disorder is quite limited
  - Prior to rational polypharmacy, attempts should have been made to find a formal, evidence-based psychotherapy practitioner for each patient
  - Both patients had pre-existing metabolic disorder symptoms
  - Despite close medical monitoring, choosing an SNRI with blood pressure issues and an atypical antipsychotic with greater weight-gain and blood glucose elevation issues was problematic
  - One patient developed a dystonia on a typical antipsychotic
  - This approach was chosen based on clinical experience with similar patients who were imminently escalating toward violence
  - This approach also was influenced by a pivotal single research study that examined a different patient population, schizophrenia
  - Use of an atypical antipsychotic approved for agitation management may have avoided the EPS
- *Possible action items for improvement in practice*
  - Be aware that psychotropic drugs with noradrenergic potential are pressor agents and may allow for subtle increases in blood pressure, which may be problematic in treatment-resistant hypertensives
  - SNRIs, NDRIs, some TCAs, and some atypical antipsychotics possess NRI properties as well
  - Be aware that there are certain atypical antipsychotics that are more metabolically detrimental compared with those that are a bit more benign
  - Choose metabolically safer agents in those patients who are
    - Already suffering from metabolic illness
    - Have a clear family history and carry genetic risks for developing metabolic illness

Tips and pearls

- Choosing an antipsychotic should be based on several factors
  - First, using approved agents for approved conditions affords some confidence in outcome, as a sufficient evidence base of at least two randomized trials exists, which have been audited by regulatory authorities
  - Second, an antipsychotic may be chosen based on tolerability
    - Some are more EPS prone, metabolically prone, sedation prone, etc.
  - Third, an antipsychotic may be chosen based on its pharmacodynamic receptor profile
    - For example, some atypicals carry SRI, NRI, 5-HT1A receptor agonsim, 5-HT2A/5-HT2C/5-HT7 receptor antagonism, which may promote more antidepressant-like and procognitive effects in theory
    - Most of the older, typical antipsychotics do not have this theoretical potential
  - Fourth, is cost
    - In one of the patient's in this case, the CATIE schizophrenia trial was popular at the time and there was much writing about using the older, less costly generics
    - Haloperidol, low dose, was used due to this and to its routine, accepted use in treating acute agitated behavior
    - Much of the data regarding atypical use for agitation was not available at the time
    - In this case, use of the cheaper generic was effective but did cause dystonia problems, which resulted in a dental emergency
  - Given this, the net cost to the public insurance he was covered by was likely increased by using the less expensive generic typical antipsychotic

Two-minute tutorial

What is rational polypharmacy for Cluster B traits?

- As there are no FDA approvals for the treatment of personality disorder, clinicians must start with a framework in mind for approach and clinical application when prescribing
- Soloff[1] proposes a dimensional approach where the prescriber must choose particular target symptoms to treat rather than the personality disorder as a whole. The clinician should focus on prescribing medications to lower cognitive-perceptual, affective, or impulsive behavioral symptoms

[1] See References.

- Others suggest an outcome-focused approach where prescribers should clearly delineate the purpose of a pharmacologic intervention for both the patient and the clinician, choose outcomes that are measurable and related to functional improvements, and foster an understanding of the underlying psychobiologic mechanisms that cause the personality symptoms
- Meta-analyses based on randomized controlled trials suggest that typical and atypical antipsychotics have a moderate effect on improving cognitive and perceptual symptoms and even larger effects on lowering anger. The antidepressants have little effect on depression and impulsive behavior, but may lower anxiety. The mood stabilizers tend to have large effects on improving impulsive behavior dyscontrol, anger, and anxiety
- Gunderson[2] suggests an algorithm that is easy to follow
  - If a patient is accurately diagnosed with BPDO, the clinician must further delineate what symptom clusters are the most important to treat pharmacologically. If the patient has mild symptoms and requests no medication management, then psychotherapy is the ongoing treatment of choice. If the patient requests medication management, then use of an SSRI is warranted, as they may be the safest and best-tolerated option, but may have some of the lowest effect sizes globally when treating BPDO
  - If a patient is exhibiting more severe symptoms and the patient or the clinician feels pharmacotherapy is warranted, then a decision must be made as to which symptom cluster is to be treated: affective, impulsive/anger driven, or cognitive/perceptual
  - For affective symptoms, mood stabilizers have the greatest effects, followed by antidepressants
  - For impulsive/anger-based symptoms, antipsychotics seem to fare better than mood stabilizers. Both are better than antidepressants
  - For cognitive/perceptual symptoms, the antipsychotics have the best effect sizes

Posttest self-assessment question and answer

Which of the following are approved for treating mood swings?

A. Fluoxetine (Prozac)
B. Lamotrigine (Lamictal)
C. Asenapine (Saphris)
D. Alprazolam (Xanax)
E. All of the above
F. None of the above

[2] See References.

Answer: F

None of the above has been approved as treatment for mood swings or mood lability as an individual symptom, or as a treatment for mood lability due to personality disorder. All of these may help decrease affective dyscontrol symptoms in clinical practice. Interestingly, the most commonly used SSRIs may have the least data and lowest effectiveness. Rapid downward mood swings into dysphoria, euphoria, or agitation are sometimes helped in an off-label manner in personality-disordered patients with all of these agents. Smaller open-label and controlled trials do exist supporting the use of antidepressants and the atypicals to a greater degree to support psychotherapy-based symptom reduction in personality-disordered patients.

References

1. Gregory RJ, Chlebowski S, Kang D, et al. A controlled trial of psychodynamic psychotherapy for co-occurring borderline personality disorder and alcohol use disorder. *Psychotherapy* 2008; 45:28–41.
2. Goldman GA, Gregory RJ. Preliminary relationships between adherence and outcome in dynamic deconstructive psychotherapy. *Psychotherapy* 2009; 46:480–5.
3. Gregory RJ, Delucia-Deranja E, Mogle JA. Dynamic deconstructive psychotherapy versus optimized community care for borderline personality disorder co-occurring with alcohol use disorders: a 30-month follow-up. *J Nerv Ment Dis* 2010; 198:292–8.
4. Goldman GA, Gregory RJ. Relationships between techniques and outcomes in borderline personality disorder. *Am J Psychother* 2010; 64:359–71.
5. American Psychiatric Association. *Diagnostic and Statistical Manual of Mental Disorders, Revised,* 4th edn. Washington, DC: American Psychiatric Association Press, 2000.
6. Swartz MS, Stroup TS, McEvoy JP, et al. What CATIE found: results from the schizophrenia trial. *Psychiatr Serv* 2008; 59:500–6.
7. Hori A. Pharmacotherapy for personality disorders. *Psychiatry Clin Neurosci* 1998; 52:13–19.
8. Stoffers J, Völlm BA, Rücker G, et al. Pharmacological interventions for borderline personality disorder. *Cochrane Database Syst Rev* 2010; 16:CD005653.
9. Soloff PH. Psychopharmacology of borderline personality disorder. *Psychiatric Clin North Am* 2000; 23:169–92.
10. Gunderson JG. *Handbook of Good Psychiatric Management for Borderline Personality Disorder,* 1st edn. Arlington, VA: American Psychiatric Publishing, 2014.

11. Links PS, Boggild A, Sarin N. Psychopharmacology of personality disorders: review and emerging issues. *Curr Psychiatry Rep* 2001; 3:70–6.

12. Ingenhoven T, Lafay P, Rinne T, Passchier J, Duivenvoorden H. Effectiveness of pharmacotherapy for severe personality disorders: meta-analyses of randomized controlled trials. *J Clin Psychiatry* 2010; 71:14–25.

The Case: Anxiety, depression, or pre-bipolaring?

The Question: When to decide if someone is truly becoming bipolar disordered

The Dilemma: Antidepressant activation can be a side effect or a sentinel event

Pretest self-assessment question (answer at the end of the case)

If a manic spell is instigated by initiation of an antidepressant, which of the following is likely to happen?

A. The induced mania will be more severe
B. The induced mania will last longer
C. The induced mania will be less severe and shorter in duration
D. None of the above

Patient evaluation on intake

- 26-year-old man with a chief complaint of being "depressed, more or less"
- Mainly experiences MDEs of varying lengths and severities, occurring since he was a teenager
- Asks for a consultation because he has legal issues concerning an altercation that occurred recently

Psychiatric history

- Significant MDEs consistent with recurrent MDD are evident
  - Some MDEs have been incapacitating and have interfered with school and work
  - Seems to have good inter-episode recovery, which allows him to return to class and work
- When in the middle of an MDE, he admits to most MDD symptoms
  - Except he does not have suicidal thoughts
  - Admits to decreased sleep, despondent thoughts and mood, low interest in activities, poor energy and cognition
  - Says his self-esteem drops as he feels disgruntled, rejection-sensitive, and is guilt-ridden for no apparent reason
- He admits to SAD symptoms where he
  - Is often nervous around new people and acquaintances
  - Experiences anticipatory anxiety and will avoid certain social events
  - The SAD appears separate from the MDEs where these anxiety symptoms occur regardless of his affective state
- The main reason for consultation is that he has a legal issue regarding drinking while driving that he feels was likely fueled by psychiatric symptoms

- At the time of the infraction, he had been started on an SSRI for the MDD and SAD symptoms
  - This caused his mood to elevate excessively and in a sustained fashion over several days
- With this, he felt invincible and that the law did not apply to him
- During this episode he was also in an altercation at a bar when he purposefully antagonized another patron
  - This is extremely out of character for his usually quiet, socially anxious demeanor
- Despite being a shy, avoidant, SAD person during this period, he lost all anxiety, fear, and avoidance tendencies
  - During these spells, he experienced a moderate amount of talkativeness, distractibility, racing thoughts, hyperactivity, hyposomnia, impulsivify (flirting, drinking more than usual, fighting) and grandiosity (becomes invincible, arrogant, back-talking, and challenging of authority [police, bystanders, etc.])
- These mood-elevating events were complicated by the fact that AUD criteria were likely met during these times
  - While in college, he admitted to heavy alcohol use on weekends
  - When depressed, he may use cannabis intermittently
- Has now completed college and has few friends in the immediate area
- Family is very supportive
- Wants to be a writer, specifically a news reporter, and is planning on applying to graduate school
- Currently presents in a euthymic state at his first office appointment

Social and personal history

- Graduated high school and college
- Is not gainfully employed but is considering graduate school now
- Drug and alcohol history as noted
- He does not smoke and uses low amounts of caffeinated drinks
- His family is supportive

Medical history

- There are no acute or chronic medical issues

Family history

- GAD is reported for his mother
- No bipolar family members

Medication history

- Via his PCP, he has had two short SSRI trials with sertaline (Zoloft) 50 mg/d and paroxetine (Paxil) 20 mg/d, both of which caused mood elevations with problematic behaviors and drinking
- Took a few doses of mood stabilizing divalproex sodium (Depakote) but was too sedated to continue its use
- Prescribed the BZ anxiolytic clonazepam (Klonopin) in the past without misuse

Psychotherapy history

- None

Patient evaluation on initial visit

- Recurring MDD since late teens with comorbid SAD are evident
- Possible hypomanic spells in last two to three years versus antidepressant-induced activating side effects versus alcohol intoxication-induced mood disorder
- All mood elevations reported seem secondary to SSRI and/or alcohol use
- He has not had a chance to be compliant with medication treatment due to side effects
- He has no suicidal ideation and no signs of psychosis
- He is euthymic now and functioning well psychosocially

Current medications

- None

Question

What does a family history of, or lack thereof, bipolar disorder mean clinically?

- Nothing, as there is no clear bearing on risk of bipolar disorder or treatment outcomes
- Risk of bipolar disorder appears clear as family, twin, and adoption studies have provided evidence for a strong genetic component to bipolar disorder
  - Particularly, twin studies demonstrated higher concordances for the disorder among monozygotic identical twins, as compared with dizygotic fraternal twins, with an estimated heritability >80%
  - People with a first-degree relative with bipolar disorder have a 13.63-fold increased risk of developing bipolar disorder themselves

Attending physician's mental notes: initial evaluation

- This patient is somewhat complex given his MDD, SAD, and AUD comorbidities

- He has had two spells consistent with hypomania symptomatology, but the origin of these symptoms might be due to the SSRI treatments, his alcohol abuse, or frank onset of bipolar illness
- He has no family history of bipolar disorder, which seems to decrease his bipolar risk 13-fold
- His multiple SSRI-induced activations are often considered to be bipolar disorder prodromes or sentinel events and are troubling
- Many bipolar patients appear to be unipolars with anxiety problems in their young adult years but progress toward bipolar disorder as they age
- He is undertreated in that he has not had a full trial of any psychotropic

Question

Which of the following would be your next step?

- He is euthymic, thus do nothing and await any symptom relapse, then choose an appropriate medicine to match his affective state
- Collect collateral information from relatives to better delineate his mood elevations to determine if he is bipolar I, II, or neither
- Start a mood chart to observe in real time any mood swings that he might develop to better delineate his diagnosis
- Issue a rating scale such as the MDQ to better delineate his bipolar diagnosis
- Start an approved mood stabilizer for presumed bipolar II disorder
- Start another antidepressant for his SAD, while watching for mood elevation in real time
- Start a BZ sedative for his SAD to avoid mood-elevating side effects that have been noted previously when he used SSRIs

Attending physician's mental notes: initial evaluation (continued)

- This patient seems to be either very sensitive to excessive mood-elevating side effects from his SSRI treatments, or he is a relatively new bipolar II disorder patient
- Collateral information suggests that his two hypomania spells were clearly preceded by SSRI use *and* excessive alcohol use
- His behavioral and legal problems occurred after the mood elevation was noted
- He has no family history of bipolar illness and these facts seem to point toward SSRI-induced hypomanic-like side effects
- However, it is also likely that these ominous "SSRI side effects" are likely signs of pre-bipolar disorder emergence, a bipolar prodrome, also known as "pre-bipolaring"
- He is currently drug and alcohol free while euthymic

PATIENT FILE

Further investigation

Is there anything else you would especially like to know with regard to treating this patient?

- Are there any bipolar II approved medications?
  - No
- Are there any well-established guidelines specifically to help in these situations of pre-bipolaring?
  - No
- Are some antidepressants safer with regard to lower risk of hypomanic escalation?
  - Yes, SSRI and NDRI (bupropion) antidepressants seem safer than TCA, MAOI, and possibly SNRI classes
- Some studies suggest that SSRI may work as well as lithium stabilization in bipolar II patients
  - However, this may be at odds with the fact that antidepressants are felt to allow patients to worsen from bipolar II to bipolar I disorder more often, or convert patients to mixed features or rapid cycling specifiers

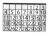

Case outcome: first interim follow-up visit three months later

- Patient is educated about his presumptive bipolar II diagnosis as a worst case scenario
- Instructed to maintain a usual sleep–wake schedule and avoid marked amounts of caffeine or alcohol
- Agrees to release information for his family so that there can be better monitoring of his treatment and symptoms between visits
- As there are no clear guidelines for treating bipolar II disorder, he is instructed about bipolar I treatment options, and that conservative approaches would consider treating him as if he were a bipolar I patient
- This might lower the chance of depressive and hypomanic relapses, and might prevent escalating to a bipolar I diagnosis in the future
- He is re-evaluated for *DSM-5* mixed features specifier, and he has not yet met the criteria

Question

What is the chance that this presumptive unipolar MDD patient will develop a bipolar disorder, or if he is a presumptive bipolar II patient, that he will worsen and progress to bipolar I disorder?

- Not much risk as these are separate disorders
- Some risk if we consider him unipolar now, as longitudinal studies suggest that 27% of severely depressed unipolar MDD patients will develop bipolar II and 19% bipolar I disorders, respectively
- Some risk if we consider him a bipolar II patient as he may escalate into a bipolar I disorder

Case outcome: first interim follow-up visit three months later (continued)

- There is clear risk of escalation from MDD to bipolar II disorder, and also from bipolar II to a full syndromal bipolar I disorder
  - If one were to assume his legal problems were to have resulted from mood elevation symptoms and not his AUD, then he would have enough psychosocial dysfunction to warrant the bipolar I diagnosis now
- Several mood stabilizing treatments are offered and initially are refused
- Between sessions, he researches the medication options and now asks to start lamotrigine (Lamictal) as it is approved for bipolar maintenance treatment and seems to have "fewer side effects" when compared to other mood stabilizers such as lithium, divalprox (Depakote), olanzapine (Zyprexa), etc.
  - There is less organ damage risk, neuromuscular side-effect risk, and metabolic syndrome risks with lamotrigine
  - He is titrated according to regulatory guidelines to 200 mg/d, over six weeks, to avoid severe rash risks
- He misses his one-month appointment but does attend at three months
  - There have been no hypomanic episodes
  - Feels moderately depressed
  - SAD continues at a mild level
  - There are no side effects
- He is taking some miscellaneous college higher-level courses and feels the depression is interfering, and requests treatment specifically for this

Question

What would you do next?

- Refer for psychotherapy; continue the lamotrigine
- Increase lamotrigine in the hope that it will treat his depression and anxiety
- Add an antidepressant in the hope that his depression and SAD will improve while minimizing hypomania escalation risk, and while he is mood stabilized
- Add a bipolar depression-approved agent such as olanzapine–fluoxetine combination (Symbyax), quetiapine (Seroquel-XR), or lurasidone (Latuda)
- Add another mood stabilizer such as lithium to his lamotrigine

Attending physician's mental notes: second interim follow-up visit at six months

- This is problematic. He did not become hypomanic using the relatively safer NDRI antidepressant approach, but it has failed to help

- He is a student with no insurance and will not agree to have psychotherapy
- Adding another antidepressant likely means stepping back into the SSRI class, where he became hypomanic twice before when he was not mood stabilized in advance

Case outcome: second interim follow-up visit at six months

- The patient moves away and takes classes two hours away at a new school, thus will come for visits every 90 days but with phone contact throughout
- As he is mood stabilized on lamotrigine, he is next titrated onto the NDRI bupropion-XL (Wellbutrin-XL) to the maximum dose of 450 mg/d while continuing lamotrigine
- This approach maximizes the antidepressant and the mood stabilizer dose
- Continues to be very depressed and anxious
- There is no clear change in symptoms
- There are no side effects and no activation to hypomania

Question

What would you do next?

- Insist he be referred for psychotherapy; continue the lamotrigine and bupropion-XL
- Increase lamotrigine in the hope that it will treat the depression and anxiety
- Add an SSRI antidepressant in the hope that the MDD and SAD will improve while minimizing hypomania escalation risk, and while he is mood stabilized
- Add a bipolar depression-approved agent such as olanzapine–fluoxetine combination (Symbyax), quetiapine(Seroquel-XR), or lurasidone(Latuda)
- Add another mood stabilizer such as lithium

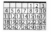

Case outcome: interim follow-up visits through nine months

- Gradually, the SSRI escitalopram (Lexapro) is started at the low 5 mg/d dose as samples were available
  - The patient had no income and no insurance
- The ineffective bupropion-XL was discontinued while maintenance lamotrigine (Lamictal) is continued
- He and his family were alerted to watch specifically for hypomania onset symptoms
- Eventually at 15 mg/d of escitalopram
  - Is still depressed and anxious
  - Develops weight gain

- ○ To which he admits he is very sensitive
- ○ Develops mild sexual side effects too
- – Asks promptly for non-SSRI options and elects to increase the lamotrigine to 300 mg/d in the hope that it will alleviate depression without adverse effects
- At the next visit, he is free of depression
  - – There are moderate reductions in SAD symptoms
  - – There is no evidence of hypomania on higher dose lamotrigine (Lamictal) monotherapy

Question

What would you do next?

- As the lamotrigine (Lamictal) 300 mg/d dose seems to have allowed depressive remission, the SSRI should be discontinued
- It is unclear if the lamotrigine worked alone to gain depressive remission, or if it worked in combination with the SSRI escitalopram (Lexapro); therefore, both should be continued
- The lamotrigine should be increased again to see if the SAD will remit as well
- Increase the escitalopram despite side effects to see if the SAD will remit
- Switch the SSRI to a novel class of antidepressants such as mirtazapine (Remeron), trazodone-ER (Oleptro), or vilazodone (Viibryd)
- Add a BZ anxiolytic to remit the SAD symptoms

Attending physician's mental notes: interim follow-up visits through nine months

- Patient seems to be mood stabilized and is solidly euthymic now
- His SAD is 50% better and it seems that he is able to control these symptoms, which he admits are not interfering with his life at this time
- He is concerned about weight gain and sexual side effects but seems to accept the benefits of his medications
- He asks to keep his medications as they are and agrees to continue the SSRI escitalopram (Lexapro)

Case outcome: interim follow-up visits through 36 months

- Now returns with some mild depressive symptoms and anxiety is also a bit worse
- SSRI is increased to the maximal approved escitalopram (Lexapro) dose of 20 mg/d
- This intervention markedly helps alleviate the MDD and SAD for many more months
- Unfortunately, toward the end of this three-year euthymic period, he returns more depressed, requiring an intervention

Question

What would you do next?

- As lamotrigine has now failed as a maintenance drug from a depression standpoint, it should be tapered off
- As escitalopram has failed to treat his depression it should be tapered off
- As lamotrigine has worked well prophylactically against mania, it should be continued
- As he has now failed three SSRIs and an NDRI, a switch to a novel class of antidepressants is warranted despite a slightly increased inherent risk in mania escalation

Case outcome: interim follow-up visits through 48 months

- The depression is now interfering with school and threatens to impede his career
- This is problematic as he has just been accepted at another premier graduate program out of state, to which he hopes to transfer
- The now ineffective escitalopram (Lexapro) is tapered off and he starts the SNRI desvenlafaxine (Pristiq), and is warned of increased manic escalation risks over the last SSRI approach
- Continues on higher-dose lamotrigine (Lamictal)
- As he is due to move, he will have less social support as he is away from his family and will have less monitoring of his symptoms as he is farther away from his psychiatric practitioner
- While away, he was "feeling well" and stops his medications
- This was followed by a depressive relapse, a self-imposed restart of his unipolar SNRI, desvenlafaxine (Pristiq), without restarting the mood stabilizer, and a more sustained hypomanic spell ensued
  - This caused him to leave school again
- Both medications were re-established
  - Euthymia and a relative lack of SAD were also re-established
- Recovered enough to move away again and take a job in another city while contemplating a return to graduate school
- While at the new location, he suffered an increase in insomnia and anxiety to a moderate degree and developed a persistent rash causing the lamotrigine to be discontinued
- With strong encouragement, he starts another mood stabilizing atypical antipsychotic agent in its place, aripiprazole (Abilify), to avoid future hypomania, and its use may effectively thwart the new anxiety and dysphoria symptoms as it is an augmentation to continuing desvenlafaxine (Pristiq) use
  - A few weeks later, the patient called reporting restlessness and more insomnia
  - From a distance this appears to be akathisia

- Starts atenolol 25 mg/d as an antidote to this EPS
- Weeks later, reports that he left his apartment due to manic level behavior; e.g., spending and legal problems that were more pronounced and sustained than previously reported
- Back in session finally, it was clear that his akathisia was actually goal directed and impulsive hyperactivity that was associated with a sense of invincibility and elevated mood
- The severity level of this mood episode is high enough for him to qualify as a bipolar I patient as he has met his first full manic criteria episode
- Again, the pattern appears to be fueled by relatively unopposed antidepressant use as the aripiprazole (Abilify) dose at the time (10 mg/d) was subtherapeutic as an anti-manic agent and not able to prevent or stop the emergence of a manic episode

Case debrief

- Many patients with bipolar disorder present in their teens with depression and anxiety
- This patient appears to have had a prodrome in a similar fashion and then experienced two sentinel bipolar events where he was sensitive to SSRI use and became hypomanic
  - These spells were brief, mild, and well circumscribed clinically
  - Both abated with SSRI cessation
- As he was a presumed bipolar II patient, there was a relative lack of guidelines, but he was treated with a mood stabilizer that allowed for no hypomania spells for many years
- This failed to treat his depression and anxiety fully at times
- To treat his remaining symptoms, an antidepressant was added in the presence of a mood stabilizer and maximized with remission of all symptoms for a few years
- Unfortunately, as the patient was out of town with a relative lack of observation and social support, his medication non-compliance increased, which apparently caused depression followed by a clear hypomanic episode
- Once stabilized, he moved again, and was noncompliant as before, escalating into hypomania and then ultimately mania
- This shows the unfortunate progression of bipolar illness toward more cycling and impairment over time

Take-home points

- There are no clear treatment guidelines for bipolar II disorder
- Clinicians must decide whether they wish to prescribe riskier anti-epilepsy or atypical antipsychotic mood stabilizers similar to

treating bipolar I patients, or if they wish to gradually treat with unipolar antidepressants and closely watch for hypomanic escalation
- Antidepressant-induced hypomania or mania episodes are likely sentinel bipolar disorder events, more so than just side effects
  - These hypomanias tend to be shorter and less severe than non-antidepressant-induced bipolar II hypomania events
  - Per the *DSM-5*, antidepressant-induced (hypo)mania episodes are now considered to be bona fide bipolar I and II events

Performance in practice: confessions of a psychopharmacologist
- *What could have been done better here?*
  - The initial, maximized, family collateral support and information gathering dissipated as the patient moved away
    - ○ Non-compliance increased, causing more bipolar cycling
    - ○ Therefore, establishing with a psychiatrist or a psychotherapist at the distant city was suggested but the patient declined
      - ▪ Perhaps this should have been more strictly enforced, thus increasing the likelihood of earlier hypomania detection
  - The atypical antipsychotic aripiprazole (Abilify) treats unipolar depression as an augmentation at relatively low doses (2–10 mg/d) and was started low in this case to avoid side effects and because the patient was depressed, not hypomanic
    - ○ Perhaps starting the dose at 15 mg/d or higher per acute mania treatment regulatory instructions would have promoted anti-manic effects and avoided the escalation
    - ○ Perhaps low-dose atypical antipsychotics are, in fact, unipolar antidepressants but without the anti-manic protection afforded to their moderate to high doses

Tips and pearls
- A majority of bipolar patients spend much more time depressed than manic
- The depressive component of bipolar disorder is often the most disabling cumulatively over time
- Therefore, reasonable yet aggressive treatment of depressed phase symptomatology is warranted
- Bipolar I treatment guidelines often suggest
  - Always use a mood stabilizer or approved atypical antipsychotic
  - If bipolar depression occurs, use an approved bipolar depression-specific treatment
    - ○ These often act as an antidepressant but with the least risk of manic escalation

- ○ Examples include olanzapine–fluoxetine combination (Symbyax), quetiapine (Seroquel), quetiapine-XR (Seroquel-XR), lurasidone (Latuda)
- ○ These often carry significant side effects such as metabolic and movement disorders
- ○ The atypical antipsychotics appear to be more antidepressant-like at lower doses and more antimanic- or antipsychotic-like at middle to higher doses
  - ▪ This likely occurs due to the fact that D2 receptor affinity is lower compared to the serotonin receptor affinities of the atypical antipsychotics
- – Unipolar antidepressants may be used in the presence of an adequately dosed mood stabilizing agent
  - ○ Must be dosed slowly and emergence of mania closely monitored
- • Conservatively, these guidelines should likely be utilized when treating bipolar II patients as well
- • Some bipolar II patients will escalate to bipolar I disorder, and therefore, following good mood stabilization guidelines may help to lower this risk of disease progression

Two-minute tutorial

What is the bipolar spectrum?

- • Based on Akiskal and Pinto's work,[1] clinicians might encounter patients meeting formal *DSM-5* diagnostic criteria noted as bipolar I or II or unspecified
  - – Otherwise, the following expanded system of bipolar spectrum symptom presentations might afford better classification and communication while treating these patients
  - – Ultimately, it must be assumed that if a patient enters in the weaker, less severe end of the spectrum, they could escalate toward the more severe end without treatment or with the administration of noncompliant or reckless prescribing practices
  - – Therefore, despite the classification system used, the primary goal should be mood stabilization
- • First, some unipolar patients may have soft symptoms suggestive of future bipolarity where they report
  - – Their mood often changes, happiness to sadness, with and without social reasons or stressors
  - – They have frequent ups and downs in mood, with and without apparent cause

[1] See References.

- They often feel guilty without a good reason
- Their feelings are rather easily hurt
- They often feel as though their future looks dark
- Ideas run through their minds so that they cannot sleep
- They often find it difficult to go to sleep because of thinking about what happened during the day
- They often feel disgruntled
  ○ In retrospect, the patient in this case experienced many of these during his *pre-bipolaring* or prodromal phase
- Second, a more formal operationalizing of the bipolar spectrum of disorders may be, theoretically, as follows
  - Bipolar I: full mania with full MDEs (like the *DSM-5* disorder)
  - Bipolar I and ½: depression with protracted hypomania (similar to the *DSM-5*'s cyclothymic disorder but with associated full MDEs instead of minor depressive episodes
  - Bipolar II: depression with hypomania (like the *DSM-5* disorder)
  - Bipolar II and ½: cyclothymic depressions (similar to the *DSM-5* cyclothymic disorder)
  - Bipolar III: antidepressant-induced mania (similar to this case initially where short and less severe manias were precipitated by SSRI use)
    ○ In the *DSM-5*, an antidepressant-induced (hypo)mania is no longer considered a drug-induced side effect but is, in fact, counted toward a bona fide bipolar I or II disorder
  - Bipolar III and ½: bipolarity masked – and unmasked – by stimulant abuse (self-explanatory)
  - Bipolar IV: hyperthymic depression (patients with persistent depressive disorder [dysthymia] but underlying traits of a hyperthymic temperament)
    ○ This latter temperament suggests that certain personality traits may lend to the development of bipolarity or be prodromal
    ○ Hyperthymic temperament or personality traits might include
      ▪ Increased energy and productivity
      ▪ Short sleep patterns
      ▪ Vivid, active, extroverted behavior
      ▪ Self-assured/self-confidence
      ▪ Strong willed
      ▪ Extremely conversational
      ▪ Tendency to repeat oneself
      ▪ Risk taking/sensation seeking
      ▪ Breaking social norms of others
      ▪ Strong libido
      ▪ Attention loving
      ▪ Low threshold for boredom

- Generous and spendthrift
- Emotion sensing
- Cheerful and jovial
- Unusual warmth
- Expansiveness
- Robust tirelessness
- Irrepressible, infectious quality in interpersonal interactions

- Of note is the new *DSM-5* mixed features specifier. If during the course of Bipolar 1 or 2 (hypo)mania, the patient experiences three or more depressive disorder symptoms, they are said to meet this specifier. In theory, this could occur in any of the bipolar spectrum areas noted above

Posttest self-assessment question and answer

If a manic spell is instigated by initiation of an antidepressant, which of the following is likely to happen?

A. The induced mania will be more severe
B. The induced mania will last longer
C. The induced mania will be less severe and shorter in duration
D. None of the above

Answer: C

Available data is minimal but suggests that antidepressant-induced mania is often less severe and of a shorter duration, assuming the offending antidepressant is stopped.

References

1. Akiskal HS, Pinto O. The evolving bipolar spectrum: prototypes I, II, III, and IV. *Psychiatr Clin North Am* 1999; 22:517–34.
2. Doran CM. *The Hypomania Handbook: The Challenge of Elevated Mood*. Philadelphia, PA: Lippincott Williams & Wilkins, 2007.
3. Stoll AL, Mayer PV, Kolbrener M, et al. Antidepressant-associated mania: a controlled comparison with spontaneous mania. *Am J Psychiatry* 1994; 151:1642–5.
4. Parker G, Parker K. Which antidepressants flick the switch? *Aust NZ J Psychiatry* 2003; 37:464–8.
5. Wehr TA, Goodwin FK. Can antidepressants cause mania and worsen the course of affective illness? *Am J Psychiatry* 1987; 144:1403–11.
6. Leverich GS, Altshuler LL, Frye MA, et al. Risk of switch in mood polarity to hypomania or mania in patients with bipolar depression during acute and continuation trials of venlafaxine, sertraline, and bupropion as adjuncts to mood stabilizers. *Am J Psychiatry* 2006; 163:232–9.
7. Amsterdam JD, Shults J. Efficacy and safety of long-term fluoxetine versus lithium monotherapy of bipolar II disorder: a randomized,

double-blind, placebo-substitution study. *Am J Psychiatry* 2010; 167:792–800.

8. Frye MA, Helleman G, McElroy SL, et al. Correlates of treatment-emergent mania associated with antidepressant treatment in bipolar depression. *Am J Psychiatry* 2009; 166:164–72.

9. Suppes T. Is there a role for antidepressants in the treatment of bipolar II depression? *Am J Psychiatry* 2010; 167:738–40.

10. Akiskal HS, Hantouche EG, Allilaire JF, et al. Validating antidepressant-associated hypomania (bipolar III): a systematic comparison with spontaneous hypomania (bipolar II). *J Affect Disord* 2003; 73:65–74.

11. Depue RA, Slater JF, Wolfstetter-Kausch H, et al. A behavioral paradigm for identifying persons at risk for bipolar depressive disorder: a conceptual framework and five validation studies. *J Abnorm Psychol* 1981; 90:381–437.

12. Taylor L, Faraone SV, Tsuang MT. Family, twin, and adoption studies of bipolar disease. *Curr Psychiatry Rep* 2002; 4:130–3.

13. Craddock N, Jones I. Genetics of bipolar disorder. *J Med Genet* 1999; 36:585–94.

14. Mortensen PB, Pedersen CB, Melbye M, Mors O, Ewald H. Individual and familial risk factors for bipolar affective disorders in Denmark. *Arch Gen Psychiatry* 2003; 60:1209–15.

15. Twiss J, Jones S, Anderson I. Validation of the mood disorder questionnaire for screening for bipolar disorder in a UK sample. *J Affect Disord* 2008; 110:180–4.

16. Rice JP, McDonald-Scott P, Endicott J, et al. The stability of diagnosis with an application to bipolar II disorder. *Psychiatry Res* 1986; 19:285–96.

17. Schwartz TL, Stahl SM. Treatment strategies for dosing the second generation antipsychotics. *CNS Neurosci Ther* 2011; 17:110–17.

18. Hantouche EG, Angst J, Akiskal HS. Factor structure of hypomania: interrelationships with cyclothymia and the soft bipolar spectrum. *J Affect Disord* 2003; 73:39–47.

The Case: The patient who was not lyming

The Question: Can Lyme disease cause depression?

The Dilemma: Managing depression and possible neuropsychiatric illness

Pretest self-assessment question (answer at the end of the case)

Regarding Lyme disease as a neuropsychiatric illness, which is most accurate?

A. Almost all patients bitten by infected Lyme disease-carrying ticks will develop an easily diagnosable rash
B. Once bitten, most patients will develop clinical Lyme disease
C. Depression as a result of Lyme disease infection is a common clinical presentation
D. Blood antibody testing is often a definitive diagnosis and should be followed by antibiotic treatment

Patient evaluation on intake

- 48-year-old woman states she has been "depressed and anxious since childhood"
- She is extremely worried she will become incapacitated and institutionalized

Psychiatric history

- Does not remember any sustained euthymia since her teenage years
- Feels as though she has fluctuated between chronic lower-level dysthymia symptoms and has had many MDEs consistent with double depression
- Now has full syndrome of MDD symptoms
  - Admits having passive and chronic suicidal thoughts but has much ideational guilt that she feels she is a bad mother and was an unreliable employee
  - Feels quite fatigued with an inability to focus or concentrate
  - Appetite is low and sleep is interrupted often
- Additionally, she has uncontrollable worry, racing thoughts, muscle tension, irritability, nightmares, feelings of dread and detachment
  - Some of these latter symptoms she attributes to being neglected, but not abused, as a child
- She admits to having BN in college
- She denies SUD symptoms

Psychotherapy history

- Attends eclectic, supportive psychotherapy often and has recently started with a new therapist
- Has no history of undergoing organized psychoanalysis, or completing a course of CBT or IPT

Social and personal history

- Graduated from college and worked as a teacher until MDD worsened two to three years ago
- Has two children but was divorced several years ago
- Has brothers who are supportive
- Smokes cigarettes and drinks a moderate amount of coffee

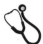

Medical history

- Denies current medical problems except she is considering being treated for a possible Lyme disease diagnosis as many family members have suffered from this after unknown exposures, although she has not been tested yet

Family history

- Mother suffered from treatment-resistant bipolar disorder and was institutionalized often
  - The patient reports much fear and currently reliving episodes related to her mother's symptomatology
  - Her mother was often absent in her life because of psychiatric institutionalization
- She has two other siblings with bipolar illness
- AUD is present in many family members

Medication history

- Currently she is taking
  - Alprazolam (Xanax) 3 mg/d (BZ)
  - Mirtazapine (Remeron) 30 mg/d (NaSSA)
  - Divalproex sodium (Depakote) 1000 mg/d (mood stabilizer)
- In her current MDE occurring over the last two years, she has failed to respond to
  - Therapeutic trials of an SSRI, citalopram (Celexa) plus various BZs
  - An atypical antipsychotic (risperidone [Risperdal]) 2 mg/d, and a mood stabilizer (lamotrigine [Lamictal] 200 mg/d) augmentation
  - A combination SSRI plus an NDRI (bupropion-SR [Wellbutrin-SR] 300 mg/d)

Patient evaluation on initial visit

- Chronic MDD symptoms with associated, or possibly comorbid GAD or PTSD for many years
- MDD progressively more resistant to treatment with each MDE, lasting longer

- Possible exposure to tick bites and Lyme disease, but patient does not recollect a bite or a rash
- She and her family are particularly concerned as other family members have suffered with Lyme disease
- Appears to be compliant with medication management and has attended psychotherapy
- Does have passive suicidal ideation, is quite despondent, but is amenable to outpatient treatment and contracts for safety
- Reports no current side effects

Current medications

- Divalproex sodium (Depakote) 1000 mg/d (mood stabilizer)
- Mirtazapine (Remeron) 30 mg/d (NaSSA)
- Alprazolam (Xanax) 3 mg/d as needed (BZ)

Question

Based on your geographic location, is Lyme disease a reasonable differential diagnosis?

- No, there is a very small deer population in my area and chances of deer tick bites are very low
- Maybe – I live in a geographic area where more cases are being reported every year
- Yes, most cases of Lyme disease are concentrated in a few areas, and most infections occur in the northeast, in the Great Lakes region, and along the Pacific coast of the United States. I live in one of these areas

Attending physician's mental notes: initial evaluation

- This patient has chronic and recurrent MDD
- Likely has comorbid GAD and PTSD, or these are at least present in a subsyndromal aspect
- There is a possibility that she has an infectious etiology as well
- These comorbidities and chronicity of her illness make her prognosis fair at best
- She has had several recent therapeutic polypharmacy trials, albeit not always dosed at maximum levels, and has had many monotherapy trials over the years
    - This also worsens her prognosis with regard to achieving remission
- She does have positive family support and initial indications suggest that she is compliant with treatment, both of which improve her prognosis

PATIENT FILE

Question

Which of the following would be your next step?

- Increase the NaSSA antidepressant mirtazapine (Remeron) to the full FDA dose of 45 mg/d to maximize its potential
- Increase the BZ alprazolam (Xanax) to a higher dose to treat her agitation and anxiety
- Check divalproex (Depakote) levels, and if warranted, increase to make this therapeutic despite the patient not having bipolar disorder
- Augment the current medications with yet another agent to enhance antidepressant response
- Refer for formal CBT or IPT manualized psychotherapy
- Confer with outside clinicians regarding Lyme disease workup and findings

Attending physician's mental notes: initial evaluation (continued)

- This patient seems to be taking standard treatment for resistant MDD
  - Good use of multiple antidepressant classes and augmentations with evidence-based agents
  - Now is on a moderate dose of an antidepressant
- However, there is concern about the use of divalproex (Depakote) as she does not appear to have a bipolar history
  - Perhaps it was prescribed for anxiolysis as she is quite agitated at times and failing to respond to BZ
- She seems very guilt-ridden and ruminative about her perceived inadequacy
  - Will need to continue to investigate if this is delusional

Further investigation

Is there anything else you would especially like to know about this patient?

- What about details concerning her past medication treatment?
  - Her doses of medications appear to be therapeutic (moderate to high dosages)
  - The divalproex is confirmed as being used for anxiety, not bipolar disorder
  - She has never misused controlled prescriptions
- What about details concerning her possible Lyme disease exposure?
  - Has lived most of her life in areas that are prevalent for Lyme disease
  - Does not recollect a tick bite
  - Does not recollect the typical "bull's eye" rash
  - States multiple family members have developed Lyme disease without known bites/rashes

- Her local internist does not feel this is Lyme disease, which has angered family members who have arranged a visit to a Lyme disease expert in another state for a second opinion, as they feel strongly that it is
- Her present MDE is chronic and has similar features compared to her previous MDEs, which would predate her possible Lyme exposure
  o The current MDE does not appear different symptomatically from her prior MDEs

Case outcome: first interim follow-up visits four and eight weeks later

- At the first follow-up visit, opts to leave the medications as given, to await her laboratory results and levels and collaboration with outside physicians
- At the follow-up visit, she acknowledges the same MDD, GAD, PTSD symptoms as in the initial office appointment and agrees to increase the mirtazapine (Remeron) antidepressant to the full 45 mg/d dose and taper off the ineffective divalproex (Depakote)
- Now recollects that her trial of lamotrigine (Lamictal) in the past was somewhat helpful and free of side effects
  - She asks if this can be restarted and it is titrated slowly per usual guidelines to avoid serious rash complications
- Reports that she is having fluctuating anxiety and agitation and reveals that she takes her alprazolam (Xanax) as needed, but sporadically
  - She may "take three tablets a day for a few days, then zero tabs, then perhaps one or two. ..."
  - It is possible that on her off-use days she is having rebound anxiety as a side effect
- She is convinced to take 2 mg/d routinely to avoid this possible rebound phenomenon, keep consistent drug levels present, and to also provide better longitudinal anxiety control
- Shortly after this follow-up visit, she begins seeing a new, psychodynamically oriented psychotherapist who felt she required inpatient psychiatric stabilization, and she was admitted for a 10-day stay

Question

What would you suggest to the inpatient psychiatrist regarding possible treatment options?

- Continue mirtazapine (Remeron) full dose as it has not had enough time therapeutically to become effective
- Continue to titrate lamotrigine (Lamictal) as it has not reached its usual effective dose as an off-label depression augmentation
- Switch the ineffective mirtazapine to a TCA or an MAOI antidepressant

- Augment the current medications with an atypical antipsychotic, lithium, or thyroid hormone
- Start ECT treatments
- Start VNS treatments
- Start TMS treatments

Attending physician's mental notes: second interim follow-up visit at three months

- Despite being a little better, the patient still has significant MDD symptoms
- She has a clinically meaningful response now in that she is not suicidal, is less anxious, and has better affective range, but she is not a 50% responder yet
- She now has side effects of increasing fatigue and sedation
  - This type of side effect makes her feel more guilty as she is "able to do less, and is less functional" as a result
- She takes medications known to have serious, long-term side effects
  - She is warned of, and monitored for, metabolic disorder, which appears not to be a problem now
  - She is warned of, and monitored for, TD/EPS, which appears not to be a problem now
  - She is warned of, and monitored for, BZ misuse, which appears not to be a problem now
  - She is warned of, and monitored for, rashes, which appear not to be a problem now

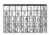

Case outcome: second interim follow-up visit at three months

- The patient returns from hospitalization taking
  - Olanzapine (Zyprexa) 7.5 mg/d (atypical antipsychotic)
  - Lorazepam (Ativan) 4mg/d (BZ)
  - Lamotrigine (Lamictal) 50 mg/d (mood stabilizer)
  - Mirtazapine (Remeron) 45 mg/d (NaSSA)
  - Zolpidem-CR (Ambien-CR) 12.5 mg at bedtime (BZRA)
- This regimen differs in that she was augmented with an atypical antipsychotic, her sedative alprazolam (Xanax) was changed to lorazepam (Ativan), and zolpidem-CR (Ambien-R) was added to improve sleep
  - The patient now has a moderately better affective range, fewer psychomotor agitation symptoms, and states an absence of suicidal thoughts
  - She is felt to be 20%–30% better after her inpatient stay

Question

What would you do next?

- Increase the dose of her olanzapine (Zyprexa) augmentation
- Switch the mirtazapine to an SSRI, which may mimic the approved olanzapine–fluoxetine combination drug (Symbyax), which is approved specifically for TRD
- As she is a partial responder and has failed many therapeutic trials, could combine with a second approved antidepressant such as bupropion (NDRI), or trazodone (SARI), or an SNRI
- As she is a partial responder with a minimal response and has failed many therapeutic trials, could augment with a stimulant or a nutraceutical
  - L-methylfolate (Deplin) 15 mg/d
  - SAMe 400–800 mg twice a day
  - N-acetyl cysteine (NAC) 1000 mg twice a day
- Continue to wait on the current regimen and PDP for full effectiveness to occur

Attending physician's mental notes: second interim follow-up visit at three months (continued)

- The patient seems to be losing some ground after her hospitalization in that she is experiencing increased guilt and recurrent negative thoughts
  - This seems triggered by the sedating side effects
- Her affect did appear better after the addition of the atypical antipsychotic, which is dosed low at this point
- Likely now is sedated by medications and needs to be addressed

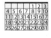

Case outcome: interim follow-up visits through six months

- To honor the patient's request for less fatigue-based side effects, she is tapered off the zolpidem-CR hypnotic agent in the hope of alleviating the morning sedation, but the lorazepam is continued for anxiolysis
- The relatively ineffective mirtazapine and lamotrigine are discontinued
- Next is switched to olanzapine–fluoxetine combination (Symbyax) and titrated to the 6 mg/50 mg/d dose
  - This combination agent is approved for TRD
  - The insomnia returns and a SARI, trazodone(Desyrel) 150 mg at bedtime, is added to the regimen to treat insomnia, but may also act as an antidepressant augmentation
- She ultimately improves and is considered a responder as she is 50% improved
  - There is less symptom severity and she starts exercising and socializing again
  - Anxiety is no longer felt to be chronic and pervasive but appears situational and more manageable

Question

What would you do next?

- Make no changes as she is a responder to her medications and PDP is ongoing and should improve her symptoms gradually with time
- Escalate the olanzapine–fluoxetine (Symbyax) combination dose to better gain remission
- Augment the current regimen with lithium or thyroid hormone to better gain remission
- Augment the current regimen with a stimulant
- Augment her current regimen with a nutraceutical

Attending physician's mental notes: interim follow-up visits through six months

- Patient is 50% better on a regimen essentially of an atypical antipsychotic, an SSRI, a BZ, and an alpha-adrenergic-1 receptor antagonizing hypnotic/SARI antidepressant
- Given her recurrent MDD, and previous attempts with at least four medication trials to obtain a response, she unfortunately is likely to relapse into MDD within the next 6 to twelve months, even if continuing current treatment, especially as she is not in full MDD remission now
- Will need to monitor her closely and intervene if relapse is pending
- It is likely worth pushing forward with more aggressive antidepressant augmentation now, to better aim for remission, which is needed to better avoid a depressive relapse

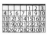

Case outcome: interim follow-up visits through nine months

- A Lyme disease expert deems patient to be suffering from this neuropsychiatric illness
- Based on this opinion, the mounting fatigue-related side effects, and pressure from family members, she stops her psychotropic regimen and starts multiple antibiotic therapy (doxycycline, rifampin, zithromax) for Lyme disease
  - MDD returns fully within a matter of weeks
  - A full course of antibiotics has failed to treat her possible Lyme disease and its secondary depression
  - She is amenable to restarting her psychotropics but again wants to avoid fatigue
- Restarts fluoxetine (Prozac) up to 40 mg/d and is started on the less-sedating atypical antipsychotic aripiprazole (Abilify) up to 4 mg/d as it is often clinically less sedating than olanzapine
  - It is an approved MDD augmentation strategy

302

- Given that the fluoxetine (Prozac) inhibits CYP450 2D6 hepatic enzymes, the aripiprazole dose is likely elevated in her plasma (likely equivalent to 8–12 mg/d)
  - This atypical antipsychotic is also approved as an adjunctive treatment for MDD at this dose range
- Restarts lorazepam (BZ) and trazodone (SARI)
- This new regimen attempts to re-create the last semi-effective regimen but with the hope of less sedation
- She experiences some MDD symptom relief again but also complains of daytime sedation
  - She will not tolerate this problem
- Trazodone (Desyrel) and lorazepam (Ativan) are lowered significantly to help resolve this sedation side effect, with reasonable results

Attending physician's mental notes: interim follow-up visits through nine months

- The atypical antipsychotics seem to be helpful in controlling her depression to a certain degree
- When the MDD improves, then the anxiety symptoms are also much better controlled
  - This suggests that her GAD and PTSD symptoms are likely subsyndromal and being driven, or escalated, by her depressive state
- Compliance issues are clear in that she *will not* tolerate fatigue-related side effects
- Will need to keep working on the medication regimen to hopefully gain a full remission of symptoms

Question

Antibiotic treatment did not alleviate her alleged Lyme disease-induced MDD. What does this mean?

- Her MDD is not from Lyme disease as her symptoms did not resolve
- Her MDD still could be from Lyme disease as this infectious illness may have caused damage to her nervous system and her MDD symptoms continue as a result

Case outcome: interim follow-up visits through 15 months

- Develops EPS (akathisia) on aripiprazole (Abilify), which is not resolved with BZ therapy
- Insists on a tapering off of the atypical antipsychotic
  - Refuses future atypical antipsychotics
  - Refuses to take other akathisia antidotes (beta-blockers, anticholinergics)

- Continues on fluoxetine (Prozac) and is sequentially augmented with stimulants, then L-methylfolate (Deplin) 15 mg/d, then combined with bupropion-XL (Aplenzin) 348 mg/d, and finally therapeutically dosed trazodone-ER (Oleptro) 300 mg/d
- As the anxiety fluctuates, she is tried on several different BZ anxiolytics for better symptom control
  - These interventions do not prevent an MDD full relapse
- She begins drinking alcohol, which has never been a clinical issue
- This abrupt misuse is successfully treated with acamprosate (Campral) 1998 mg/d
  - This glutamate metabotropic receptor antagonizing drug unfortunately did not help lower her anxiety, despite anecdotal reports suggesting it has anxiolytic activity
  - This medication was also paired with a harm-reduction, stage-of-change, motivational-interviewing therapeutic approach
- Rehospitalization occurs as she becomes incapacitated and more suicidal
  - A family member makes contact and states that he had never disclosed this to the patient, but also has had chronic depression and was successfully treated with ECT many years ago
  - After informed consent, the patient undergoes ECT treatment while on the inpatient service

Case debrief

- This patient presented in a highly treatment-resistant state
- She was suffering from comorbid depression and anxiety
- There was a likelihood that she also suffered from active Lyme disease, but this was ultimately treated and ruled out as a primary cause of her depressive symptoms
- This patient's treatment course was interrupted in several ways
  - Non-compliance with medications
  - Inability to tolerate mild side effects
  - Strife with family members and other providers regarding her diagnosis
    - These punctuated her partial response periods with depressive relapses
    - She never gained remission
  - She was noncompliant at pivotal points, which caused relapses, and many attempts were made to create a psychotropic regimen that would be effective with less fatigue-related side effects
- The patient underwent ECT and again was deemed a 50% responder, but over the next few years suffered relapses into MDD

- She engaged in three-times-a-week PDP and a year-long course of DBT, which appears to have helped her to sustain a response more successfully for more substantial periods, but has never achieved a sustained symptom remission
- She finally underwent a course of TMS, which remains a maintenance treatment
  - This neuromodulation approach was free of side effects for her
  - She has not achieved remission but likely has reached the best sustained response so far with regard to her TRD

Take-home points

- Patients with TRD are more apt to attain only partial symptom relief and to relapse frequently into MDEs
- Frequent medication regimen adjustments are warranted to attempt to gain remission and to hopefully delay relapses
- Sometimes treatment regimens are interrupted by outside forces (family, friends, outside providers) and have to be navigated acutely
- Side-effect management in chronic depression often becomes more important than obtaining symptom reduction
  - If a patient will not stay on a medication at therapeutic doses, they cannot obtain good outcomes
  - In psychopharmacologic practice, it often is not about choosing the right medication but the art of keeping the patient on a good medication
- Comprehensive and intensive psychotherapy may also be utilized to better treat patients with TRD
- Infectious organic CNS insults, like Lyme disease, should be considered in TRD cases
  - In this case, Lyme disease may have been a fully plausible explanation, especially if there was a more acute onset of MDD symptoms over the last few years since exposure and if there were positive laboratory findings
  - Lyme disease might also have been more likely if her current MDE came with a "different flavor" or different, novel symptomatology compared to her previous MDEs
  - However, this episode presented with symptoms similar to her previous MDEs
  - This patient's chronic depression since childhood made Lyme disease a less likely etiology, but worthy of a workup regardless

Performance in practice: confessions of a psychopharmacologist

- *What could have been done better here?*
  - Psychiatrists are often not up-to-date on medical illness comorbidities

- Clinicians have become better regarding metabolic disorder detection and management, but likely not in infectious illnesses such as Lyme disease
- Some areas of the country have much higher infection rates and prevalence of Lyme disease
- Clinicians in these endemic areas should be up-to-date on Lyme disease as it can mimic depression, anxiety, and dementia to a certain degree
  - Lyme disease patients tend to have many somatic symptoms
  - This type of presentation also occurs in the depressed–anxious patient population
- As this patient was partially treated by an atypical antipsychotic, could atypicals with less sedation be utilized to improve adherence?
  - Aripiprazole was used instead of olanzapine (Zyprexa) at one point, but to no avail
  - Perhaps ziprasidone (Geodon) could have been tried
  - Lurasidone (Latuda) was not available at the time, but this could be an option as a possibly less-sedating medication
  - Alternatively, atypical antipsychotic-induced fatigue could have been challenged by using a stimulant such as methylphenidate (Ritalin) or a wakefulness-promoting agent such as modafinil (Provigil)
  - These combinations could provide a "win–win" situation in that fatigue may have lessened, improving her medication compliance, and could have acted as an augmentation strategy to improve her MDD
  - Controversially, consider if adding a DA-enhancing stimulant makes clinical sense when the patient was taking a D2 receptor blocking atypical antipsychotic
- *Possible action items for improvement in practice*
  - Review the epidemiology of Lyme disease in your geographic area
  - Review its etiology, diagnosis, and treatment standards

Tips and pearls

- As in this case, sometimes treating the MDD often alleviates or lowers the impact of comorbid anxiety disorders
- It is unclear then if the TRD is creating or driving the anxiety symptoms or if the agents used to treat the MDD treat the anxiety primarily as well
- In treatment-resistant cases, aggressive psychotherapy may be helpful in both further symptom reduction and at least improving quality of life issues
- Device-based neuromodulation treatments should always be considered in TRD

– Introducing initial informed consent earlier in the course of TRD treatment as a later possibility likely keeps the shock of hearing about ECT, brain pacemakers, and brain magnets lower, and patients may be more accepting of these treatments when they are truly warranted (. . . pun intended)

Neuropsychiatric moment

Primer on Lyme disease

Causes, incidence, and risk factors

- Lyme disease is caused by a bacterium (*B. burgdorferi*)
- Ticks carry this bacterium and bite mice or deer, which become infected as an animal vector
- Humans get the disease when bitten by an infected tick
  - Deer ticks can be so small that they are almost impossible to see
  - Many people with Lyme disease never even see a tick
- The first case was reported in 1975 in Connecticut, and has spread to most of the northeast and now to some mid-Atlantic, mid-West, and Pacific coast states
- Lyme disease is usually seen during the late spring, summer, and early fall

Symptoms

- There are three stages of Lyme disease
  - Stage 1 is called primary Lyme disease
  - Stage 2 is called secondary Lyme disease or early disseminated Lyme disease
  - Stage 3 is called tertiary Lyme disease or chronic persistent Lyme disease
- Not everyone infected with the bacterium becomes clinically ill
  - Most bitten patients do not develop the infection
  - If a person does become ill, the first symptoms resemble the flu and include
    ○ Chills
    ○ Fever
    ○ Headache
    ○ Lethargy
    ○ Muscle pain
  - There may be a "bull's eye" rash
    ○ A flat or slightly raised red spot at the site of the tick bite
    ○ Often there is a clear area surrounding the center of the bite with another red ring beyond that
    ○ It can be larger than one to three inches wide

- Symptoms in people with early infection and then later stages of the disease include
  - Fatigue
  - Low grade fevers, "hot flashes", or chills
  - Night sweats
  - Sore throat
  - Swollen glands
  - Stiff neck
  - Migrating arthralgias, stiffness, and less commonly, frank arthritis
  - Myalgia
  - Chest pain and palpitations*
  - Abdominal pain, nausea*
  - Diarrhea
  - Sleep disturbance*
  - Poor concentration and memory loss*
  - Irritability and mood swings*
  - Depression*
  - Back pain
  - Blurred vision and eye pain
  - Jaw pain
  - Testicular/pelvic pain
  - Tinnitus
  - Vertigo
  - Cranial nerve disturbance (facial numbness, pain, tingling, palsy, or optic neuritis)
  - Headaches
  - Lightheadedness
- Headache, stiff neck, sleep disturbance,* and problems with memory and concentration* are findings consistently associated with more chronic neurologic Lyme disease
- Other symptoms associated with Lyme disease have been identified, although these have not been consistently present in patients
  - Numbness and tingling*
  - Muscle twitching
  - Photosensitivity
  - Hyperacusis

Notice many of these symptoms are associated with DSM-5 diagnosed depressive and anxiety disorders.

Signs and tests

- A blood test can be obtained to check for antibodies to the bacterium that causes Lyme disease
  - The most commonly used test is the ELISA for Lyme disease

- A western blot test is done to confirm initial ELISA results
- These tests do confirm that a patient was bitten with the introduction of the Lyme disease-causing bacterium but do not necessarily prove a present or ongoing infection
- There is some controversy regarding the accuracy of these two standard tests
  - These antibody tests can confuse Lyme disease antibodies with antibodies created by other complications in the body, including those created in reaction to non-Lyme disease bacteria
  - Some feel that a negative test result cannot guarantee that Lyme disease antibodies do not exist in a given patient
- Not as well known, but very effective, is the PCR test for Lyme disease
  - This PCR test confirms in real time that Lyme disease bacteria are present in the body
  - The PCR test is relatively new and is designed to confirm that Lyme disease bacterial DNA is present
  - A positive PCR test is a greater guarantee that a patient has active Lyme disease
- The latest diagnostic test is the Lyme C6 peptide ELISA
  - It is a Lyme disease ELISA test but appears to be more accurate than previous ELISA approaches
- A physical examination may show joint, cardiac, or neurological problems in people with advanced Lyme disease

Treatment

- Everyone who has been bitten by a tick should be watched closely for at least 30 days
- Most people who are bitten by a tick do not get Lyme disease
- A single course of antibiotics (doxycycline, amoxicillin, cefuroxime) may be offered to someone soon after being bitten by a tick, if all of the following are true
  - The person has a tick that can carry Lyme disease attached to their body
    ○ This usually means that a nurse or physician has looked at and identified the tick
  - The tick is thought to have been attached to the person for at least 36 hours
  - The person can begin taking the antibiotics within 72 hours of removing the tick
  - The person is over eight years old or is not pregnant or breastfeeding
- A full course of antibiotics is used to treat people who are proven to have Lyme disease
  - The specific antibiotic used may depend upon the stage of the disease and the symptoms

Prognosis

- If diagnosed in the early stages, Lyme disease can be cured with antibiotics
- Without treatment, complications involving the joints, heart, and nervous system can occur
- Rarely, a person will continue having symptoms that can interfere with daily life
- Some people call this post-Lyme disease syndrome
  - There is no effective treatment yet for this
- Advanced stages of Lyme disease can cause long-term joint inflammation (Lyme arthritis) and heart arrhythmias
- Nervous system (neurological) problems are also possible, and may include
  - Decreased concentration
  - Memory disorders
  - Nerve damage
  - Numbness
  - Pain
  - Paralysis of the face muscles
  - Sleep disorders
  - Vision problems

Pharmacodynamic moment

Atypical antipsychotics and anti-H1 receptor antagonism-induced sedation

- There are now many atypical antipsychotics available for use
- They may be divided into those with higher or lower EPS rates
- They may be divided into those with higher or lower rates of weight gain, hyperlipidemia, or hyperglycemia
- Blocking H1 receptors has been well known to cause sedating side effects since psychotropics, such as the TCAs and phenothiazine-based typical antispychotics, were first approved in the 1950s
  - Therefore, the atypical antipsychotics may also be divided into those with more or less sedation, higher or lower antihistamine activity, respectively
- The atypical antipsychotics are not immune to this pharmacodynamic property either
- Based on affinity for each atypical antipsychotic for antagonizing the H1 receptor, clinicians may be able to predict sedation rates from this class of psychotropics

Table 20.1. Atypical antipsychotics and antihistamine receptor antagonism

Atypical (Ki-value provided by manufacturer where higher values equal lower affinities)	Affinity for H1
Lurasidone (Latuda)	1000+
Iloperidone (Fanapt)	473
Aripiprazole (Abilify)	61
Ziprasidone (Geodon)	47
Olanzapine (Zyprexa)	7
Risperidone (Risperdal)	5.2
Paliperidone (Invega)	3.4
Quetiapine/norquetiapine (Seroquel)	4.41/1.15
Asenapine (Saphris)	1

*Table reproduced with permission of K. Bedynerman MD, SUNY Upstate Medical University

- This table shows the least antihistaminergic atypical antipsychotic at the top and increased anti-H1 receptor antagonism activity at the bottom
- Therefore, sedating side effects should increase in theory as you progress down the table
- If a patient is sedated on an agent lower in the table, then the clinician could switch to an atypical antipsychotic higher up in the table that is less sedating
- This is complicated
  - Antihistaminergic activity is associated with sedation. Some atypical antipsychotics possess increased noradrenergic activity (quetiapine, ziprasidone), which can promote wakefulness
  - Other atypical antipsychotics antagonize NE alpha-1 receptors (iloperidone), which may cause fatigue in addition to the antihistamine effects
  - Tables can help guide clinicians but clinicians must be aware that they do not exist in a vacuum and many of our psychotropics possess multiple pharmacodynamic properties

Pretest self-assessment question and answer

Regarding Lyme disease as a neuropsychiatric illness, which is most accurate?

A. Almost all patients bitten by infected Lyme disease-carrying ticks will develop an easily diagnosable rash
B. Once bitten, most patients will develop clinical Lyme disease
C. Depression as a result of Lyme disease is a common clinical presentation
D. Blood antibody testing is often a definitive diagnosis and should be followed by antibiotic treatment

Answer: D
A sizeable minority of patients do not recognize they have been bitten and a majority of patients will not develop clinical Lyme disease. Depression is a controversial complication of Lyme disease and great variability among infected patients is common. The combination of living in a highly tick-infested geographic area, exhibiting clinical signs and symptoms, and use of blood testing is fairly accurate (albeit not perfect) in diagnosing Lyme disease.

References

1. http://www.ncbi.nlm.nih.gov/pubmedhealth/PMHT0025348/. Accessed July 15, 2011.
2. Wormser GP, Dattwyler RJ, Shapiro ED, et al. The clinical assessment, treatment, and prevention of Lyme disease, human granulocytic anaplasmosis, and babesiosis: clinical practice guidelines by the Infectious Diseases Society of America. *Clin Infect Dis* 2006; 43:1089–134.
3. Feder HM Jr., Johnson BJ, O'Connell S, et al. A critical appraisal of "chronic Lyme disease." *N Engl J Med* 2007; 357:1422–30.
4. Halperin JJ, Shapiro ED, Logigian E, et al. Practice parameter: treatment of nervous system Lyme disease (an evidence-based review): report of the Quality Standards Subcommittee of the American Academy of Neurology. *Neurology* 2007; 69:91–102.
5. http://www.ilads.org/lyme/treatment-guideline.php. Accessed July 15, 2011.
6. Rush AJ, Trivedi MH, Wisniewski SR, et al. Acute and longer-term outcomes in depressed outpatients requiring one or several treatment steps: a STAR*D report. *Am J Psychiatry* 2006; 163:1905–17.
7. Schwartz TL, Siddiqui UA, Raza S, Costello A. Acamprosate calcium as augmentation therapy for anxiety disorders. *Ann Pharmacother* 2010; 44:1930–2.
8. Bedynerman K, Schwartz TL. Utilizing pharmacodynamic properties of second generation antipsychotics to guide treatment. *Drugs of Today* 2012; 48:283–92.

The Case: Hindsight is always 20/20, or attention deficit hyperactivity disorder

The Question: What to do when a primary anxiety disorder is fully treated and inattention remains

The Dilemma: Residual inattention may be difficult to treat

Pretest self-assessment question (answer at the end of the case)

How does an alpha-2a receptor agonist really improve attention?

A. It lowers brainstem NE output similar to its antihypertensive effects
B. It promotes DA activity in the DLPFC secondarily
C. It lowers GABA activity, which allows greater glutamate activity in the thalamus
D. It allows fine tuning of cortical pyramidal glutamate neurons to improve signal to noise ratios in frontocortical information processing

Patient evaluation on intake

- 31-year-old man with a chief complaint of anxiety of "different types"
- Patient states that he "has been successful in graduate school, has financial worries, but states that he worries and is tense most of the time"

Psychiatric history

- Has been anxious for many years, mostly since college and now graduate school
- Working part-time and going to school part-time and feels "torn in many directions"
- Generally is tense, restless, irritable, and worries about things even outside school and work
  - When legitimate stressors diminish, the anxiety lowers, but is still present and discouraging
- This causes him to be argumentative and temperamental most of the time
- He says he is active and likes to stay busy all of the time, but he wonders if "he is doing too much, as he has no time for all of the things" he wants to do

Social and personal history

- Graduated high school, college, and is enrolled in a graduate-level training program for family counseling
- Gainfully employed now in a clinical setting
- Married and without children
- Does not use drugs or alcohol

Medical history

- There are no medical issues but is allergic to penicillin

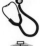

Family history

- Father has AUD
- Distant family members have probable bipolar disorder

Medication history

- There was serendipitous anxiety relief when his PCP placed him on hydroxyzine (Vistaril) 50 mg/d for an allergic skin reaction
  - This helped to "calm him down" but was only temporary
- Has taken the SSRI paroxetine (Paxil) 40 mg/d but had a difficult time balancing its anxiolytic effects and its sexual side effects
  - Felt that he was less anxious at these higher doses of this SSRI, but this was too problematic from a tolerability point of view
  - Next changed to the slow-release preparation at a lower dose (paroxetine-CR 25 mg/d), which better balanced efficacy and tolerability
- Next, he responded to a radio advertisement for an anxiety research study and he was placed on an SGRI antiepileptic, tiagabine (Gabitril), as an augmentation strategy, which he found moderately beneficial at a dose of 12 mg/d

Psychotherapy history

- Patient has seen a few psychotherapists for both supportive psychotherapy and PDP
- He reports having psychological issues regarding his father, who was abusive and an alcoholic
  - Psychotherapy has been very helpful
  - There is no *DSM-5* evidence of PTSD despite this history

Patient evaluation on initial visit

- Patient suffers from chronic GAD symptoms that fluctuate over time
- Clear stress-based, adjustment disorder-driven causes of anxiety are superimposed over a baseline of persistent GAD symptoms
- Despite these symptoms, he is coping fairly well at work and in relationships
- Has been compliant with medication management, but has somewhat fragmented care in that he was seeing different providers who were monitoring his individual medications separately
- Does not appear to be at risk for any suicidal attempts
- Experiences minor sexual side effects and fatigue from his current medications

Current medications

- Hydroxyzine (Vistaril) 50 mg/d (antihistamine anxiolytic)
- Paroxetine (Paxil-CR) 25 mg/d (SSRI)
- Tiagabine (Gabitril) 12 mg/d (SGRI)

Question

In your opinion, does this combination of medications make clinical sense?

- Yes
- No

Attending physician's mental notes: initial evaluation

- This patient has chronic GAD without many comorbidities
- His GAD exacerbations are often triggered by social stressors
- He is motivated, bright, and compliant
- His medication regimen is interesting, and even though it was provided by three different clinicians, it makes rational sense
  - First, the paroxetine-CR was causing side effects at higher doses, thus augmenting with other agents while keeping paroxetine-CR at a low therapeutic dose makes clinical sense
  - Second, hydroxyzine (Vistaril/Atarax) was being used as an anti-allergy medication, but it is approved as an antihistaminergic anxiolytic
  - Third, tiagabine (Gabitril) is an anti-epilepsy medication that has failed monotherapy trials in GAD and PTSD, but has some supportive data as an augmentation strategy for TRA when combined with SSRIs
    - It is a GAT1 GABA reuptake inhibitor that functions to increase endogenous synaptic GABA levels
    - Idiosyncratically, this may cause seizures in non-epileptics who are prescribed this medication in off-label situations
  - Fourth, this regimen facilitates serotonin by blocking the SERT, or reuptake pump, antagonizes histamine activity at the H1 receptor, and facilitates GABA by blocking GAT1 transporters
    - All of these mechanisms are complementary, do not overlap in pharmacodynamic redundancy, and look to manipulate neural pathways involved in the etiology of anxiety

Question

Which of the following would be your next step?

- Increase the paroxetine (Paxil-CR)
- Increase the tiagabine (Gabitril)
- Increase the hydroxyzine (Vistaril)

- Augment the current medications with a fourth agent such as an NRI, a 5-HT1A receptor partial agonist, or a BZ anxiolytic
- Consider him a partial responder on this regimen, which is unacceptable, and streamline and convert him to a less complicated regimen with an SNRI, TCA, or MAOI monotherapy

Attending physician's mental notes: initial evaluation (continued)

- The combination the patient presents with is a good one, covering many mechanisms of action that are individual, yet complementary
- There is a significant family history of addiction, so avoiding BZs makes sense
- He has room to increase any one of his three current medications, but this will likely exacerbate his sexual and fatigue-based side effects further, which the patient will not appreciate

Further investigation

Is there anything else you would especially like to know about this patient?

- What about details concerning his past trauma history?
  - Grew up in less than ideal circumstances with an alcoholic and verbally abusive father
  - Denies overt reliving symptoms but clearly has hyperarousal (worry, muscle tension) thought currently to be from GAD
  - Denies avoidant or phobic behavior
  - Feels psychotherapy has been very helpful
- What about details regarding personality style and coping skills?
  - The patient is socially engaging, hard working, and very active
  - If he is not working, he is exercising and being active
  - Never seems to sit still as he has always been a busy person
  - Keeping busy and exercising allows him to remain calm and more focused
  - Feels he would be distracted and less attentive if he did not have time to exercise

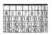

Case outcome: first interim follow-up visit four weeks later

- Declines escalating the SSRI due to sexual side effects
- Felt tiagabine (Gabitril) dosing is reasonable but mildly fatiguing
- As hydroxyzine (Vistaril/Atarax) is the lowest therapeutically dosed of the three, he opts to increase this up to 100 mg/d at the risk of daytime sedation
  - Returns acknowledging the same symptoms as his first appointment
  - States that he is too tired on the increased hydroxyzine dose to continue it

Question

Do you find hydroxyzine a reasonable anxiolytic?

- Yes, for short-term, adjustment-based anxiety symptoms
- Yes, for longitudinal anxiety treatment
- Yes, especially for use in patients who cannot risk taking a BZ anxiolytic, i.e., addictive patients
- Yes, for treating GAD and agitation but not for PD or OCD
- No

Attending physician's mental notes: second interim follow-up visit at two months

- This was easy in that escalating the SSRI seems to be helping gradually
- He is now about 50% better with global improvement in his GAD symptoms and agrees to continue the SSRI and off-label SGRI
- Will need to discuss with him long-term maintenance on the SSRI and also some pharmacologic antidotes if his sexual side effects become intolerable or threaten poor medication adherence in the future
- Tiagabine (Gabitril) has a limited evidence base where switching from an SSRI to tiagabine monotherapy may maintain efficacy while alleviating SSRI sexual dysfunction

Case outcome: second interim follow-up visit at two months

- The patient is tapered off hydroxyzine altogether and begrudgingly agreed to try a higher dose of paroxetine (Paxil-CR) at 37.5 mg /d while continuing the tiagabine (Gabitril) 12 mg/d
  - A moderate reduction in anxiety symptoms occurs
  - There were greater sexual side effects noted
  - Can see the benefit of the increased SSRI dosing
- Felt to be 20%–30% better compared to the last appointment

Question

If he continues toward full symptom remission, but develops major sexual side effects, what would you do?

- Just switch to tiagabine (Gabitril) monotherapy
- Lower the SSRI and try a less sexual side effect-prone drug, such as bupropion-XL (Wellbutrin-XL), trazodone-ER (Oleptro), mirtazapine (Remeron), vilazodone (Viibryd)
- Add bupropion-XL (Wellbutrin-XL) at doses of 300 mg/d or more to the SSRI/SGRI combination to alleviate his sexual dysfunction
- Add buspirone (BuSpar) to alleviate his sexual dysfunction

- Add sildenafil (Viagra) to alleviate his sexual dysfunction
- Lower the SSRI and switch to a BZ as they have lower incidence of sexual side effects

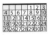

Case outcome: interim follow-up visits through five years

- The patient completes graduate school and finds a permanent job in his field of choice
- Reports much new performance anxiety and hyperarousal around this
- There is now stress in other areas of his life as well, but these create more dysphoria and despondency suggesting possible onset of depressive illness
- Tolerates the same medication regimen with good effects until late in his fifth year of treatment when the adjustment issues and his GAD symptoms begin to escalate
- Begins seeing his psychotherapist again, and is unwilling to increase his SSRI any further

Question

What would you do next?

- Nothing, as the psychotherapy should address his adjustment disorder issues
- Augment the current tiagabine plus paroxetine-CR combination with a third agent
- Switch his currently failing combination to an SNRI

Attending physician's mental notes: interim follow-up visits through five years

- Patient has received a fair amount of anxiety stabilizing treatment from his current two medications (SSRI plus SGRI) for many years
- While there are certainly adjustment disorder issues here, he does genuinely have increased GAD symptoms
- His therapist provides PDP, thus giving him a course of CBT for his performance anxiety is unlikely to help now, as disturbing transference issues should be avoided
- As he is comfortable on his current medications, adding a third agent to re-establish his remission makes sense

Case outcome: interim follow-up visits through six years

- The patient considers much of his newer stress and dysphoria to arise from performance anxiety in his new work
- Starts propranolol (Inderal) up to 30 mg/d as needed, to use specifically for performance anxiety symptoms, and he does well

- For the baseline GAD symptoms, he continues on tiagabine (Gabitril) and paroxetine-CR (Paxil-CR) but is augmented next with L-methylfolate (Deplin) 7.5 mg/d
  - Ideally this can boost the anxiolytic effects of his SSRI and help avoid the need to increase the SSRI further, thus avoiding sexual side effects

Note: L-methylfolate (Deplin) is an approved medical food that may boost the effectiveness of antidepressants in treating depression. Why might this work in anxiety disorders?

- SSRIs treat both depression and anxiety, so should L-methylfolate (Deplin) augmentation
- L-methylfolate theoretically enhances the one-carbon metabolic cycle, which lends to the ability of neurons to make more monoamines, such as serotonin
- L-methylfolate's ability to escalate serotonin levels allows SSRIs to be more effective in that SERT inhibition now accounts for more synaptic serotonin availability when compared to those levels prior to augmentation
  - Essentially, the SSRI now has more serotonin to work with
  - This mechanism theoretically should enhance serotonin antidepressant or anxiolytic efficacy in TRD or TRA
- The patient does not respond to the L-methylfolate (Deplin) augmentation and it is discontinued
- Switches to a combination strategy where the 5-HT1A partial receptor agonist-approved GAD anxiolytic, buspirone (BuSpar) 30 mg/d, is added to the SSRI paroxetine-CR (Paxil-CR) while the SGRI tiagabine (Gabitril) is tapered off and deemed to be ineffective at this point
  - Around this time, warnings that tiagabine may induce seizures in certain non-epilepsy patients also led to the decision to not escalate it further and to discontinue its use
- The combination of buspirone/paroxetine-CR failed to obtain remission

Question

What would you do next?

- Insist he change to a CBT therapist
- Augment with an alpha-2-delta calcium channel blocking antiepileptic medication such as gabapentin (Neurontin) or pregabalin (Lyrica)
- Deem that his SSRI is also ineffective and switch to an SNRI
- Deem that his SSRI is also ineffective and switch to a BZ

Attending physician's mental notes: interim visits through year six

- This patient is appearing to have more significant TRA now
- He is being treated by a competent psychotherapist and is compliant with his medications
- He is very agitated at times, which is interfering with his work
- Would like to use an as-needed BZ while we work out a longer-term strategy, but worries about addiction given his family history
- Failed an SSRI, a 5-HT1A receptor partial agonist, an antihistamine anxiolytic, and an SGRI

Case outcome: interim follow-up visits through six years (continued)

- The patient agrees to taper off paroxetine-CR (Paxil-CR) and is started on an SNRI, duloxetine (Cymbalta), and is titrated to 60 mg/d
  - Its escalation further is limited by side effects of frequent headaches and lightheadedness that do not dissipate with time
- During this time, he is allowed 0.5 mg as needed and uses the BZ GABA-A receptor PAM, alprazolam (Xanax), with close monitoring for misuse
  - Misuse does not occur and the anxiolytic is clinically effective while awaiting the SNRI to become more effective
- At the 60 mg/d monotherapy SNRI dose, the patient states that his GAD symptoms are well controlled but not in remission
  - Still has fluctuating bouts of tenseness, irritability, and worry, regardless of situational stress
  - No longer requires the as-needed alprazolam and it is discontinued
- In addition, states that one of the main residual complaints is inattention, inability to focus on longer tasks. This leads to actual and perceived performance problems at work, raising his anxiety and dysphoria further
  - Interestingly, while physically injured recently and unable to exercise for a few weeks, he realized he is routinely hyperactive
  - Reflects that he has been this way "since he was a kid"

Question

Does this patient have ADHD that was missed in the initial evaluation?

- No, GAD has indecisiveness, inattention, poor concentration, and psychomotor agitation are key symptoms that can look identical to ADHD
- No, the ADHD was not diagnosed in his elementary school years and is not valid as an adult diagnosis as such

- Yes, his GAD has likely been treated to remission, his adjustment disorders have resolved, and these residual symptoms are likely comorbid ADHD that went undiagnosed for years
- Maybe, but it does not matter as inattention as a residual symptom of GAD or from comorbid ADHD may be treated by similar medications

Attending physician's mental notes: interim visits through year six (continued)

- The patient's history, in retrospect, makes a good case for long-standing inattention, which likely predates the GAD onset
- Despite adequate GAD treatment and resolution of social stressors, he is inattentive and not at his peak of possible wellness
- It would be a win–win situation if an augmentation agent could be utilized that might lower his remaining anxiety and also treat his inattentive symptoms
- As his SNRI, duolextine (Cymbalta), has full ability as an NRI, using an ADHD-approved NRI such as atomoxetine (Strattera) would be redundant and likely not be helpful
- Owing to intolerability, his current SNRI cannot be increased to gain better NRI effects
- Adding bupropion-XL (Wellbutrin-XL) might act in a novel manner as a DRI and redundantly as an NRI, would not risk addiction, but again is partially redundant given his SNRI use
- Adding a stimulant or wakefulness-promoting agent may work well for inattention, but escalate his anxiety as a side effect and further risk addiction
- Adding an alpha-2 receptor agonist, such as guanfacine-ER (Intuniv) (approved for child and adolescent ADHD) might allow for an improvement in ADHD-driven inattention or dampen anxiety further, secondarily improving inattention
  - There would be little risk of addiction or escalating his anxiety
  - This drug is also an antihypertensive, hence low blood pressure may be a risk

Case debrief

- GAD is one of the most common anxiety disorders
- GAD is one of the highest comorbidities to occur in those suffering with adult ADHD
- A win–win situation occurs in this comorbidity when the SNRI class of medications is able to treat the anxiety with its SNRI dual mechanism of action, and treat the ADHD symptoms specifically with the SNRI's NRI mechanism
  - In this case, the patient experienced a partial ADHD and GAD clinical response, but not remission

- In order not to escalate this patient's GAD symptoms or risk addiction, stimulants were avoided by using the ADHD medication, guanfacine-ER (Intuniv)
- This was added to his duloxetine (Cymbalta) and titrated to 2 mg/d
- If the patient had comorbid depression (instead of GAD) and ADHD, then a stimulant augmentation might be ideal as it would be less likely to aggravate anxiety (which would not be present), and might carry with it good antidepressant and procognitive effects
- In this patient, low-dose guanfacine-ER improved his attention, concentration, and anxiety to where he was deemed to be in remission from both GAD and ADHD

Take-home points

- There are several ways to treat GAD
- Psychotherapy, SSRI, SNRI, 5-HT1A receptor partial agonism, anti-H1 receptor antagonism, and GABA-A receptor PAM are all mechanistic ways with solid evidence bases with regard to treating GAD symptoms
- Like depression, GAD can become more treatment resistant and the use of combination and augmentation strategies may be utilized in a method similar to that of treating depressive disorders, i.e., rational polypharmacy
- When combining/augmenting, clinicians should use drugs with different mechanisms of action instead of redundant mechanisms, as this may theoretically increase effectiveness and avoid additive side effects
- Some off-label medications may have limited data to support their use, but understanding each medication's mechanism of action gives theoretical backing and permission to use it as long as the prescriber documents the rationale behind its use
- In this case, the SGRI mechanism of tiagabine (Gabitril) would be suggestive for anxiolysis as other medications that facilitate GABA activity (i.e., BZs) help anxiety as well

Performance in practice: confessions of a psychopharmacologist

- *What could have been done better here?*
  - Instead of using polypharmacy approaches with a limited evidence base (e.g., SGRI), consider using solid approved monotherapies earlier for GAD, such as buspirone (BuSpar), Venlafaxine-ER (Effexor-XR), duloxetine (Cymbalta), etc.
  - Instead of considering adult ADHD as a diagnosis of exclusion, evaluate this symptom complex earlier in care
    - Perhaps use of a rating scale, such as the ASRS would help
- *Possible action items for improvement in practice*
  - Research typical comorbidities and presentations for adult ADHD patients

– Research diagnostic rating scales and instruments that may aid in diagnosing ADHD in adults

Tips and pearls

- Antihypertensives are often used in psychopharmacology practice
- Prazosin, an andrenergic alpha-1 receptor antagonist, is gaining popularity for use in treating nightmares associated with PTSD
- Propranolol, a beta-adrenergic receptor antagonist, has been a standard approach in treating performance-type SAD for many years
  - It may also aid in treating and preventing PTSD if used quickly after exposure to traumatic events
- Clonidine and guanfacine, both adrenergic alpha-2 receptor agonists, have been used for treating childhood ADHD, off-label, for many years
  - Clonidine, especially, has been used in an off-label manner to treat agitation and insomnia associated with anxiety disorders as well
  - Slow-release preparations of clonidine and guanfacine are approved for childhood ADHD now (Kapvay and Intuniv)

Mechanism of action moment

Why does adrenergic alpha-2 receptor agonism treat ADHD symptoms?

- Stimulating presynaptic alpha-2 receptors in the LC, with the use of approved antihypertensive medications within this pharmacological family of medicines (e.g., guanfacine [Tenex] and clonidine [Catapres]), dampens adrenergic tone by reducing NE release, and thus causes a lowering of blood pressure
- Dampening of peripheral sympathetic, noradrenergic tone makes sense from an anxiolytic point of view in that palpitations, diaphoresis, tremulousness are driven by the sympathetic nervous system and diminished by certain antihypertensives
  - However, this mechanism may not explain how these drugs treat ADHD, where good cortical noradrenergic tone is actually needed to treat ADHD symptoms
- The slow-release preparations of these medications are now approved for childhood ADHD (e.g., guanfacine-ER [Intuniv] and clonidine-ER [Kapvay])
  - When prescribed for ADHD, they hypothetically stimulate postsynaptic alpha-2 receptors on cortical glutamate pyramidal neurons, instead of those located presynaptically in brainstem regulatory centers that control blood pressure
  - Centrally in the DLPFC, these noradrenergic agonist drugs hypothetically affect postsynaptic cortical heteroreceptors in that they bind to alpha-2 NE heteroreceptors located upon glutamate neurons

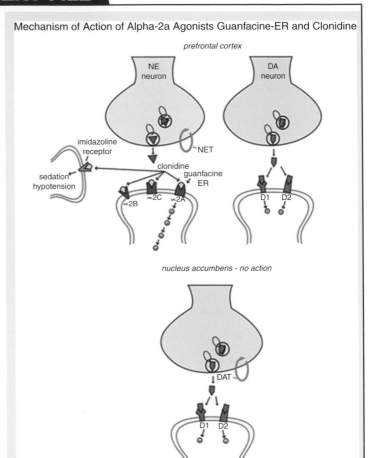

Mechanism of Action of Alpha-2a Agonists Guanfacine-ER and Clonidine

Figure 21.1. Mechanism of action of alpha-2a agonists guanfacine and clonidine.

- Alpha-2 adrenergic receptors
  - Are present throughout the CNS, including the prefrontal cortex, but do not have high concentrations in the nucleus accumbens
  - In particular, are believed to mediate the inattentive, hyperactive, and impulsive symptoms of ADHD, while other alpha-2 adrenergic receptors may have other functions

- Clonidine is an alpha-2 adrenergic receptor agonist that is non-selective, and binds to alpha-2a, -2b, *and* -2c receptors
  - It also binds to imidazoline receptors, which contribute to its more sedating and hypotensive effects as well
  - Although clonidine's actions at alpha-2a receptors make it a therapeutic option for ADHD, its actions at other receptors may increase side effects
  - The slower-release preparation of clonidine (Kapvay) is approved for ADHD, keeping drug plasma levels lower and helping mitigate these side effects
- Guanfacine-ER (Intuniv) is a more selective alpha-2a receptor agonist, and thus has therapeutic efficacy with a reduced side-effect profile as it does not stimulate the alpha-2b and -2c receptors as much as clonidine products do
- In Figure 21.2A, a DLPFC glutamate pyramidal neuron is depicted
- Situated on this neuron's spine is an alpha-2a adrenergic heteroreceptor and a D1 dopaminergic receptor
- These are both connected via cAMP to cation channels called HCN channels
- If DA and NE act in concert and are in balance, binding their respective receptors, then the HCN channels are opened to the appropriate size allowing the pyramidal glutamate neuron to fire efficiently – not too much and not too little
- If millions of these cortical neurons fire efficiently and in synchrony, adequate attention and concentration theoretically occur
- In ADHD, patients may have an imbalance in this cortical system, which allows inefficient processing with subsequent inattention
- In situations such as those with inattention due to ADHD, or even anxiety, these HCN channels may be out of balance
- In Figure 21.2B, endogenous NE may bind to an alpha-2a heteroreceptor and this will in turn close down its associated HCN channel
  - This allows the glutamate pyramidal neuron to retain some of its internal electrical signal (it maintains or improves its signal to noise ratio) and to become focused on its own firing
  - If this occurs, in millions of these neurons, the DLPFC may become more efficient and allow for better focus and concentration symptomatically
- It is at these alpha-2a receptor sites where ADHD medications such as clonidine-ER and guanfacine-ER may exert their anti-ADHD mechanism of action

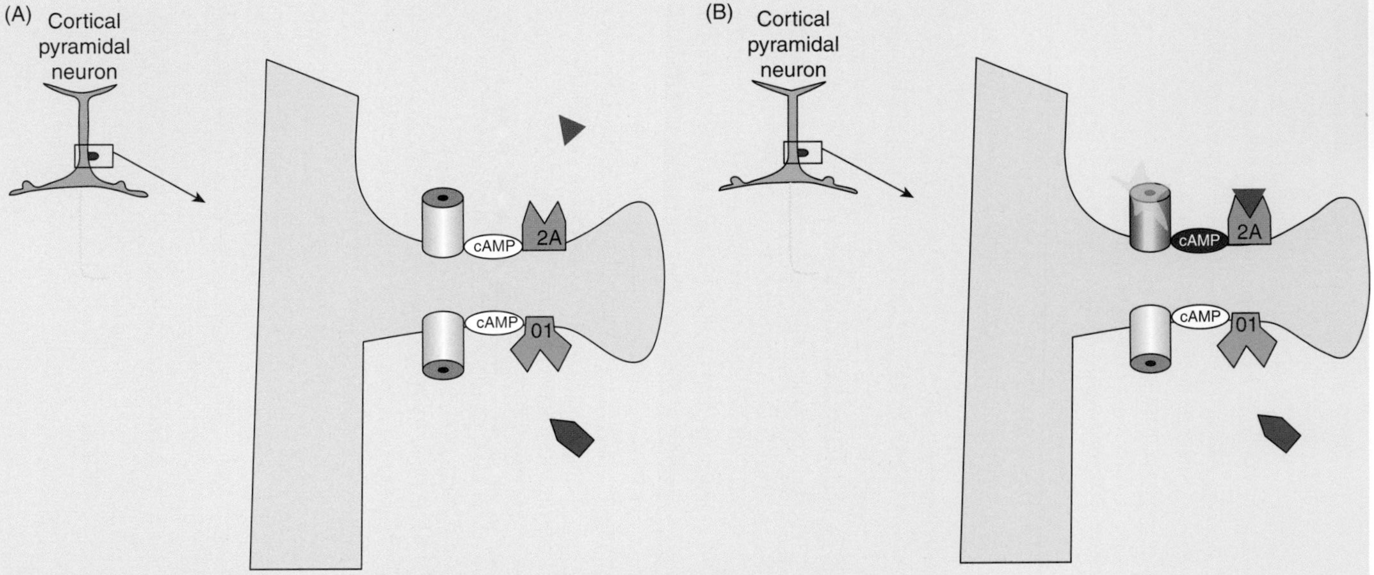
(A)
Cortical
pyramidal
neuron
cAMP
2A
cAMP
01
(B)
Cortical
pyramidal
neuron
cAMP
2A
cAMP
01

Figure 21.2. The pyradimal glutamate neuron: structure and mechanism of action of receptors.

Two-minute tutorial

Using antihypertensives in psychiatric practice

- Clinicians have to be aware and competent in their use
  - This may be achieved by reading each drug's approved package insert or by reviewing relative prescribing textbooks
- All antihypertensives are *antihypertensive;* therefore, a key therapeutic effect in patients with elevated blood pressure includes a lowering of the problematic blood pressure
  - However, in psychiatric care, many of our patients treated with antihypertensives are actually normotensive, so that lowering their blood pressure may not be desired
- A standard of care likely should involve routine blood pressure monitoring in the office setting of the psychopharmacologist because
  - Many of our antidepressant medications that elevate NE may increase blood pressure
  - Many of our medications that increase weight gain may increase blood pressure
  - Many of our medications that antagonize alpha-2a or alpha-1 receptors may lower blood pressure
- These three things likely encompass most prescribing practices, and therefore, should drive better use of blood pressure monitoring

Clinical pearls should include

- In those patients who are normotensive, provide adequate informed consent and start at low doses of the antihypertensive drug being used
- Warn of common side effects: lightheadedness, dizziness, orthostasis, and syncope
- Suggest patients start treatment on a day where they can afford to lie down and not drive, if they need to combat fatigue or hypotensive side effects
- Initially suggest patients also increase fluids and salts if these side effects occur
- Start at a lower than normal dose when compared to patients suffering from essential HTN, and titrate more slowly to avoid side effects
- Consider teaching the patient to self-monitor at home with a commercially available automated blood pressure cuff/system
- A win–win scenario may occur if the patient is hypertensive from an idiopathic or iatrogenic point of view
  - For example, if the patient becomes hypertensive on an SNRI (iatrogenic) or comes to your practice with essential HTN

(idiopathic), then use of an antihypertensive becomes warranted for the HTN *and* for their ADHD, insomnia, or anxiety
- Clinicians, in these cases, may treat HTN and psychiatric symptoms simultaneously

Posttest self-assessment question and answer

How does an alpha-2a receptor agonist really improve attention?

A. It lowers NE output similar to its antihypertensive effects
B. It promotes DA activity in the DLPFC secondarily
C. It lowers GABA activity, which allows greater glutamate activity in the thalamus
D. It allows fine tuning of cortical pyramidal glutamate neurons to improve signal to noise ratios in cortical information processing

Answer: D

As depicted in the figures in this case, specifically for inattention symptoms, these antihypertensive, alpha-2 noradrenergic receptor agonists act upon heteroreceptors. They modulate glutamate pyramidal neurons originating in the frontal cortex. In synchrony with other pyramidal neurons, alpha-2 receptor agonists improve signal to noise ratios and may fine tune neuronal firing, thus improving attention and concentration. Lowering NE tone for HTN reasons would not help attention. This is a separate mechanism of action. Alpha-2 agonists do not promote DA activity; rather they act in concert with endogenous DA activity, which occurs at the D1 receptor also situated on glutamate neurons. The alpha-2 agonists do not manipulate GABA in order to modulate glutamate neurons.

References

1. Stahl SM. Novel therapeutics for depression: L-methylfolate as a trimonoamine modulator and antidepressant-augmenting agent. *CNS Spectr* 2007; 12:739–74.
2. Jensen PS, Hinshaw SP, Kraemer HC, et al. Bottom of form ADHD comorbidity findings from the MTA study: comparing comorbid subgroups. *J Am Acad Child Adolesc Psychiatry* 2001; 40:147–58.
3. Schatz DB, Rostain AL. ADHD with comorbid anxiety. A review of the current literature. *J Atten Disord* 2006; 10:141–9.
4. Schwartz TL, Nasra G, Ashton A, et al. An open-label study to evaluate switching from SSRI or SNRI to Tiagabine to alleviate antidepressant-induced sexual dysfunction in generalized anxiety disorder. *Ann Clin Psychiatry* 2007; 19:25–30.
5. Schwartz TL, Nihalani N, Simionescu M, Hopkins G. History repeats itself: pharmacodynamic trends in the treatment of anxiety. *Curr Pharmaceut Design* 2005; 11:255–64.

6. Vaiva G, Ducrocq F, Jezequel K, et al. Immediate treatment with propranolol decreases posttraumatic stress disorder two months after trauma. *Biol Psychiatry* 2003; 54:947–9.

7. Hoehn-Saric R, Merchant AF, Keyser ML, Smith VK. Effects of Clonidine on anxiety disorders. *Arch Gen Psychiatry* 1981; 38:1278–82.

8. Hollifield M, Mackey A, Davidson J. Integrating therapies for anxiety disorders. *Psychiatr Ann* 2006; 36:329–38.

9. Stahl SM. *Stahl's Essential Psychopharmacology*, 4th edn. New York, NY: Cambridge University Press, 2013.

10. Stahl SM. *Stahl's Essential Psychopharmacology: The Prescriber's Guide*, 5th edn. New York, NY: Cambridge University Press, 2014.

11. Belkin M, Schwartz TL. Alpha-2 receptor agonists for the treatment of posttraumatic stress disorder. *Drugs in Context*. 2015; 4:212286.

The Case: This one's too hot, this one's too cold. . .this one is just right

The Question: What to do when patients cannot tolerate low-dose atypical antipsychotics

The Dilemma: Activation or sedation, not sure what you are going to get when taking the atypical antipsychotics

Pretest self-assessment question (answer at the end of the case)

In which of the following clinical situations is ECT felt to be robustly effective?

A. MDD with psychotic features
B. MDD
C. OCD
D. Schizophrenia
E. A and B
F. A, B, and C
G. All of the above
H. None of the above

Patient evaluation on intake

- 18-year-old man states he has been "depressed all year"
- He has been reasonably successful in high school, enjoys athletics, has a girlfriend, and should be happy
- He is not, he is despondent to the point of being suicidal

Psychiatric history

- Reports increasing MDD symptoms over the last several months
  - Cannot sleep without medication
  - Is fatigued and cannot concentrate at school, and is allowed to attend for half days as a result
  - Reports marked guilt as he is letting others down
  - He is convinced he will never get better
  - Admits daily suicidal thinking that so far he has not acted on, but states it is "a struggle every day"
  - Experiences intrusive "images" where he sees himself hurting himself or others that he deems separate from his suicidal thinking, which he states are "clearly his own thoughts"
    ○ These images started shortly after the depression began
- These MDD symptoms started after a break up with a girlfriend, but never remitted, even as his social life improved

- He has long-standing feelings that people do not like him and has low self-esteem despite being a well-rounded and accomplished teenager, as he was picked on for being overweight as a child
  - He is not overweight now
- There is no evidence of sustained manic episodes, anxiety disorder, eating disorder, or SUD, confirmed by corroborative history and diagnostic rating scales
  - Interestingly, his previous provider had diagnosed him with bipolar disorder and ADHD
  - He transitioned to this provider on a stimulant, a mood stabilizer, and an antidepressant

Social and personal history

- Due to graduate high school on time this year but has had academic accommodations given his MDD
- Parents are married and supportive
- Has no siblings
- Does not abuse substances, nicotine, or caffeine

Medical history

- There are no medical issues

Family history

- There is no family history of bipolar disorder or schizophrenia
- Uncles may have AUD
- Aunts may have MDD

Medication history

- First took an SSRI, fluoxetine (Prozac) 20 mg/d, without effect, one and a half years ago
  - This did not alleviate MDD symptoms and next was augmented with the atypical antipsychotic aripiprazole (Abilify) 5–10 mg/d
  - This caused a marked increase in suicidal thinking and symptoms consistent with EPS-based akathisia
- Since this time, he has been taking
  - Escitalopram (Lexapro) 10 mg/d (SSRI)
  - d/l-amphetamine salts (Adderall) 15 mg/d (stimulant)
  - Divalproex sodium-ER (Depakote-ER) 750 mg/d (mood stabilizer)

Psychotherapy history

- Sees a clinical social worker routinely for supportive psychotherapy

- He is given supportive, problem-oriented psychotherapy, and has a good rapport with this provider
- He looks forward to sessions

Patient evaluation on initial visit

- Patient suffers from a single, severe, and possibly psychotic MDD
- He sees images that look like "videos playing" vividly in front of him
  - These are intrusive and ego-dystonic
  - Tries to avoid thinking of these images
  - They sound like obsessive, intrusive images consistent with OCD but could be ruminations or even psychotic visual hallucinations
- He has a blunted affect, concrete thoughts, and mild thought slowing
  - This could be from MDD
  - Also need to consider these as negative symptoms, that his obsessive images are frank hallucinations, and that this is a schizophrenia prodrome
- Has been compliant with medication management and psychotherapy
- Suicidal thinking is readily apparent, serious, and problematic
- There is no evidence of bipolarity

Current medications

- Escitalopram (Lexapro) 10 mg/d (SSRI)
- d/l-amphetamine salts (Adderall) 15 mg/d (stimulant)
- Divalproex sodium-ER (Depakote-ER) 750 mg/d (mood stabilizer)

Question

Do you think his obsessive images are from MDD or OCD?

- OCD as they are intrusive images that appear in the distance, instead of being generated internally, and he does not interact with them
- OCD as they often depict a loss of control and violence toward himself or others, which he does not identify with and they horrify him
- MDD as these images started after the MDD and increased as his MDD escalated
- MDD as these images were never present when euthymic
- Neither; these are paranoid in nature and may be early schizophrenia or schizoaffective disorder
- Neither as they are likely induced by his stimulant
- Not sure as all of these are plausible

Attending physician's mental notes: initial evaluation

- This patient has a risky, severe MDD given his symptoms and suicidal thinking

- The images appear to be intrusive, obsessive images, or depressive ruminations rather than psychotic ones
- Negative and cognitive symptoms appear consistent with vegetative MDD
- His medication regimen is interesting and cannot be explained easily
  - There are no defined (hypo)mania spells, based on careful interview with patient and family
  - Rating scales suggest no current mania, nor mixed features
  - The inattention and poor concentration symptoms seem consistent with inattentive ADHD
    - Patient feels he has always been this way but is worse over last one to two years
    - Parents and school records suggest no problems academically or behaviorally in elementary school that would be consistent with ADHD
    - Stimulant has not helped and may have made him worse
    - If he has bipolar disorder, he should be stabilized on the divalproex (Depakote) but might be destabilized on the antidepressant and stimulant, which could be problematic
    - The inattention and cognitive dysfunction currently are likely due to depression, agitation, and not ADHD

Question

Which of the following would be your next step?

- Discontinue the mood stabilizer, divalproex (Depakote)
- Discontinue the stimulant, d/l-mixed amphetamine salts (Adderall), and increase the SSRI antidepressant
- Discontinue all but the SSRI, augment it with an atypical antipsychotic, admit to an inpatient psychiatric unit

Attending physician's mental notes: initial evaluation (continued)

- The medication combinations the patient presents with are not effective. They may even be worsening the patient's original MDD symptoms
- The patient is horribly depressed but resilient enough to maintain some schooling and some friendships
- He is suicidal, but has many psychosocial supports and an extensive safety plan that has successfully avoided inpatient hospitalization
- He either has psychotic MDD or MDD with comorbid OCD

PATIENT FILE

Further investigation

Is there anything else you would especially like to know about this patient?

- Could the obsessional/psychotic images be organic?
  - There is no history of head injury
  - There is no evidence of migraine or seizure activity
  - He is forthcoming about random experimentation regarding illicit drugs but does not seem to have had any acute use to explain these symptoms
  - Blood laboratory tests, EEG, and MRI were negative
- What about details regarding his personality style and coping skills?
  - The patient has been socially engaging
  - Seems a bit dependent on his family and perhaps enmeshed
    - It is unclear if this is his usual personality pattern or
    - If owing to MDD causing a regression into more severe personality traits or
    - If owing to the sick role he has accommodated due to his severe MDD
  - Does not appear to have affective dyscontrol, mood swings outside those triggered by his depressive state
  - Often is rejection sensitive with some avoidant traits due to being picked on as a youngster
  - Does not seem to meet clear criteria for a personality disorder diagnosis, but has certain dependent/avoidant traits that are troublesome

Case outcome: first interim follow-up visits one to two weeks later

- All medications except for the SSRI escitalopram (Lexapro) are discontinued
- The SSRI is increased to 20 mg/d because
  - The 10 mg/d dose was not effective
  - The intrusive images are felt to be obsessional, and often high-dose SSRIs are needed to alleviate OCD symptoms
- A SARI, trazodone (Desyrel) 50–100 mg at bedtime, is given to treat insomnia
  - Insomnia is an acute risk factor for suicide
  - Aggressive treatment here may lower risk of suicide and avoid an inpatient stay
  - He immediately sleeps better and his suicidal ideation is reduced
  - This off-label use of an SARI may also provide MDD augmentation treatment

Question

If his images are from OCD, how long should a clinician wait for an SSRI to become effective?

- A few weeks at the minimum therapeutic dose, just like treating other anxiety disorders
- Several weeks at the minimum dose as OCD responds more slowly than other anxiety disorders
- Several weeks at a high dose are often required to adequately treat OCD
- A dozen weeks at a high dose is often required to adequately treat OCD

Attending physician's mental notes: second interim follow-up visit at three to four weeks

- Several more weeks may be needed for the SSRI to take effect
- What if these symptoms are psychotic?
  - SSRI sometimes treat depressive psychosis, but an antipsychotic may be warranted
- Atypical antipsychotics are often used in OCD patients who fail to respond to adequate dose and duration of SSRI treatment
  - This patient has not had an adequate dose and duration of his high-dose SSRI yet, but waiting several weeks may be too risky
  - Using an atypical antipsychotic now could speed his response to his SSRI
  - It may also decrease his agitation acutely

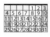

Case outcome: second interim follow-up visit at three to four weeks

- The patient is no better
  - Depressed and suicidal still
  - His intrusive images continue
  - He is "fed up waiting to get better" and is not sure "how much more he can take"
  - He and his parents ask if there is anything more to do outside waiting for his SSRI to become effective
- Inpatient admission is considered
- Outpatient collaboration of providers and number of visits is increased instead

Question

What would you do?

- Admit to an inpatient setting and modify treatments there
- Await for 20 mg/d escitalopram (Lexapro) to become effective while increasing psychosocial supports and safety planning

- Increase escitalopram (Lexapro) to 30 mg/d, which is super-dosed and off-label, but may be warranted and helpful in treatment-resistant OCD
- Add an atypical antipsychotic
- Add a BZ

Case outcome: interim follow-up visits through four to six weeks later

- An atypical antipsychotic is added to his escitalopram (Lexapro) 20 mg/d and the trazodone (Desyrel) 50–100 mg at bedtime
  - Ziprasidone (Geodon) 20 mg twice a day is started
    - ○ The first few days is taken without food, to lower its bioavailabilty by half and to hopefully avoid akathisia similar to what occurred with the prior aripiprazole (Abilify) trial
    - ○ This is changed to with food to obtain full bioavailability and allow further dose titration after a few days
    - ○ This atypical antipsychotic is chosen, as similar to aripiprazole, ziprasidone tends to minimize weight gain and metabolic disorder side effects relative to other atypical antipsychotics
      - ▪ This teenager is sensitive to his weight and does not want to gain weight
- There is too much sedation
  - Asks for a medication change
  - This increases his despondency, as he knows titration will take longer and that he feels more worthless as he sleeps more and is even less productive and worthwhile
- The atypical antipsychotic ziprasidone is tapered off and the atypical antipsychotic lurasidone (Latuda) is started instead
  - A similar strategy due to absorption and bioavailability is employed, where he takes it without food for a few days
    - ○ This keeps the initial dose and EPS risk lower
  - Next, it is taken with food; however, unlike ziprasidone, lurasidone is therapeutic in treating his psychosis at 40 mg/d
  - Similar to ziprasidone, this newer atypical antipsychotic also carries a lower risk of weight gain and metabolic disorder compared to other agents in the class
- However, family calls to report that he is worse in between sessions
- There is more agitation, sleep is worse, and he gets shivers and sweats with some palpitations and headaches now
  - This is not like the activating and akathisia side effects where he was restless on aripiprazole (Abilify) and fluoxetine (Prozac)

- This is felt to be mild serotonin syndrome from the current SSRI, escitalopram, SARI, trazodone, and his recently added atypical antipsychotic, lurasidone (Latuda)
  - The latter interacts at 5-HT2A, 5-HT1A, and 5-HT7 receptors
- Lurasidone (Latuda) is lowered to 40 mg/d *without* food (likely 20 mg equivalent bioavailability) and the side effects resolve
- Several days later in an attempt to obtain better efficacy with the atypical antipsychotic, he is rechallenged with 40 mg/d with food and the same side effects return

Question

How can you tell akathisia from mild serotonin syndrome?

- Akathisia is either internal or external restlessness where the patient feels as though he or she needs to move incessantly, usually without other systemic side effects present
- Mild serotonin syndrome, or toxicity, can have restlessness that is often attributed to anxiety and agitation
  - The symptoms are often described as a clinical triad of abnormalities
    - Cognitive effects: headache, agitation, hypomania, mental confusion, hallucinations, coma
    - Autonomic effects: shivering, sweating, hyperthermia, HTN, tachycardia, nausea, diarrhea
    - Somatic effects: myoclonus (muscle twitching), hyperreflexia (manifested by clonus), tremor

Attending physician's mental notes: interim follow-up visits through six weeks

- Patient is still depressed, suicidal with intrusive images
- Failed an SSRI plus three separate atypical antipsychotic augmentations, all due to different side effects: akathisia, sedation, mild serotonin toxicity
- Several weeks of high-dose SSRI has not improved symptoms
- Outpatient personal and psychiatric support maximized in attempts to keep him safe and avoid a psychiatric hospitalization

Case outcome interim follow-up visits through 10 weeks

- Lurasidone (Latuda) is discontinued and the mild serotonin toxicity resolves
- As the differential diagnosis is still MDD with psychosis versus MDD plus OCD, or even mixed features, use of an atypical antipsychotic is still warranted
- He is started on the fourth atypical antipsychotic, asenapine (Saphris)

- Takes subtherapeutic 5 mg sublingual initially as this drug has a more sedating profile, which previously disturbed him while taking ziprasidone previously
- This agent is known less for its akathisia and more for its sedating side effects
- Metabolically, its trial data suggests minimal weight gain or metabolic problems over the long term, comparatively speaking
- Trazodone (Desyrel) is discontinued and the asenapine (Saphris) increased to 10 mg sublingual, at bedtime to avoid oversedation in the mornings
  - Asenapine (Saphris) is usually dosed twice daily
  - In this case, as the patient is sensitive to sedation, it is felt better to leave all until bedtime to improve tolerability
  - Asenapine's half-life is 24 h; thus, theoretically, it should allow for antipsychotic effects dosed once a day
  - It is the only atypical antipsychotic requiring sublingual dosing because the drug is not absorbed after swallowing whole as it cannot become activated
- Tolerates escitalopram (Lexapro) 20 mg/d plus asenapine (Saphris) 10 mg/d and seems to appreciate getting to a combination that does not bother him or make him worse
  - He appears less despondent and more hopeful
- Still is very depressed with intrusive images and asks for more aggressive medication options
  - Offered an escalation of the escitalopram SSRI to an off-label 30 mg/d as extra high doses of SSRI are warranted in some OCD patients
  - Offered a higher dose of the atypical antipsychotic asenapine again as a boost for his OCD, MDD, or as an antipsychotic in case his images are frank hallucinations
    - Chooses to increase the SSRI to 30 mg/d

Case debrief

- The patient has clear MDD with risky suicidal features
- He was treated with aggressive medication changes to better treat these symptoms and improve tolerability of his regimen
- His diagnosis was complicated by intrusive images
  - When first reported, appeared to be classic obsessions as described in *DSM-5*
  - However, clearly these were externally experienced like psychotic visual and auditory hallucinations that developed after his MDD began

- Despite the medication changes and maximized psychosocial supports, the patient continued to be suicidal and eventually his safety could not be guaranteed
- The patient did not want to go to an inpatient hospital and astutely asked if there were any treatments that were faster that could be used to lower his symptoms to avoid a hospital stay
  - Round the clock observation was arranged by family members at home
  - Outpatient ECT was arranged
    - ○ The patient received seven treatments over two to three weeks
    - ○ Tolerated these procedures well with the usual post-ECT fatigue and anterograde amnesia
- MDD symptoms based on the IDS lowered from severe depression (43) to remission (3)
- He continues escitalopram (Lexapro) 30 mg/d, asenapine (Saphris) 10 mg/d, and weekly supportive psychotherapy
- He has no side effects, including the absence of EPS, weight gain, and metabolic disorder
- In retrospect, he is more definitively diagnosed with psychotic MDD as OCD tends not to respond to ECT treatments, where typically only anecdotal case reports support its use

Take-home points

- Psychotic MDD often has guilt-based delusions, but sometimes hallucinations may be the principal psychotic symptom, as in this case
- Atypical antipsychotics are plentiful and numerous
  - They are all equally effective for psychosis in schizophrenia but have unique side-effect profiles that may affect individual tolerability
- Sometimes, several atypical antipsychotics must be tried in sequence to obtain the best balance of efficacy and tolerability
- ECT is very effective in treating psychotic MDD

Performance in practice: confessions of a psychopharmacologist

What could have been done better here?

- Simply escalating and waiting for high-dose SSRI effectiveness may have avoided side effects associated with trials of a myriad of atypical antipsychotics
- Occasionally depressive psychoses respond to SSRI alone
- Despite his young age of 18, ECT could have been provided earlier

Possible action items for improvement in practice

- Research the differential diagnostic dilemmas between MDD with psychosis versus OCD
- Research the use of ECT in young adults

Tips and pearls

- Atypical antipsychotics appear to be roughly equal in efficacy in treating schizophrenia and in many cases of bipolar mania
- Atypical antipsychotics are not equal in treating depressive disorders, as at present, only olanzapine, quetiapine, aripiprazole, brexpiprazole and lurasidone are approved for depressive disorder treatment
- Atypical antipsychotics are relatively understudied in the treatment of anxiety disorders and there are no approvals
- Choose an atypical antipsychotic based on approval status, evidence base availability, and its purported mechanisms of action
- Otherwise, it is often wise to choose based on side effect profiles
  - Sedating or not
  - Weight-gain-promoting or not
  - EPS-prone or not
  - QTc prolongation-promoting or not

Two-minute tutorial

Acute suicide risk

Chronic risks

- The most consistent demographic risks include being male, over 45 years old, white, living alone, and having a chronic medical illness where the patient perceives poor health
- Completed suicides are most likely in older men who use more lethal means
  - These patients often have an associated mood disorder and substance abuse
- Suicidal ideation is common and has been reported to occur in up to a third of the population in general
- It is estimated that there are 18 suicide attempts for every completed suicide
- Women have a higher rate of attempted suicide but much lower rates of completion
- Men are four times more likely to complete suicide
- Suicide is higher among whites and Native Americans than among African Americans, Hispanics, or Asians
  - 73% of all suicides in the United States are committed by white men
- The strongest overall predictor for suicide is the presence of psychiatric illness
  - MDD and AUD are the most frequently made diagnoses in persons who commit suicide
  - More than 90% of all persons who commit suicide have a diagnosable psychiatric illness

- 5% of suicides occur in patients with chronic medical illnesses
- Other patients at risk for suicide include those diagnosed with schizophrenia, borderline personality, antisocial personality, bipolar disorder, persistent depressive disorder, SUD, narcissistic personality disorder, and anxiety disorder

Acute risks predictive of future suicide attempt include*

- Severe anxiety (92%) or panic attacks (80%)
- Depressed mood (80%)
- Recent loss of close relationship (78%)
- Alcohol or substance abuse (68%)
- Hopelessness (64%)
- Helplessness (62%)
- Worthlessness (29%)
- Global insomnia (46%)
- Partial insomnia (92%)
- Anhedonia (43%)
- Chronic deteriorating medical illness (41%)
- Inability to maintain job or student status (36%)
- Recent onset of impulsive behavior (29%)
- Recent diagnosis of a life-threatening illness (e.g., cancer, AIDS) (9%)
  - Interestingly, 69% of patients do not admit suicidal thoughts prior to attempt
  - 67% of patients have no previous suicidal behaviors

*Percentage of patients exhibiting acute symptoms prior to suicide attempt

Summary

- Both chronic demographics and acute suicide risks should be assessed in treatment planning
- Any prescribed medication in these cases should be chosen based upon tolerability and safety in overdose for these at-risk patients
- Psychotropics may actually lower some of these acute risk variables and save lives
  - Lithium has regulatory data and indication for lowering suicidal thinking in bipolar disorder
  - Clozapine has similar findings in schizophrenia
  - BZ sedatives may actively lower insomnia or anxiety (acute predictive risk factors) within single doses or within a few days of dose escalation
    - Limited quantities should be issued in case of overdose
    - Likely should not be used in alcohol-or opiate-misusing patients
  - Atypical antipsychotics may act similarly
    - Limited quantities should be issued due to potential QTc prolongation in case of marked overdose

- ○ Some atypical antipsychotics cause akathisia more than others
  - Adding this side effect to insomnia and agitation might provoke more suicide risk
  - Proper warning, informed consent, and provider access likely would mitigate this

Posttest self-assessment question and answer

In which of the following clinical situations is ECT felt to be robustly effective?

A. MDD with psychotic features
B. MDD
C. OCD
D. Schizophrenia
E. A and B
F. A, B, and C
G. All of the above
H. None of the above

Answer: E

ECT is one of the most effective acute treatments for MDD. It is noted to be an excellent treatment for psychotic MDD as well. There is some evidence to suggest that ECT can help in schizophrenia, perhaps with certain negative symptoms, and those suffering from schizoaffective conditions. There is little evidence to support its use in OCD.

References

1. Stahl SM. *Stahl's Essential Psychopharmacology*, 4th edn. New York, NY: Cambridge University Press, 2013.
2. Stahl SM. *Stahl's Essential Psychopharmacology: The Prescriber's Guide*, 5th edn. New York, NY: Cambridge University Press, 2014.
3. Citrome L. Lurasidone for schizophrenia: a review of the efficacy and safety profile for this newly approved second-generation antipsychotic. *Int J Clin Pract* 2011; 65:189–210.
4. Stahl SM. Antidepressant treatment of psychotic major depression: potential role of the sigma receptor. *CNS Spectr* 2005; 10:319–23.
5. Megna J, Schwartz TL, Siddiqui U, Herrara-Rojas M. Obesity in adults with serious and persistent mental illness: a review of postulated mechanisms and current interventions. *Ann Clin Psychiatry* 2011; 23:131–40.
6. Boyer EW, Shannon M. The serotonin syndrome. *N Engl J Med* 2005; 352: 1112–20.
7. Dunkley EJ, Isbister GK, Sibbritt D, Dawson AH, Whyte IM. The Hunter serotonin toxicity criteria: simple and accurate diagnostic decision rules for serotonin toxicity. *QJM* 2003; 96:635–42.

8. Citrome L. Asenapine for schizophrenia and bipolar disorder: a review of the efficacy and safety profile for this newly approved sublingually absorbed second-generation antipsychotic. *Int J Clin Pract* 2009; 63:1762–84.

9. Marazziti D, Consoli G. Treatment strategies for obsessive-compulsive disorder. *Expert Opin Pharmacother* 2010; 11:331–43.

10. Hall RC, Platt DE, Hall RC. Suicide risk assessment: a review of risk factors for suicide in 100 patients who made severe suicide attempts: evaluation of suicide risk in a time of managed care. *Psychosomatics* 1999; 40:18–27.

11. American Psychiatric Association. *Diagnostic and Statistical Manual of Mental Disorders Revised*, 4th edn. Washington, DC: American Psychiatric Association Press, 2000.

12. Bedynerman K, Schwartz TL. Utilizing pharmacodynamic properties of second generation antipsychotics to guide treatment. *Drugs of Today* 2012; 48;283–92.

The Case: Schizophrenia patient needs sleep

The Question: What if patients are not responsive to benzodiazepine sedative–hypnotic agents?

The Dilemma: Non-benzodiazepine hypnotics may or may not work if patients have been taking benzodiazepines routinely

Pretest self-assessment question (answer at the end of the case)

Which of the following antidepressants is also formally approved for treating insomnia?

A. Quetiapine
B. Diphenhydramine
C. Hydroxyzine
D. Trazodone
E. Amitriptyline
F. Doxepin
G. All of the above
H. None of the above

Patient evaluation on intake

- 36-year-old man states he "cannot sleep"
- He is all "worked up" and his "head is all wrong at night"

Psychiatric history

- Has been seen in practice over the last 10 years
- Was admitted after two psychotic episodes
- During these discrete spells he was noted to
  - Be hyper-religious in a paranoid manner
  - Be responding to internal stimuli
  - Experience occasional catatonic stupors
- There is a baseline of mild negative symptoms where he
  - Is concrete in his thoughts and abstractions
  - Laughs at odd times
  - Talks loudly and at close interpersonal space
- There are no other psychiatric comorbidities including substance misuse, mania, depression, or anxiety disorder

Social and personal history

- Graduated high school
- Works in the family business, which is considered a sheltered work environment, otherwise has not been gainfully employed
- Single and has no close friendships outside extended family and church members

- Has been involved and seems accepted in community volunteer activities
- Does not misuse substances, nicotine, or caffeine

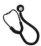

Medical history

- There are no medical issues
- He is routinely screened for metabolic disorders in conjunction with his PCP and currently is healthy

Family history

- There is no family history of schizophrenia
- Grandparents may have suffered MDD and GAD on both sides

Medication history

- During the first two psychotic episodes he was placed on antipsychotics with remission of psychotic symptoms but with continued residual negative symptoms
  - The typical antipsychotic, haloperidol (Haldol) 10 mg/d for the first psychotic episode
  - The atypical antipsychotic, risperidone (Risperdal) 4 mg/d and the BZ clonazepam (Klonopin) 1 mg/d during the second episode
    ○ This atypical antipsychotic was used to lower the psychotic symptoms, hopefully improve the negative symptoms, lower acute EPS risk and the longitudinal TD risk
- Remained without psychosis over the last decade on this last set of medications and now presents as a new patient because his psychiatrist has retired

Psychotherapy history

- Attended supportive psychotherapy routinely throughout the last 10 years
- Enjoys meeting his therapist
- Looks forward to sessions although he is concrete and not psychologically minded regarding the perceived benefits
  - He cannot identify how therapy helps him

Patient evaluation on initial visit

- Patient suffers from undifferentiated schizophrenia with paranoid and catatonic features
  - These terms are obsolete in the *DSM-5* but do seem to quickly and accurately describe this patient's schizophrenic presentation over the years

- Over last several years, suffers only negative symptoms, making him appear more a residual schizophrenic
- There are no other complaints regarding the schizophrenia now and he would like to continue his medications as given

Current medications

- Risperidone (Risperdal) 4 mg/d (atypical antipsychotic)
- Clonazepam (Klonopin) 1 mg/d (BZ)

Question

Over the last several years, this patient has suffered from only negative symptoms. What do you think will happen next?

- He will remain a residual schizophrenic for the rest of his life
- He will likely have a paranoid or catatonic relapse sometime
- He will likely develop psychiatric comorbidities such as MDD or an anxiety disorder

Attending physician's mental notes: initial evaluation

- This patient has had two schizophrenic psychotic episodes after a classic prodrome
- He is now doing well due to excellent medication and visit compliance, as well as his family's support
- Suspect that if his medications are maintained, he will continue only with negative symptoms
- Will likely have to contend with movement or metabolic disorder side effects over time

Question

Which of the following would be your next step?

- Do nothing as his medications are optimal
- Lower his atypical antipsychotic slightly as he has been quite stable and this might lower his risk for long-term side effects
- Lower the BZ sedative anxiolytic as he is not anxious or agitated anymore

Attending physician's mental notes: initial evaluation (continued)

- The combination of medications the patient is taking is currently effective and without side effects
- As this was his first office visit, it may make sense to develop and maintain a solid rapport instead of making medication changes to a seemingly good regimen

- It makes sense to keep in mind that reducing his antipsychotic to its minimally effective dose and lowering his anxiolytic may be worth considering for future visits

Further investigation

Is there anything else you would especially like to know about this patient?

- Some of the patient's negative symptoms seem atypical
  - He tends to talk loudly
  - He speaks in close proximity to people
  - He often has an odd affect and odd prosody of speech
  - In discussions with his family at the initial visit, "he has always been that way"
    - He has had few friends, but has been content
    - He has not exhibited anxiety about missing a clear, distinct peer group
    - After his positive symptoms developed, these premorbid social interaction deficits have remained the same but have been labeled as "negative symptoms" instead of his premorbid personality style
- Were these negative symptoms really present since childhood?
  - It is unlikely that these negative schizophrenia symptoms were a 20-year prodrome
  - The patient may have a developmental disorder such as an ASD which predates his first psychotic break
  - He does not meet ASD criteria formally
  - His IQ is likely low-average, e.g., 85–100, but has never been formally tested
  - There are no clear chromosomal abnormality stigmata nor maternal infectious exposure stigmata
  - He is a likeable, straightforward, socially awkward, talkative man

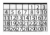

Case outcome: first interim follow-up visits through six months

- Clinically continues without change
- Risperidone (Risperdal) is lowered to 3 mg/d to avoid long-term movement disorder and metabolic risk, and due to the fact that he has been largely asymptomatic
- Later reports an increase in anxiety over interpersonal interactions and states he now has insomnia
- There are no re-emergent positive psychotic symptoms
- Clonazepam (Klonopin) is increased to 2 mg/d taken at night to cover these anxiety and insomnia symptoms, with good effect
- Later, risperidone (Risperdal) is lowered to 2 mg/d without incident

Question

Can traditional BZ sedative–anxiolytics be used as sedative–hypnotics too?

- No, these are separate approvals and only sedative–hypnotics should be used to treat insomnia
- No, sedative–anxiolytics are less sedating and tend not to promote sleep
- Yes, both classes are BZs, which are PAMs at the GABA-A receptor and may promote fatigue, somnolence, and induce sleep
- Yes, although off-label, the sedative–anxiolytics are less sedating than the sedative–hypnotics, but increasing the dose of the anxiolytic is often accompanied by increasing sedation and ultimately hypnosis

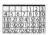

Case outcome: second interim follow-up visits through 12 months

- There is no psychosis but an increase in insomnia is reported again
  - This stresses the patient as he is worrying about his lack of sleep and has the clinical feel of classic, primary insomnia
  - He is more irritable
  - He dislikes doing his usual activities as he is tired and not his usual self
  - He enjoys things less as such
  - He has no other worries outside his pending insomnia every night
- Denies depression feelings and reports there are no acute stressful events at home or work
  - There is a possibility that the insomnia is the sentinel symptom of a depressive episode or a third psychotic episode

Question

What would you do next?

- Increase the risperidone (Risperdal) back to 4 mg/d as everything was working well before the dose reduction
- Switch his current atypical antipsychotic to one that is more sedating and dose at night
- Continue escalating the clonazepam (Klonopin) anxiolytic for better effect
- Add an approved sleep-inducing agent in addition to his current regimen

Case outcome: second interim follow-up visits through 12 months (continued)

- Instead of escalating clonazepam (Klonopin), the patient is placed on the BZRA approved sleeping agent, zolpidem (Ambien) 10 mg at bedtime, with no effect
- It is doubled, off-label, with no effect
- Clonazepam (Klonopin) is increased to 3 mg/d without effect

- Eventually, he agrees to switch from risperidone (Risperdal) to another atypical with a more sedating, sleep-inducing profile
  - He is titrated on to quetiapine (Seroquel) up to 400 mg/d, the minimal effective dose for psychosis
  - Zolpidem (Ambien) 20 mg at bedtime is discontinued as it was ineffective
  - Clonazepam (Klonopin) is reduced gradually back to 1 mg/d as it was ineffective at higher doses
  - He begins sleeping better

Question

Why did the BZRA zolpidem (Ambien) not work, but the atypical quetiapine (Seroquel) did help his insomnia?

- Some drugs will not work in certain individual patients
- The moderate-dose BZ (clonazepam [Klonopin]) was already facilitating GABA-A receptor activity, likely desensitizing GABA-A receptors in the CNS sleep centers so that the added BZRA agent, zolpidem, was less likely to be effective as it works mechanistically in a similar fashion and faced pre-existing GABA-A receptor desensitization
- Quetiapine (Seroquel) is an effective atypical antipsychotic with strong anthistamine activity. This H1 receptor antagonism-induced fatigue and somnolence through a non-GABAergic mechanism and hence was more effective
- Quetiapine (Seroquel) has properties where noradrenergic alpha-1 receptors are antagonized, inducing sleepiness as a side effect
- Quetiapine (Seroquel) has serotonin (5-HT2A) receptor antagonism and this may promote deeper, more efficient sleep architecture on EEG

Attending physician's mental notes: interim visits through 18 months

- The patient now has symptoms more consistent with anxiety and a hypochondriacal thought process. He seems to be getting nocebo (essentially placebo-induced adverse effects) effects
- He may have had hallucinations telling him to "freeze" but he denies this upon questioning
- The freezing spells have stopped
- He seems genuinely disapproving of another trial of atypical antipsychotics
- It is possible that the multifactorial activity of the atypical antipsychotics at different receptor sites is causing him random, ill-defined side effects
- He is sleeping well, which is a relief

Case outcome: interim follow-up visits through 18 months

- The patient does well and sleep improves, but now starts to gain weight on quetiapine (Seroquel) and also begins to have many somatic symptoms and "freezing spells"
  - These spells happen once or twice a week where he may be sitting on the couch and either becomes catatonic or panicky and "freezes" where he feels he cannot move
- Both clonazepam (Klonopin) and quetiapine (Seroquel) are increased to 3 mg/d and 600 mg/d, respectively, as this is a presumed recurrence of catatonic psychosis
  - He does not worsen, but he does not respond
  - Becomes overly sedated especially in the morning
- Quetiapine (Seroquel) is tapered off as it is ineffective now and oversedating
  - Next fails a subtherapeutic trial of ziprasidone (Geodon) due to many odd somatic complaints, possibly nocebo effects
  - Then fails a subtherapeutic trial of aripiprazole (Abilify) due to many odd somatic complaints
  - He recollects that haloperidol (Haldol) was helpful in the past and asks if it, or a similar medicine, can be taken now

Question

What would you do next?

- Continue sequentially trying the atypical class of antipsychotics
- Return to use of a typical antipsychotic
- Continue trying to treat the somatic symptoms with sedatives and/or antidepressants

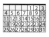

Case outcome: interim follow-up visits through 24 months

- Patient is engaged in a discussion about typical versus atypical antipsychotics
  - He has lost faith in the atypical antipsychotics and views them as having more anxiety and somatic symptom-inducing side effects
  - The last atypical antipsychotic is discontinued and he is titrated onto thiothixene (Navane), a thioxanthene-based high-potency (affinity) typical antipsychotic
  - At 4 mg/d he is no longer "freezing" and the usual negative symptoms continue, but he no longer has somatic anxiety
  - Continues clonazepam (Klonopin) now at 2 mg/d
  - Needs no sleep-inducing medications
- Presents later with an unfortunate return of his marked insomnia

Question

What would you do next?

- Use an antipsychotic combination by adding quetiapine (Seroquel) back into his regimen as it was successful before
- Increase the partially effective BZ clonazepam (Klonopin) further
- Add a different BZRA hypnotic agent
- Add an antihistamine at night to improve his sleep
- Add a melatonergic sleep agent at night

Attending physician's mental notes: interim follow-up visits through 24 months

- For the insomnia, escalating GABAergic drugs failed to help last time
- Adding an atypical antipsychotic with strong antihistamine (and other pharmacodynamic) properties was quite effective previously
- Do not want to add quetiapine (Seroquel) back as he was developing metabolic problems on it last time, and often antipsychotic polypharmacy is frowned upon clinically
- An over-the-counter antihistamine hypnotic could be issued, such as diphenhydramine or doxylamine
- A prescription TCA-based antihistamine could be added, such as doxepin (Silenor/Sinequan)
- The thiothixene (Navane) is working well; it likely should be augmented with a sleeping pill that is not GABA-based, such as melatonergic ramelteon (Rozerem) or onexin inhibiting suvorexant (Belsomra)

Case outcome: interim follow-up visits through 24 months (continued)

- The MT1/MT2 receptor agonist hypnotic (ramelteon [Rozerem]) became available and is prescribed at 8 mg at bedtime, to no avail
  - It was used off-label next at 16 mg at bedtime, without effect, and was discontinued
- Doxepin, initially approved as a TCA at doses of 150–300 mg/d, was re-evaluated at lower doses as a non-addictive, H1 receptor antagonist hypnotic agent
  - Therefore, doxepin (Silenor) was prescribed at the usual 6 mg at bedtime dose
- The patient was also maintained on his typical antipsychotic and low-dose BZ

Case debrief

- The patient suffers from schizophrenia
- Generally experiences good psychotic symptom control

- He continued with either premorbid ASD symptoms, or schizophrenia-induced negative symptoms throughout
- Like many schizophrenics, he developed side effects that needed to be managed
- He also developed the comorbidity of insomnia and hypochondriacal thinking that needed to be managed
- Typical of an illness that may last decades, sometimes dealing with comorbidities and secondary illnesses is the focus of schizophrenia patient care
- He sleeps well now, usually with 6 mg/d of doxepin (Silenor), but has permission to double the dose in an off-label manner for breakthrough insomnia
- It is likely in this case that the routine use of his GABAergic BZ anxiolytic caused his BZ and BZRA hypnotics not to be effective due to tachyphalaxis or tolerance. His GABA-A receptors theoretically became insensitive due to similar mechanistic agents being used
- Attempts to use a non-GABAergic hypnotic that is melatonin enhancing, e.g., ramelteon (Rozerem), made clinical sense as it has a different mechanism of action, but this failed
- Knowledge of quetiapine's (Seroquel) H1 receptor antagonism and its effectiveness in treating the patient's insomnia earlier guided the choice to a formal antihistamine hypnotic (Doxepin [Silenor]) in the end, with successful results
  - Theoretically, the TCA doxepin should have much less metabolic syndrome and TD/EPS side effects to contend with compared to the previously used atypical antipsychotic quetiapine

Take-home points

- Insomnia is a common symptom in schizophrenia
- This is sometimes due to paranoia, agitation, or a circadian rhythm phase shift, as some schizophrenics become nocturnal
- Often, atypical antipsychotics possess the pharmacodynamic properties to treat insomnia as they induce somnolence through H1 receptor antagonism and promote deeper sleep through 5-HT2A receptor antagonism. Some antagonize noradrenergic alpha-1 receptors to induce somnolence as well
- If this monotherapy approach fails, approved hypnotic agents that act through GABA, melatonin, or histamine systems may be utilized to improve sleep
- To treat insomnia, clinicians should be aware of on- and off-label medications that antagonize H1 receptors, alpha-1 receptors, onexis receptors or agonize MT1/MT2 receptors or GABA-A receptors

- Finally, a new class of hypnotic agent has been approved, called suvorexant (Belsomra), which antagonizes orexin receptors
  - Agonism of orexin receptors promotes and stabilizes normal wakeful states
  - Therefore, blocking orexin receptor activity may destabilize wakefulness and promote sleep
  - It could have been used as an alternative in this case

Performance in practice: confessions of a psychopharmacologist

- *What could have been done better here?*
  - The patient was doing well on the very first atypical antipsychotic, perhaps this should never have been changed
  - More aggressive anxiolysis through even higher-dosed BZs could have been utilized to overcome the desensitization or tolerance
  - A referral to short-term psychotherapy (perhaps CBT) may have been utilized to treat the somatic anxiety and insomnia
  - Be aware that insomnia may be an independent risk factor indicative of a pending relapse into psychosis
- *Possible action items for improvement in practice*
  - Research the rates of development of TD and metabolic disorder over long- term care in schizophrenia to better determine the risks and benefits of using certain atypical antipsychotics versus high-potency typical antipsychotics as in this case; manipulating his effective atypical may have started the cascade of medication changes
  - Research clinical rationale for utilizing typical antipsychotics in an era dominated by atypical antipsychotic use
  - Research and become more familiar with typical and atypical antipsychotics that possess potential hypnotic pharmacodynamic profiles

Tips and pearls

- Primary insomnia is prevalent and common even in non-psychiatric patients
- Primary insomnia may be comorbid with both mental and medical disorders
- Insomnia may also be secondary to one of these primary disorders
- Interestingly, in the *DSM-5* there is no longer the need to debate if insomnia is primary or secondary. Insomnia disorder can now be listed as a separate disorder of concern along with other psychiatric conditions being treated, if it is a focus of treatment
- Insomnia is often a side effect of prescribing antidepressants and stimulants
- Insomnia is often a residual untreated symptom of many psychiatric disorders
- Insomnia is a risk factor for acute suicidal behavior, depressive, manic, or psychotic relapse

- Routine monitoring and aggressive treatment of insomnia is warranted
- Monotherapy using the safest agent first is suggested
- Escalating treatment of insomnia, including the use of polypharmacy, may be needed in severe cases

Two-minute tutorial

GABA-A receptors and the positive allosteric modulation of the BZs

- GABA-A receptors become activated once endogenous GABA molecules bind to them
- This allows a conformational change in an adjacent chloride channel, opening an ion pore, allowing negatively charged chloride ions to enter the neuron and hyperpolarize it, and inhibit it from firing
- Studies with the BZ diazepam (Valium) in animal models suggest
  - GABA must be bound at the GABA-A receptor for the drug to work
  - Diazepam, when bound simultaneously, actually increases the affinity of the GABA-A receptor for endogenous GABA in the synapse
  - This facilitates increased GABA/GABA-A receptor binding rates and ultimately allows more chloride channels to open, or open more frequently
  - This effect, when a drug binds a receptor and facilitates its usual activity, is called PAM
  - In the case at hand, this action may lower anxiety or improve sleep translationally
  - Facilitating GABA-A receptor activity in the sleep-inducing centers of the brain (VLPO) will increase sleepiness. Enhancing GABA tone in the limbic system may lower anxiety. Depending on the neuroanatomic preference of these drugs (their affinity for certain receptor subtypes in specific brain areas), clinicians may see a difference in anxiolytic versus hypnotic propensity

GABA-A receptors: desensitization, tachyphylaxis, and tolerance

- After repeated use of alcohol, barbiturates, or BZs, which all bind at the GABA-A receptor, it is often noted that clinical effectiveness may diminish over time or that increasing doses of these agents are required to obtain the same clinical effect found upon initial dosing
- This is called tachyphylaxis or tolerance from a pharmacological point of view
  - The term tolerance is more often used clinically
- The present case may demonstrate this effect, as the patient was taking chronic, moderate-dose clonazepam (Klonopin), which appeared to require greater doses over time to maintain clinical anxiolytic effectiveness

- Additionally, a cross-tolerance may have developed as he was a non-responder to the GABA-A receptor PAM sleeping agent, zolpidem (Ambien), even at double the approved dose
- It was as if the patient's GABA-A receptors in his sleep centers did not respond to the zolpidem hypnotic agent, likely as his GABA-A receptors were desensitized
- Or in this case, as GABA-A PAM did not improve sleep, the histaminergic system was next manipulated to improve sleep

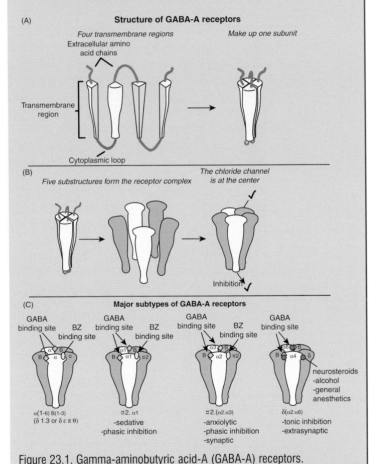

(A) **Structure of GABA-A receptors**

Four transmembrane regions
Extracellular amino acid chains
Make up one subunit

Transmembrane region

Cytoplasmic loop

(B) Five substructures form the receptor complex
The chloride channel is at the center

Inhibition

(C) **Major subtypes of GABA-A receptors**

GABA binding site / BZ binding site

α(1-6) β(1-3)
(δ 1.3 or δ ε π θ)

ϱ2. α1
-sedative
-phasic inhibition

ϱ2.(α2.α3)
-anxiolytic
-phasic inhibition
-synaptic

δ(α2.α6)
-tonic inhibition
-extrasynaptic

neurosteroids
-alcohol
-general anesthetics

Figure 23.1. Gamma-aminobutyric acid-A (GABA-A) receptors. **A**: Shown here are the four transmembrane regions that make up one subunit of a GABA-A receptor. **B**: There are five copies of these subunits in a fully constituted GABA-A receptor, at the center of which is the chloride channel, or pore. **C**: Different types of subunits can combine to form a GABA-A receptor.

Why does this happen?

- The subunits shown in the Figure 23.1 include six different alpha isoforms, three different beta isoforms, three different gamma isoforms, delta, epsilon, pi, theta, and three different rho isoforms
- The ultimate type and function of each GABA-A receptor subtype will depend on which subunits it contains (Figure 23.1C)
  - BZ-sensitive GABA-A receptors (middle two) contain gamma- and alpha- (1 through 3) subunits and preferentially respond when a patient takes a BZ
  - BZ-sensitive GABA-A receptors containing alpha-1 subunits are involved in sleep induction (second from left), while those that contain alpha-2 and/or alpha-3 subunits are involved more in reducing anxiety (second from right)
  - GABA-A receptors containing alpha-4, alpha-6, gamma-1, or delta subunits (far right) are BZ insensitive
- Tolerance to BZ after chronic, repeated exposure may occur when BZ-sensitive gamma subunits are replaced by the individual neuron with more insensitive subunits, i.e., alpha-4 or -6 subunits
- Likely, neurons interpret excessive GABA-A PAM as a novel and toxic situation
  - As the brain strives to maintain homeostasis in the face of BZ use, neurons expressing GABA-A receptors likely react when transcription factors become active in neuronal nuclei, turning certain genes off (those that produce gamma subunits) and turning certain genes on (those that make alpha subunits)
  - The net effect over time is that more alpha subunit-based GABA-A receptors are made instead of gamma subunit-based receptors, and sent to the neuronal surface
  - These newer GABA-A receptors are now more often insensitive to BZs that are ingested, and patients may either require higher doses of BZ, or frankly, will stop responding to them

Posttest self-assessment question and answer

Which of the following antidepressants is also formally approved for treating insomnia?

A. Quetiapine
B. Diphenhydramine
C. Hydroxyzine
D. Trazodone
E. Amitriptyline
F. Doxepin

G. All of the above
H. None of the above
Answer: F
Doxepin (Sinequan) is an antidepressant and also approved at much lower doses as a hypnotic (Silenor). At these low doses, the cardiotoxic and anticholinergic side effects and risks are generally avoided. EKG and plasma level monitoring is not required. Trazodone and amitriptyline are approved antidepressants often used off-label to induce sleep. Hydroxyzine is an antihistamine anxiolytic that may be used off-label as a hypnotic. Quetiapine is an atypical antipsychotic that may induce sleep but is not formally approved as a hypnotic.

References

1. Stahl SM. *Stahl's Essential Psychopharmacology*, 4th edn. New York, NY: Cambridge University Press, 2013.
2. Stahl SM. *Stahl's Essential Psychopharmacology: The Prescriber's Guide*, 5th edn. New York, NY: Cambridge University Press, 2014.
3. Citrome L. Lurasidone for schizophrenia: a review of the efficacy and safety profile for this newly approved second-generation antipsychotic. *Int J Clin Pract* 2011; 65:189–210.
4. Miller DD. Atypical antipsychotics: sleep, sedation, and efficacy. *Primary care companion.* J Clin Psychiatry 2004; 6:3–7.
5. Chemerinski E, Ho BC, Flaum M, et al. Insomnia as a predictor for symptom worsening following antipsychotic withdrawal in schizophrenia. *Compr Psychiatry* 2002; 43:393–6.
6. Masand PS, Schwartz TL, Wang X, et al. Prescribing conventional antipsychotics in the era of novel antipsychotics: informed consent issues. *Am J Ther* 2002; 9:484–7.
7. Sadock BJ, Sadock VA. *Kaplan and Sadock's Synopsis of Psychiatry: Behavioral Sciences/Clinical Psychiatry*, 10th edn. Philadelphia, PA: Lippincott Williams & Wilkins, 2007.
8. Lavoie AM, Twyman RE. Direct evidence for diazepam modulation of GABA-A receptor microscopic affinity. *Neuropharmacology* 1996; 35:1383–92.

The Case: The man with greasy hands needs fine tuning

The Question: What to do with a bizarre side effect

The Dilemma: Fine tuning polypharmacy treatment

Pretest self-assessment question (answer at the end of the case)

Which of the following evidence-based antidepressant augmentations likely has the least side-effect burden?

A. SAMe

B. Lithium carbonate

C. Aripiprazole

D. Thyroid hormone

Patient evaluation on intake

- 52-year-old man cannot sleep
- He has been "in a funk" for about a year after he had difficulty at his work site

Psychiatric history

- The patient has been emotionally well his whole life
- About a year ago, developed vision problems due to diabetes, which interfered with his ability to work safely at his job site as an assembly line worker
- He was placed on lighter duty and then ultimately laid off due to bad economic times
- At the time of his transition to light duty, he began experiencing psychiatric symptoms as follows
  - Insomnia
  - Dysphoria and irritability
  - Increasing anhedonia
  - Poor concentration
  - Poor appetite
  - Feelings of worthlessness and hopelessness
  - Fatigue
  - He denied suicidal thoughts, or psychotic, manic, anxiety, and substance misuse symptoms

Social and personal history

- Married with five adult children
- Takes care of his grandchildren often and might be considered a primary caregiver
- Has tenth grade education

- Gainfully employed as an assembly line worker for many years until recently
- Most of his friends, support, and identity as an autoworker were disrupted when he was forced to leave work
- He does not abuse substances, nicotine, or caffeine

Medical history

- Suffers from DM2 with worsening vision, renal function, and neuropathy in his feet
- Has HTN and hyperlipidemia
- He has good attendance and follow-up with his PCP and currently has these metabolic disorders well controlled

Family history

- One son has bipolar disorder and substance abuse problems
- Mother suffered from MDD
- AUD is present in multiple family members at each generation

Medication history

- PCP started him on the SSRI sertraline (Zoloft) 50 mg/d three weeks ago
  - Sleep is starting to improve somewhat and there is less noticeable irritability
  - Complains now that his hands feel "greasy and tacky"
    ○ Feels like he has residual car "motor oil on them" all the time
    ○ Washes his hands to no avail
    ○ There are no rashes or skin changes on examination

Psychotherapy history

- Started supportive psychotherapy several weeks ago
- Attendance is good
- Feels better after sessions but this is short lived

Patient evaluation on initial visit

- Patient suffers from new-onset MDD
- He is somewhat better but dislikes the side effects in his hands as they "feel greasy"

Current medications

- Sertraline (Zoloft) 50 mg/d (SSRI)
- Insulin sliding scale
- Atorvastatin (Lipitor) 40 mg/d

- Metoprolol (Toprol-XL) 100 mg/d
- Metformin (Glucophage) 2000 mg/d

Question

Greasy hands? Is that a real side effect?

- No, it is hypochondriacal, hysterical, or a nocebo side effect
- No, it is not listed in the regulatory package insert for sertraline
- Yes, a web search reveals that two to three other patients have posted similar experiences
- Yes, it is likely a paresthesia, and these occur in 1% of patients taking sertraline
- Yes, it is a side effect because the patient says it is, and it bothers him

Attending physician's mental notes: initial evaluation

- This patient has an index episode of MDD that is moderate in severity
- This was likely initiated due to an interpersonal loss and social stressor when his working career ended beyond his control
- He may be starting to respond to his inaugural SSRI at this time, but has a strange side effect where his hands feel greasy, or as if they were immersed in liquid
- He does not appear to have any comorbid psychiatric conditions
- He has some chronic medical problems but they appear stable and well controlled
- He is not felt to be suicidal

Question

Which of the following would be your next step?

- Do nothing as his SSRI is starting to become effective after three weeks of use
- His side effects are strange but minor; convince him to tolerate his medication longer
- Increase the SSRI for better effect
- Change to an alternate SSRI in the hope of continuing this early efficacy but without the paresthesia
- Change classes to a different family of antidepressant
- Add an anti-paresthesia medication such as gabapentin (Neurontin)
- Refer for specific IPT, which is well studied for depression when caused by interpersonal role change such as a loss of work

Attending physician's mental notes: initial evaluation (continued)

- The patient is somewhat better after three weeks of SSRI treatment, but this equates to 20% better at most, as only two MDD symptoms are minimally better

- If patient can tolerate his side effect a bit more and given this initial small response, it may make sense to increase his current SSRI, sertraline (Zoloft) further

Further investigation

Is there anything else you would especially like to know about this patient?

- Could there be any other cause to the strange sensations in his hands?
  - Physical examination reveals no clear skin changes or deformities
  - He has full range of motion, no arthritic changes
  - He has no history of cervical injury or pain
  - None of the medications are known to cause this kind of side effect
  - There is no evidence of carpal tunnel or other entrapment syndrome
  - Discussions with his PCP confirms these findings
  - He has leg pain and neuropathy from his diabetes, it is possible that these hand pressure sensations are the start of diabetic neuropathy in his upper extremities that presented coincidentally with the start of his SSRI

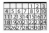

Case outcome: first interim follow-up visits through three months

- Agrees now to increase the SSRI sertraline (Zoloft) to 100 mg/d and to tolerate the side effect of greasy hands as it is explained that it may be a rare side effect or part of his DM2
- Later feels better but qualifies this as being less ruminative, less tense, and sleeping better, but still often feels amotivated and dysphoric
- The SSRI dose is raised to 150 mg/d and he returns with moderate, sustained improvement in these symptoms and he feels his appetite is better

Question

Do the SSRIs have a dose–response curve where greater doses treat a greater number of symptoms?

- No, according to regulatory information, there is no additional benefit between low, moderate, and high doses of SSRI when used to treat MDD
- No, studies suggest that low doses of SSRI successfully inhibit the SERT, indicating that further inhibition is likely not needed for greater antidepressant response
- Yes, in clinical practice, many clinicians claim that higher doses usually aid in more symptom reduction

- Yes, textbooks and a recret meta-analysis suggest higher dosing on an individual basis to deliver the highest effectiveness
- Possibly, as regulatory trials often contain 300–400 subjects and are statistically designed to show that all doses are superior to placebo but not necessarily to each other
  - They are not designed with enough subjects, i.e., 1500 or enough statistical power to show discrete differences between low, middle, and higher doses

Case outcome: interim follow-up visits through four months

- The patient appreciates his improvements so far and states his hands are not as problematic
- Agrees to final maximization of sertraline (Zoloft) up to 200 mg/d
- Appears to have resolution of a few MDD symptoms and others are felt to be moderately improved
- Now is considered a responder but not in remission from the maximal dose SSRI monotherapy

Question

What would you do next?

- Switch to a new SSRI
- Switch to an antidepressant that is not an SSRI
- Combine his current SSRI with a non-SSRI antidepressant
- Augment his current SSRI
- Refer for MDD-specific IPT

Case outcome: interim follow-up visits through six months

- Patient continues the SSRI and agrees to combine with the NDRI bupropion-XL (Wellbutrin-XL) starting at 150 mg/d
  - There is an initial boost in energy and alertness, but that falters after two weeks
- Bupropion-XL is increased to the minimum effective approved monotherapy dose of 300 mg/d
  - There is no additional benefit now but he is tolerating it well
- The bupropion-XL is increased to the maximum approved dose of 450 mg/d
  - Sertraline (Zoloft) is lowered down to 100 mg/d
    - This is done partially as the 200 mg/d dose was not felt to be robustly different from the 100 mg/d dose clinically, in retrospect
  - Additionally, sertraline is a weak to moderate CYP450 2D6 hepatic enzyme inhibitor
    - Bupropion is also a 2D6 inhibitor and a substrate

- ○ Bupropion at doses greater than 450 mg/d are known to cause seizures
- – This patient is not in a contraindicated group, but his sertraline is lowered to attempt to keep his bupropion plasma levels below theoretically dangerous levels
- – Despite this, he returns with intention hand tremors and tinnitus side effects. Interestingly, his hand paresthesias have dissipated
- – He stops smoking unexpectedly

Question

How did this patient stop smoking unexpectedly? Without trying?

- Some patients just stop
- Some bupropion preparations are approved as antidepressants (Wellbutrin-IR, -SR, -XL) and one is approved and marketed as a smoking cessation agent (bupropion-SR [Zyban])
- Most often when used with smoking cessation, bupropion-SR is paired with a behavioral intervention of determining a smoking cessation date, identifying triggers for smoking relapse, and preparing for change
- Sometimes patients lose the drive to smoke without these behavioral interventions, suggesting a purely neurochemical anti-smoking effect

Attending physician's mental notes: visits through six months

- This appeared initially to be a simple, moderate episode of MDD
- The patient is now resistant to SSRI plus NDRI combination therapy and only is a responder, not a remitter
- There are increasing side-effect problems and tolerating high doses of the NDRI was not possible
- There were some vegetative symptom improvements while on the NDRI

Case outcome: interim follow-up visits through nine months

- The problematic bupropion (Wellbutrin-XL) is discontinued
- He is maintained on the sertraline (Zoloft) 100 mg/d as it has given him a solid, sustained response
- Next, he is augmented with the approved ADHD medication atomoxetine (Strattera), and this off-label approach is explained to the patient in that
  - It may be warranted as some of his residual MDD symptoms include poor memory, concentration, and inattention
  - Atomoxetine is approved for treating inattention and poor concentration associated with ADHD and these symptoms appear similar to some of his MDD symptoms

- Atomoxetine is an NRI, which is one of bupropion's mechanisms of action and might be used in the hope of continuing better effectiveness with less tremor and tinnitus

Question

What could you have done instead of using this off-label augmentation to obtain the same mechanism of action of SRI plus NRI?

- Switching to an SNRI, such as duloxetine (Cymbalta), venlafaxine-ER (Effexor-XR), desvenlafaxine (Pristiq), or levomilnacipran (Fetzima), would accomplish the same dual mechanism of action in a monotherapy
- Add a noradrenergic TCA, such as desipramine (Norpramin), protriptyline (Vivactil), or nortriptyline (Pamelor), in order to add NRI properties to his current SSRI

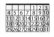

Case outcome: interim follow-up visits through nine months (continued)

- Patient now takes sertraline 100 mg/d and atomoxetine 80 mg/d
  - There are minimal to no side-effect complaints now
  - He is perhaps 70% better overall, reporting improvements in every residual symptom
  - Has bouts of low energy, poor memory, and concentration
  - Atomoxetine is a CYP450 2D6 substrate and his plasma levels may be higher than his oral dose suggests, due to sertraline's concomitant use
- He is leery of adding a third prescription antidepressant agent as he has been side effect free
- Nutraceuticals are discussed as an option and he agrees to augment the given two medications, based upon a recent literature search suggesting that SAMe 800–1200 mg/d can augment SSRI with minimal side effects, as it is an over-the-counter product found in the vitamin section of most pharmacies
- He is titrated to 800 mg twice a day
- He returns and states that his MDD symptoms are in remission and he is without any adverse effects

Case debrief

- The patient suffered from a single episode of MDD that was moderate in intensity
- He was a partial responder to SSRI monotherapy

- With assurance, he was able to tolerate the SSRI, and over time, his initial paresthesia-like side effects resolved and he was able to carry through with a full therapeutic SSRI trial
- He was a responder to SSRI plus NRI augmentation
- He remitted with the addition of SAMe

Take-home points

- In treating MDD, starting with aggressive SSRI monotherapy can be effective
- With recent approvals for atypical antipsychotic augmentations for MDD, sometimes clinicians forgo clinically reasonable and now classic combinations such as adding bupropion or buspirone
- If NRI facilitation is not tolerated with the bupropion product line, there are other NRI-possessing agents in the armamentarium that may be added instead
- Certain nutraceuticals (vitamins, minerals, cofactors, supplements) are beginning to develop an evidence base that contains in its literature some moderate-sized, randomized, and controlled studies
- These agents often have a more benign side-effect profile and might be used effectively to foster remission in those patients who are 70%–80% less depressed, but require final fine tuning, or improvement, of tenuous residual symptoms without imposing a major side-effect burden

Performance in practice: confessions of a psychopharmacologist

- *What could have been done better here?*
  - Instead of three medications being used to foster remission, perhaps an SNRI monotherapy may have worked if started initially instead of the SSRI
  - IPT, if available, would have been an ideal, side-effect-free approach
- *Possible action items for improvement in practice*
  - Research the availability and evidence base for nutraceutical use in treating MDD
  - Review textbooks to remember and maintain how antidepressant combinations and augmentations act mechanistically so that polypharmacy is rational with regard to agent selection

Tips and pearls

- SAMe has initial controlled data suggesting it can act as an augmentation in MDD
- Another nutraceutical, L-methylfolate, also has controlled data suggesting effectiveness at 15 mg/d

- St. John's Wort might be an alternative
- N-acetyl cysteine (NAC) 1000 mg twice daily is another alternative
- Before advocating or utilizing a nutraceutical, review the apparent literature for its stringency

Two-minute tutorial

A primer on SAMe

- SAMe is easier to say than its official chemical name, S-adenosyl methionine
- SAMe, folate, vitamin B_{12}, and homocysteine are linked in the one-carbon cycle that is often memorized in the first year of medical school, usually after the Krebs cycle is learned
- Many students who plan on going into psychiatry have worked out that memorizing these pathways is a way to graduate medical school and that knowledge of these metabolic pathways will never, ever be needed in psychiatry!
  - This would be an error in judgment now
- SAMe is found throughout the human body, with particularly high concentrations in the liver, adrenal glands, and pineal gland
- It is uniformly distributed in the brain, where it serves as the major donor of methyl groups required in the synthesis of neuronal messengers and membranes that have been implicated as being abnormal in mood disorders
- The antidepressant efficacy of SAMe has been studied in randomized controlled trials involving depressed adults in Europe and the United States, utilizing both parenteral and oral formulations
- Several potential mechanisms of antidepressant action have been theorized
  - It functions primarily as a methyl donor in a variety of biochemical reactions, including the methylation of catecholamines. Here, SAMe may promote greater synthesis and production of NE, DA, and 5-HT. This effect may be called trimonoamine modulation and provides a greater quantity of neurotransmitter for antidepressants to facilitate, possibly improving effectiveness
  - SAMe has been proposed to increase serotonin turnover, inhibit NE reuptake, and augment dopaminergic activity
  - Other investigations have suggested the presence of antidepressant mechanisms based on SAMe's effects on brain neurotrophic activity, inflammatory cytokines, cell membrane fluidity, and bioenergetics, suggesting that SAMe may nurture neuronal plasticity and network formation

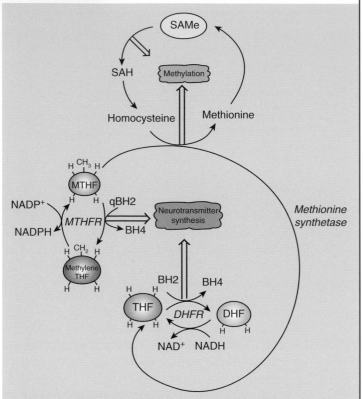

Figure 24.1. Trimonoamine modulation (TMM) of L-5-methyl-tetrahydrofolate (MTHF) and S-adenosyl-methionine (SAMe): methylation and neurotransmitter synthesis.

- SAMe regulates and promotes methylation as discussed, and its formal pathway is depicted in Figure 24.1
- The reactions that produce, utilize, and regenerate SAMe could be considered the "SAMe cycle"
  - First, SAMe-dependent methylase enzymes use SAMe as a substrate to produce S-adenosyl homocysteine
  - Next, this is hydrolyzed to homocysteine and adenosine by S-adenosyl homocysteine hydrolase and the homocysteine recycled back to methionine through transfer of a methyl group from 5-methyltetrahydrofolate methionine synthetase enzymes
  - This methionine can then be converted back to SAMe, completing the cycle
  - Regulation of this cycle can affect modulation of catabolic enzymes, monoamine transporters, and receptors, and thus is another means to regulate monoamine activity and theoretically improve MDD symptoms

Posttest self-assessment question and answer

Which of the following evidence-based antidepressant augmentations likely has the least side-effect burden?

A. SAMe
B. Lithium carbonate
C. Aripiprazole
D. Thyroid hormone

Answer: A

SAMe, as an over-the-counter CAM, likely has the least day-to-day side-effect burden and no known end organ damage risk compared to prescription medication augmentation strategies. Its evidence base, however, is less than that of the other agents. Lithium has end organ damage associated with renal dysfunction and hypothyroidism. The atypical antipsychotic, aripiprazole, is associated with TD and possible metabolic syndrome. Thyroid augmentations may be associated with inducing atrial arrhythmias such as flutter or fibrilliation that often require cardioversion.

References

1. Stahl SM. *Stahl's Essential Psychopharmacology*, 4th edn. New York, NY: Cambridge University Press, 2013.
2. Stahl SM. *Stahl's Essential Psychopharmacology: The Prescriber's Guide*, 5th edn. New York, NY: Cambridge University Press, 2014.
3. Schwartz TL, Storman L, Thase M. Treatment outcomes with acute pharmacotherapy/psychotherapy Depression. In: Schwartz TL, Petersen T, eds. Treatment Strategies and Management, 1st edn. New York, NY: Informa, 2006.
4. Papakostas GI, Mischoulon D, Shyu I, Alpert JE, Fava M. *S*-adenosyl methionine (SAMe) augmentation of serotonin reuptake inhibitors for antidepressant nonresponders with major depressive disorder: a double-blind, randomized clinical trial. *Am J Psychiatry* 2010; 167:942–8.
5. Mischoulon D, Rosenbaum JF. *Natural Medications for Psychiatric Disorders: Considering the Alternatives*. Philadelphia, PA: Lippincott Williams & Wilkins, 2008.
6. Roje S. S-adenosyl-L-methionine: beyond the universal methyl group donor. *Phytochemistry* 2006; 67:1686–98.
7. Loenen WA. S-adenosylmethionine: jack of all trades and master of everything? *Biochem Soc Trans* 2006; 34:330–3.
8. Chiang PK, Gordon RK, Tal J, et al. S-adenosylmethionine and methylation. *FASEB J* 1996; 10:471–80.
9. Weissman MM, Markowitz JC, Klerman G. *Comprehensive Guide To Interpersonal Psychotherapy*. New York, NY: Basic Books, 2000.

10. Papakostas GI, Shelton RC, Zajecka JM, et al. L-methylfolate as adjunctive therapy for SSRI-resistant major depression: results of two randomized, double-blind, parallel-sequential trials. *Am J Psychiatry* 2012; 169:1267–74.

11. Müller WE. Current St. John's wort research from mode of action to clinical efficacy. *Pharmacol Res* 2003; 47:101–9.

The Case: The combative business woman

The Question: What to do when a patient becomes abruptly psychotic

The Dilemma: The age-old functional versus organic differential diagnosis argument

Pretest self-assessment question (answer at the end of the case)

What are common causes of abrupt-onset psychosis?

A. Stimulant intoxication
B. Medically induced delirium
C. Alcohol or BZ withdrawal
D. Paranoid schizophrenia
E. A and B
F. A, B, and C
G. All of the above

Patient evaluation on intake

- 50-year-old woman with no chief complaint
- Spouse calls and states that she is "speaking nonsense" and describes soft neurological signs of ataxia and unstable gait

Psychiatric history

- This patient has had long-standing MDD and GAD symptoms since her twenties
- Suffers from MDD that is chronic and fluctuating
- Suffers from GAD that is comorbid and worsens toward frank agitation if MDD symptoms escalate
- She employs defenses consistent with idealization–devaluation, splitting, and has some element of affective dyscontrol but does not meet full personality disorder criteria
- Currently is experiencing the best control of her psychiatric symptoms over the last few years
  - The MDD and GAD symptoms are at a minimum and residual symptoms are not impairing her at work, home, or socially
- She has not had a medication change in a long time and was her usual self until four days ago

Social and personal history

- Graduated from college and has an advanced business degree
- Is an upper-level administrator in a local business firm
- She is in her third marriage, now with a supportive husband
- Has two adult sons

- Drinks coffee in the morning, rarely has alcohol, does not smoke or use illegal drugs
- Has no legal history or any episodes of acting in a violent manner

Medical history

- Hyperlipidemia
- GERD
- Hypothyroidism (euthyroid for many years)

Family history

- Feels her mother was depressed but never diagnosed
- There is no family history of psychotic disorders

Medication history

- Has taken antidepressants from every major class
- Has taken mood stabilizing anticonvulsants as augmentation strategies
- Has taken numerous sedative–anxiolytics and hypnotics
- Has not been augmented with atypical antipsychotics, stimulants, lithium, or thyroid hormone

Psychotherapy history

- Eclectic, supportive psychotherapy intermittently attended for several years
- Followed by three years of short-term intensive PDP
- Has not needed psychotherapy in two years as she has been functioning and coping very well

Patient evaluation via initial phone call

- The patient is being seen for routine, outpatient medication management of nearly remitted MDD and GAD every 90 days
- Is also seen biannually for programing of a VNS device, to which she had a good antidepressant response
- Was her usual self until four days ago when her husband called in distress from their home in the early evening
- Reportedly, she is now confused, disoriented, and speaking in nonsensical terms
- She is reported to be off balance while walking
- She is anxious and agitated
- There is no previous history of these behaviors, signs, or symptoms
- There is no evidence of acute stress, intoxication, or withdrawal from medications

Current psychiatric medications

- Nortriptyline (Pamelor) 100 mg/d (last outpatient level 78 ng/dL) (TCA)

- Clonazepam (Klonopin) 2.5 mg/d (BZ)
- Escitalopram (Lexapro) 20 mg/d (SSRI)
- L-methylfolate (Deplin) 15 mg/d (nutraceutical)
- Eszopiclone (Lunesta) 3 mg at bedtime (BZRA)
- Modafinil (Provigil) 100–200 mg/d as needed for fatigue (wakefulness agent)
- VNS pulse generator

Current medical medications

- Levothyroxine (Synthroid) 100 mcg/d
- Lansoprazole (Prevacid) 15 mg/d
- Niacin (Niaspan) 1000 mg/d

Question

In your clinical experience, is it likely that this patient's MDD or GAD would cause this acute change in mental status?

- Yes
- No

Attending physician's mental notes: initial phone evaluation

- It took years of psychotherapy, medication management, and VNS therapy to get this patient to her baseline best with regard to MDD and GAD
- She has been very stable, very compliant, without any behavioral issues
- She has no history of this type of presentation

Question

Which of the following would be your next step?

- As this is a phone call, see her at the office
- As this is an acute event with soft neurological signs, send her to the emergency room
- Increase her sedative, clonazepam (Klonopin) to ease her agitation
- Have her take her hypnotic, eszopiclone (Lunesta), now and go to bed early

Attending physician's mental notes: initial phone evaluation (continued)

- This patient seems to be in an acute confusional state where she clearly is distressed
- She has experienced no previous symptoms similar to this and now really cannot communicate what is happening to her
- She does not appear to be intoxicated or in withdrawal from her clonazepam, eszopiclone, or modafinil, and her spouse confirms she has been taking her medications per usual

- He also states that she has had no other medications prescribed or changed by other medical providers for any of her medical conditions, ruling out a new drug–drug interaction elevating any of her psychotropics' plasma levels

Case outcome: via telephone

- Spouse is instructed to bring patient to local emergency room to be evaluated for this acute neurological event
- She is seen and evaluated by emergency room staff

Further investigation

Is there anything else you would especially like to know about this patient?
- What did the emergency room determine?
  - Her vital signs were normal initially
  - She had not been hydrating well and may be dehydrated
  - Brain CT scan revealed no abnormalities
  - She developed a fever of 104°F while being worked up in the emergency room
  - Urinalysis suggested infection
  - Blood work next showed urosepsis
  - She was placed on ciprofloxacin IV, 400 mg IV every 8 h and admitted for further evaluation

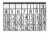

Case outcome: first interim follow-up six hours later

- Patient went to sleep on the medicine inpatient unit
- Six hours later, husband calls to state he went home and went to bed; it is now midnight and the patient has been texting him
  - Part of what she is texting states that "she has to get out" and they are "out to get me"
  - The other part is nonsensical
- This is reported to the inpatient internal medicine team in real time
  - They call for consultation and report that she is combative and refusing all medications now
  - On-call team wonders if she is paranoid like this often, and if this is part of her depression

Question

How would you answer?

- Yes, sometimes depressives become psychotic acutely
- Yes, sometimes depressives become psychotic acutely, but not in this case, as in 30 years she has not presented as such

- Yes, but only if she has taken excessive modafinil or stopped taking clonazepam or eszopiclone abruptly, causing an intoxication or a withdrawal effect. However, there is no evidence to support this now
- No, patients with MDD, bipolar disorder, or even schizophrenia typically do not go from non-psychotic to psychotic in a few hours' time
- No, she has confusion and orientation problems and these are not part of MDD, GAD, bipolar, or schizophrenia diagnostic criteria, but is more consistent with delirium

Attending physician's mental notes: six hours later

- The patient is frankly paranoid, agitated, even combative now
- Symptoms have fluctuated to different degrees over the last several hours, where she has acted normally at some times, psychotic at others
- There is no prescription misuse issues and she unlikely has made mistakes following her medication regimen, which has been stable for a few years
- There has been no recent MDD, stressors, and no indications that this was an overdose or suicide attempt
- Acute onset of clouded sensorium, confusion, behavioral change, and psychosis meets *DSM-5* criteria for delirium
- Even though they have begun treating her urosepsis with antibiotics, she is still infected, febrile, and she is likely "sundowning" with a worsening of delirium symptoms now in the evening

Question

What would you advise the medical team, as far as treating her cognitive and behavioral symptoms of delirium?

- Behaviorally, ask the husband to come in and possibly bring items from home to better orient the patient to self
- Ask the nursing staff to frequently introduce themselves, the patient's hospital location, and reason for being there to orient the patient to time and place
- Return her glasses so she can see better to avoid sensory deprivation
- Start a low-dose typical antipsychotic such as haloperidol (Haldol)
- Start a low-dose atypical antipsychotic such as risperidone (Risperdal)

Attending physician's mental notes: interim follow-up information through 72 hours

- This presentation was not due to MDD or GAD and was secondary to urosepsis, dehydration, and possible anticholinergic-induced delirium
- This was managed appropriately per guidelines
  - The underlying cause was detected and treated
  - Behavioral techniques were used to manage aggression and paranoia
  - Pharmacological treatments were refused but actually not needed
  - Physical restraints were not needed

- Her complicated psychotropic regimen was assessed and altered to avoid making the delirium worse
- Will see patient in a few weeks and likely reinstate her usual medications systematically to her usual successful regimen to make sure she does not begin an MDD or GAD recurrence

Case outcome: interim follow-up information through 72 hours

- Patient refuses oral risperidone (Risperdal) 0.5–1 mg dose and becomes selectively mute
- A nurse was stationed in the medical room for constant observation
- Nurse employed behavioral techniques (see previous case)
- This, as well as having the husband present, calmed the patient and she slept without further incident
- Awakens in the next morning without any abnormal mental state findings
- Later becomes afebrile and the infection is clearing
- The norriptyline (Pamelor) level came back elevated at 176 ng/ml and it was lowered
  - This level is considered potentially toxic
  - It likely elevated due to dehydration as her usual levels are half this amount and she is on no CYP450 2D6 inhibitors
  - EKG was normal
  - This TCA has anticholinergic potential that might worsen or prolong delirium, and lowering it makes clinical sense regardless
- The wakefulness agent/stimulant, modafinil, is discontinued as there are case reports noting it may cause psychosis and delirium, although this often occurs at drug initiation
- The BZ clonazepam and BZRA eszopiclone are continued to avoid sedative withdrawal effects and to prevent complicating her already delirious presentation
- The SSRI sertraline is continued to avoid SSRI discontinuation syndrome and to prevent complicating her already delirious presentation
- L-methylfolate (Deplin) is continued
- The patient is discharged home in a normal mental state the next day

Case outcome: interim follow-up visits through 80 hours

- The patient went home in the afternoon and went to sleep after her hospital stay
- Awoke the next day appearing slightly confused, repeatedly stating that she has to "get out"
- Attempts to leave the house in a nightgown and husband tries to passively restrain her inside the house and coerce her to get dressed
- Became verbally aggressive, began throwing objects, physically forced herself out of the house

- She was selectively mute, unresponsive again
- Ambulance was called and she reluctantly, but docilely returned to the emergency room where she presented as paranoid, refusing all treatment, and refusing to talk
- Agitation reached a dangerous level at one point where she received injections of the BZ sedative lorazepam (Ativan) 2 mg and typical antipsychotic haloperidol (Haldol) 5 mg
- She calmed down and slept
- Emergency room called for consultation and stated that the urosepsis had been successfully treated. As a result, the paranoia now "appeared psychiatric" and not due to delirium. They requested that the patient be admitted to a psychiatric unit

Attending physician's mental notes: interim follow-up information through 72 hours (continued)

- Again, this fluctuating and acute-onset presentation is not suggestive of this patient's usual psychopathology
- It does appear to be getting worse in regard to the new-onset psychosis, but the confusion and waxing/waning of consciousness are still present, indicating delirium has returned
- Was refusing medicine again at home; she could now be in sedative withdrawal
- The antibiotic ciprofloxacin has known CYP450 3A4 interactions; could she have a delirium now secondary to a drug toxicity?

Question

What would you tell the emergency room team now?

- The clinical picture is still textbook delirium and that likely her urosepsis was incompletely treated and infection may have returned
- She may have a new medical issue causing this and IV or IM lorazepam (Ativan) should be given as she is refusing oral clonazepam tablets. This should treat or rule out a sedative withdrawal etiology
- Sometimes delirious symptoms may continue for a few days after medical treatment is given and these remaining psychiatric phenomenon should be treated with low-dose antipsychotics for a few more days
- A drug interaction check shows no problems among her current medications (including ciprofloxacin), but there should be a re-evaluation for new medical insults causing an escalation in her delirium

If there is continued debate between providers over this presentation being a functional psychosis versus an organic, medically induced delirium, what would you suggest?

- A CT scan was performed acutely at admission the first time. It showed no acute hemorrhage or tumor, but cannot initially rule out ischemic

infarctions or microembolic events. Her VNS pacemaker can be turned off, and an MRI of the brain conducted if the MRI can be set up safely to avoid heating the VNS pacemaker wires
- A lumbar puncture can be performed to rule out infection or inflammatory processes in the CNS that cannot be detected by CT scan or MRI
- An EEG can be performed, and if diffuse slowing is noted, then this is reasonably indicative of delirium and not psychiatric disorder

Case outcome: interim follow-up information through 92 hours

- An EEG is performed and shows bifrontal diffuse slowing with occasional beta intrusions, suggesting ongoing delirium
- IV ciprofloxacin is restarted to make sure urosepsis is cleared
- No other clear medical cause is determined as yet
- Patient is placed on 0.5–1.5 mg/d of the typical antipsychotic haloperidol (Haldol) that can be given via multiple routes of administration, which is advantageous if she refuses oral tablets again

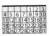

Case debrief

- This patient has a clear history of chronic MDD and GAD, which finally became responsive to PDP, medication polypharmacy, and VNS adjunctive therapy
- A near-remission status was maintained for two to three years
- She became acutely confused with altered consciousness, and then frankly paranoid, in a fluctuating course over one to three days, which is uncharacteristic
  - Given her history of no previous similar exacerbations of depression or any substance misuse
  - Or of other psychiatric disorders associated with psychosis, e.g., schizophrenia, bipolar disorder, or MDD
  - The clinical picture most accurately reflects an acute medical delirium
- This was adequately treated at first by detecting the underlying medical cause, second with behavioral interventions, and third with pharmacologic intervention
- A noninvasive EEG was performed, helping clear up the debate over the dilemma of delirium versus a new functional psychotic event
- The delirium symptoms gradually cleared over the next few days with continued antibiotics, haloperidol, and supportive care

Take-home points

- Acute onset of mental status changes within hours is often drug-induced or a medical delirium
- Confusion and a waxing of consciousness is usually not associated with other major psychiatric disorders

- Consultation and liaison between multiple providers is often needed to successfully diagnose and treat the medical and psychiatric components of delirium

Performance in practice: confessions of a psychopharmacologist

- *What could have been done better here?*
    - Not sure; this case was fairly successful
        - Every now and then, clinicians do things correctly the first time
- *Possible action items for improvement in practice*
    - Research the diagnosis and treatment of delirium in guidelines, review articles, or textbooks
    - Even psychiatrists and psychopharmacologists who do not typically specialize in the interface of psychiatry and internal medicine, called "consultation-liaison psychiatry," may be asked to consult on behalf of their outpatients in similar fashion
        - This type of information is covered on psychiatric board recertification examinations for all psychiatrists!
    - Research typical dosing strategies for both typical and atypical antipsychotics when treating delirium, as dosing is often with lower doses and for shorter durations
    - Become aware of psychotropics that are prone to intoxication effects or withdrawal effects that can mimic delirium
    - Realize that medically or surgically admitted patients may have their psychotropics discontinued, setting them up for withdrawal delirium

Tips and pearls

- Haloperidol (Haldol) is considered the gold standard antipsychotic for use in behavioral management of delirium
- It is a clean drug in that it has very little pharmacodynamic properties outside D2 receptor antagonism
    - There is little to no antihistamine sedation to cloud the mental state further
    - There is little to no anticholinergic potential as far as worsening memory or increasing delirious psychotic features
- It can be given orally or with an IM injection
- It should not be given directly via IV push, as it is known to prolong QTc intervals and place patients at risk for ventricular arrythmia. A slow IV drip may be used with appropriate cardiac monitoring in rare cases
- Guidelines suggest obtaining pre- and post-antipsychotic initiation EKGs, as many typical and atypical antipsychotics prolong QTc intervals in these already compromised medical patients
- Atypical antipsychotics may be used as they have lower EPS rates, but have less of an evidence base regarding dosing

- Risperidone (Risperdal) likely has the most supporting data
- The high-potency typical antipsychotic haloperidol (Haldol) may cause akathisia, which may appear as delirium agitation worsening and lead to a reflexive increase in haloperidol to treat the agitation, further causing more EPS
  - The atypical antipsychotics have less likelihood of akathisia and may be favored for this reason
- However, the atypical antipsychotics are not as selective in that they often have marked pharmacodynamic properties outside D2 receptor antagonism, which may cloud or alter the mental state further
  - For example, olanzapine (Zyprexa) has anticholinergic properties
  - Quetiapine has antihistamine properties
- The risk of TD is minimal as delirium is often treated for a few days to a few weeks at most, using doses lower than that used to treat schizophrenia

Two-minute tutorial

Delirium primer

- Delirium is a sudden-onset and fluctuating course consisting of confusion, altered consciousness, distractibility, and behavioral change due to an underlying medical condition that causes altered brain functioning. It is usually reversible but carries a high mortality rate as patients are often experiencing organ system failure at some level
- Delirium is rarely caused by psychiatric illness, but cases of "manic delirium" are reported in severe cases of bipolar mania
- Typical causes include
  - Alcohol or sedative drug withdrawal
  - Drug intoxication or withdrawal
  - Electrolyte or other body chemical disturbances
  - Infections such as urinary tract infections or pneumonia (more likely in people who already have brain damage from stroke or dementia)
  - Poisons
  - Surgery
- Psychiatric symptoms include
  - Disorganized thinking
    - Speech that does not make sense (incoherent)
    - Inability to stop speech patterns or behaviors
  - Emotional or personality changes
    - Anger
    - Agitation
    - Anxiety
    - Apathy
    - Depression
    - Euphoria

- ○ Irritability
- Common tests used to determine the cause of delirium include
  - Blood ammonia levels
  - Blood chemistry (comprehensive metabolic panel)
  - Blood gas analysis
  - Chest X-ray
  - CSF analysis
  - Creatine kinase level in the blood
  - Drug, alcohol levels (toxicology screen)
  - EEG
  - Head CT scan
  - Head MRI scan
  - Liver function tests
  - Mental status test
  - Serum magnesium
  - Thyroid function tests
  - Urinalysis
  - Vitamin B1 and B12 levels
- Key treatment variables include
  - Ideally, patient should be located in a pleasant, comfortable, non-threatening, physically safe environment
  - Stopping or changing medications that worsen confusion, or that are not necessary, may improve mental function significantly
  - Medications that may worsen confusion include
    - ○ Alcohol
    - ○ Analgesics, especially opioids such as codeine, hydrocodone, morphine, or oxycodone
    - ○ Anticholinergics
    - ○ CNS depressants
    - ○ Cimetidine
    - ○ Illicit drugs
  - Disorders that contribute to confusion should be treated. These may include
    - ○ Anemia
    - ○ Decreased oxygen (hypoxia)
    - ○ Heart failure
    - ○ High carbon dioxide levels (hypercapnia)
    - ○ Infections
    - ○ Kidney failure
    - ○ Liver failure
    - ○ Nutritional disorders
    - ○ Psychiatric conditions (such as depression)
    - ○ Thyroid disorders

- Avoid sensory deprivation. Some patients with delirium may benefit from using hearing aids, glasses, etc., and frequent orientation

Posttest self-assessment question and answer

What are common causes of acute-onset psychosis?

A. Stimulant intoxication
B. Medically induced delirium
C. Alcohol or BZ withdrawal
D. Paranoid schizophrenia
E. A and B
F. A, B, and C
G. All of the above

Answer: F

This case emphasized the acute psychotic onset of a medical delirium, but drug intoxication and withdrawal may produce a similar picture. Schizophrenia usually is accompanied by a prodrome and gradually escalating psychotic symptoms that occur over weeks to months, and therefore this option is incorrect.

References

1. Bressi C, Porcellana M, Marinaccio PM, Nocito EP, Magri L. Short-term psychodynamic psychotherapy versus treatment as usual for depressive and anxiety disorders: a randomized clinical trial of efficacy. *J Nerv Ment Dis* 2010; 198:647–52.

2. Driessen E, Cuijpers P, de Maat SC, et al. The efficacy of short-term psychodynamic psychotherapy for depression: a meta-analysis. *Clin Psychol Rev* 2010; 30:25–36.

3. American Psychiatric Association. *Diagnostic and Statistical Manual of Mental Disorders, Revised*, 4th edn. Washington, DC: American Psychiatric Association Press, 2000.

4. Sadock BJ, Sadock VA. *Kaplan and Sadock's Synopsis of Psychiatry: Behavioral Sciences/Clinical Psychiatry*, 10th edn. Philadelphia, PA: Lippincott Williams & Wilkins, 2007.

5. American Psychiatric Association. *Practice Guideline for the Treatment of Patients with Delirium*. Washington, DC: American Psychiatric Publishing Inc., 1999.

6. Inouye SK. Delirium and other mental status problems in the older patient. In: Goldman L, Ausiello D, eds. *Cecil Medicine*, 23rd edn. Philadelphia, PA: Saunders Elsevier, 2007.

7. Schwartz TL, Masand PS. The role of atypical antipsychotics in the treatment of delirium. *Psychosomatics* 2002; 43:171–4.

8. Schwartz TL, Dewan MJ, Lamparella V, Armenta W. Sustained manic delirium. *J Pharm Technol* 2000; 16:147–50.

The Case: The man with a little bit of everything

The Question: What to do when a patient does not meet full diagnostic criteria for anything

The Dilemma: Categorical versus symptomatic treatment

Pretest self-assessment question (answer at the end of the case)

Which of the following are most accurate about gabapentin and its ability to treat psychiatric symptoms?

A. It alleviates mania
B. It alleviates panic attacks
C. It alleviates obsessive compulsive symptoms
D. It reduces alcohol consumption
E. A and C
F. B and D
G. All of the above

Patient evaluation on intake

- 27-year-old man states he is in between graduate school assignments and "has some concerns"
- Has been depressed and anxious but is most concerned about his alcohol use

Psychiatric history

- Became increasingly anxious two years ago and was placed on the SSRI sertraline (Zoloft)
  - Was experiencing bouts of generalized worries but these episodes would last weeks but never more than a few months
  - Would have minor panic attacks, but not major disabling ones. Sometimes these are triggered by stressors but many happen unexpectedly
  - He states he is socially anxious at times, but this occurs more often in academic circles compared to social circles
  - As a teenager, he had obsessive needs to have symmetry and to wash his hands, but has not had these symptoms since his late teens
  - He denies PTSD
- Alludes to being depressed at times
  - Sleep is disrupted unless he takes the BZRA zolpidem-CR (Ambien-CR)
  - Experiences fatigue, amotivation, and admits to some low points where he has contemplated suicide
  - These may last a few days to a few weeks

- Will have bouts of increased activity and less need for sleep
  - Denies mood elevation at these times, and these episodes usually begin when he takes on new tasks, jobs, interpersonal situations
  - He does feel more capable but denies any grandiosity or invincibility feelings at these times
  - These last from days to weeks depending upon his life events
- The alcohol use increased over the last few weeks to the point of four- to five- day binges of excessive alcohol drinking where, for the first time, he started drinking in the morning
  - Never has been a daily drinker but admits to binges on weekends
    - Has had no legal, medical, or social consequences as a result
    - Does admit that once he has four to five drinks he often drinks several more and loses control of his ability to stop drinking
  - Admits that he has tried to cut back on drinking, would get annoyed if asked to stop, feels guilt now about his excessive use, and on his last binge he drank an "eye-opener" drink in the morning
    - After he tried to quit, he felt compelled to start drinking on the first morning of attempted sobriety
  - Increased tolerance over the years is noted but has never experienced alcohol withdrawal
  - Suicidal thinking escalates now when heavily intoxicated and the most recent alcohol binge scared him and convinced him to seek help

Social and personal history

- Graduated from college and is working on a doctorate in the humanities
- Has a girlfriend and has sustained meaningful relationships without difficulty
- Drinks coffee in the morning, and only smokes cigarettes when drinking alcohol

Medical history

- Denies medical problems

Family history

- Thinks one of his grandmothers suffered from MDD
- Mother takes an SSRI but he cannot recollect which one, and he is unclear if she is depressed, anxious, or both
- He has no family members with schizophrenia or bipolar disorder

Medication history

- Has been treated with two SSRIs by his PCP

- In college he took paroxetine (Paxil) 20 mg/d but was drinking and smoking most of the time so is unclear if it helped, or not
- Sertraline (Zoloft) has been used over the last year, ranging from 50 mg/d to 100 mg/d
  - 50 mg/d is partially ameliorative of his symptoms at best
  - 100 mg/d made him anxious and agitated
- The BZRA zolpidem (Ambien) 10 mg at bedtime has been used for insomnia but became ineffective due to tolerance
- Zolpidem-CR (Ambien-CR) was next used and is effective now
- Alprazolam (Xanax) 1 mg/d has been used as needed for anxiety

Psychotherapy history

- Has not had psychotherapy outside visiting a counselor a few times in college

Patient evaluation on initial visit

- The patient presents with a mixture of subsyndromal depression and anxiety
- Has brief, discrete periods of activity elevation that seem driven by anxiety in new situations
  - Possibly hypomania
- Now has a problematic, acute escalation in his drinking pattern, which left him temporarily more depressed and even suicidal
- Seems motivated to change his drinking pattern, but would like to address his depression and anxiety symptoms as well

Current psychiatric medications

- Zolpidem-CR (Ambien-CR) 6.25–12.5 mg at bedtime as needed for insomnia (BZRA)
- Alprazolam (Xanax) 0.5–1 mg/d as needed for anxiety (BZ)
- Sertraline (Zoloft) 50 mg/d (SSRI)

Question

Do any of these medications concern you regarding this patient's comorbidities?

- Yes, given his alcohol misuse, his BZRA (zolpidem-CR) should be tapered off
- Yes, given his alcohol misuse, his sedative–anxiolytic (alprazolam) should be tapered off
- Yes, his SSRI (sertraline) should be discontinued due to history of possible mood elevations and hypomania

- No, he seems to be partially treated and some patients may require dose escalation for better symptom control

Attending physician's mental notes: initial evaluation

- Seems to have minor depression and minor anxiety symptoms but does not meet a full *DSM-5* categorical diagnosis for any disorder
- Has bouts of increased goal-directed activity that seem to be driven more by anxiety in new social situations, but hypomania must be considered as he may underreport the severity and duration of these episodes
- He appears to be binge drinking and is starting to gain consequences and repercussions from his drinking. He has a few *DSM-5* AUD symptoms, perhaps placing him in the mild to moderate category of severity
- Will have to have three or four subsyndromal *DSM-5* symptom clusters, but they have added up to cause enough psychological distress that he wants to be treated now

Question

Which of the following would be your next step?

- Discuss with the patient which target symptoms (anxiety, depression, insomnia, hypomania, alcohol use) are most impairing and select a medication based upon this rationale
- Focus on alcohol sobriety as this has the highest risk for causing suicide in this patient
- Focus on mood stability as he might be a bipolar II or cyclothymic disorder patient
- As he has no definitive categorical disorder, refer for psychotherapy to address his long-term dynamic issues, anxiety and depression symptoms
- Refer for psychological testing to better delineate his symptoms

Attending physician's mental notes: initial evaluation (continued)

- He is distressed and now motivated for active change
- Views his alcohol use as a problem and being "out of control" and relates some of it to self-medicating his stress, anxiety, and depressive symptoms
- Bouts of increased energy seem to be driven by novelty in new social situations and tasks, which may be a personality trait, a response to

anxiety, but differentially do not seem to be a sustained mood elevation or bipolar disorder phenomenon
- Sees the alcohol use as the main issue and insomnia as the second most impairing target symptom
- The use of excessive alcohol, a BZ, and a BZRA hypnotic are troubling
  - There is no evidence of misusing these controlled medications, but he is at higher risk for becoming addicted to them or accidentally overdosing
  - They are marginally effective now anyhow

Case outcome: initial visit

- Patient is educated about his working diagnosis being complicated due to his minor levels of several symptom clusters, his clear AUD, and that picking an approved monotherapy may be difficult
- He is educated about the conflict of interest in that he presents being worried about alcohol misuse and is also on two addictive sedative-type medications
- Admits he has used them concurrently with alcohol in the past, but has not dose-escalated his prescription medications on his own
- Feels his lower-dose SSRI, sertraline (Zoloft), is partially effective and asks to keep it as it is and not to "give up on it"
- Agrees to taper off his potentially addictive zolpidem-CR and alprazolam with minimal resistance, assuming that his insomnia can be controlled by another regimen

Further investigation

Is there anything else you would especially like to know about this patient?
- Can anyone corroborate his history with regard to his possible hypomania spells?
  - Family members deny noticing any of these
  - There is no evidence of mood elevation, euphoria, expansive thoughts during these spells
  - There have been no impulsive, dangerous, or risky behaviors associated with these

Question

What would you prescribe in addition to continuing the sertaline (Zoloft) SSRI?
- Add another antidepressant with more sedating qualities, such as a SARI (trazodone [Desyrel], trazodone-ER [Oleptro]), a NaSSA (mirtazapine [Remeron]), to offset the agitation he developed on higher-dose SSRI and better treat his insomnia
- Add an atypical antipsychotic that is more sedating in nature

- Add a 5-HT1A receptor partial agonist anxiolytic, buspirone (BuSpar)
- Add an antiepileptic agent such as gabapentin (Neurontin), divalproex sodium (Depakote), or topiramate (Topamax)
- Add an alcohol cessation medication such as acamprosate (Campral), naltrexone (ReVia), or disulfiram (Antabuse)

Case outcome: first interim follow-up visit one week later

- Agrees to lower the controlled medications
- Attempt is made to select a medication that may control a majority of his target symptoms in one monotherapy
- Off-label gabapentin (Neurontin) is chosen for this reason as it has some peer-reviewed trial data supporting its use
  - In SAD
  - In PD
  - In insomnia, as there is evidence that it may promote more restorative slow wave sleep and has sedating clinical side effects
  - In alcohol-dependent and-abusing patients for
    - Detoxification as an adjunctive treatment
    - Alcohol withdrawal adjunctive treatment
    - Reducing alcohol consumption
    - Improving alcohol cessation
  - A similar agent, pregabalin (Lyrica) has strong data supporting its use in GAD but carries a C-V mild addiction propensity label in the United States per the FDA
    - In the United States, possibly addicting drugs are given a class labeling based upon severity of risk
    - C-I drugs are highly addictive and most often are illegal, e.g., cocaine
    - C-II drugs include stimulant medications and opioid pain medications
    - C-V drugs would be of the least addictive potential
  - Both agents are neuronal alpha-2-delta ion channel inhibitors that were initially approved as adjunctive treatment in epilepsy, but have gained more popularity in the treatment of neuropathic pain disorders and FM
  - Pregabalin also has a sedating side-effect profile, which may be utilized to induce sleep as a therapeutic effect instead of an adverse effect

Case debrief

- This patient does not have a clear categorical diagnosis outside AUD
- In the *DSM-5*, there continues to be the categorical use of the intoxication and withdrawal diagnoses, but the use of "abuse" and "dependence" has been removed

- Instead, the term for AUD is employed to describe patients who overuse this substance and develop consequences in psychosocial functioning
- If two or more symptoms of abuse/dependence are noted, then the patient would be classified as suffering from mild AUD
  - Four or more symptoms is moderate AUD
  - Six or more symptoms is severe AUD
- The depression, anxiety, and insomnia are problematic and likely fuel some of his excessive alcohol use. These are viewed as adjustment disorders and that he has limited coping skills to manage new stressors at times
- He tapered off his sedative and hypnotic after being placed on gabapentin (Neurontin) 900 mg/d in divided doses for one week
- He continued his sertraline (Zoloft) 50 mg/d
- He returned, stating that he was sleeping well and that his mood and anxiety were gradually and constantly improving
- He remained alcohol sober
- He had mild headaches as the only side effect
- He was returning to graduate school shortly, wanted to continue both medications, and had set up an appointment with a psychodynamically oriented psychotherapist there

Take-home points

- Some patients do not have bona fide *DSM-5* categorical disorders. In this case, the patient may have had AUD, other specified depressive disorder (recurrent brief depression), other specified anxiety disorder, adjustment disorder, *and* insomnia disorder
- They do have impairing symptoms, target symptoms, that can be quantified and treated psychopharmacologically
- In these cases, instead of choosing several medications to treat each individual *DSM-5* minor entity or each clinical subsyndromal symptom cluster, attempt to choose a single medicine that may be able address multiple phenomenological symptom clusters

Performance in practice: confessions of a psychopharmacologist

- *What could have been done better here?*
  - Would a monotherapy of a non-SSRI be helpful?
    - Perhaps, in that he had two low therapeutic-dose trials of SSRIs. He may also have been better served by using an SNRI, SARI, or NaSSA monotherapy

- ○ Using a more sedating antidepressant with antihistamine properties could possibly treat his dysphoria, worry, and insomnia
  - − Could his BZ have been more adequately dosed?
    - ○ His sedative–anxiolytic was dosed low and increasing it may have been able to better treat his anxiety and insomnia
    - ○ This might be considered risky given his excessive AUD patterns
- • *Possible action items for improvement in practice*
  - − Research the risks of sedative dose escalation and abuse in non-addictive patients and those with previous or current addictive histories
  - − Research non-addictive treatment options for treating anxious and insomnic patients who suffer from comorbid addictions
  - − Research strategies for treating resistant anxiety and resistant insomnia

Tips and pearls

- • Non-addictive strategies for treating target symptoms of anxiety include
  - − Antihistamines
    - ○ Hydroxyzine (Vistaril/Atarax)
  - − Serotonergic agents
    - ○ Buspirone (BuSpar)
    - ○ SSRI
    - ○ SNRI
    - ○ SARI
    - ○ SPARI
  - − Antiepileptics
    - ○ Gabapentin (Neurontin)
    - ○ Pregabalin (Lyrica)
    - ○ Topiramate (Topamax)
  - − Antipsychotics
    - ○ Typical
      - ▪ Chlorpromazine (Thorazine)
      - ▪ Perphenazine (Trilafon)
    - ○ Atypical
      - ▪ Sedating atypical antipsychotics
        - ♦ Quetiapine (Seroquel)
        - ♦ Olanzapine (Zyprexa)
        - ♦ Asenapine (Saphris)

- Non-addictive strategies for treating target symptoms of insomnia include
  - Antihistamines
    - ○ Doxepin (Silenor)
    - ○ Diphenhydramine (Benadryl)
    - ○ Doxylamine (Unisom)
  - Sedating antidepressants
    - ○ TCA (imipramine, amitriptyline, clomipramine, doxepin)
    - ○ NaSSA
  - Antiepileptics
    - ○ Gabapentin (Neurontin)
    - ○ Pregabalin (Lyrica)
    - ○ Tiagabine (Gabitril)
  - Melatonin agonists
    - ○ Ramelteon (Rozerem), tasimelteon (Hetlioz)
  - Antipsychotics
    - ○ Typicals
      - ▪ Sedating typical antipsychotics
      - ▪ Chlorpromazine (Thorazine)
      - ▪ Thioridazine (Mellaril)
    - ○ Atypicals
      - ▪ Sedating atypical antipsychotics
        - ♦ Quetiapine (Seroquel)
        - ♦ Olanzapine (Zyprexa)
        - ♦ Asenapine (Saphris)

Mechanism of action moment

Focus on alpha-2-delta calcium channel blockade

- Two antiepileptic/antineuropathic pain medications utilize this unique mechanism of action
  - Gabapentin (Neurontin)
  - Pregabalin (Lyrica)
- Blockade of neuronal calcium channels has the net effect of dampening neuronal firing
- If this occurs in
  - Peripheral pain neurons, then pain lessens
  - Cortical neurons, then synchronous epileptiform waves diminish
  - Sleep-promoting center neurons, then delta wave sleep increases
  - The limbic system, then anxiety symptoms diminish and alcohol use may diminish

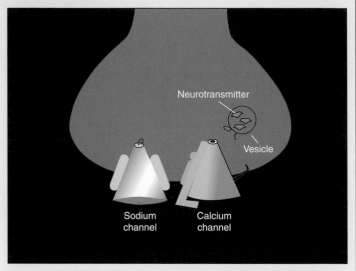

Figure 26.1. Sodium and calcium ion influx channels of a neuron.

- If the neuron experiences minor excitatory depolarization from synaptic input, sodium channels open, allowing further neuronal depolarization
- This secondary depolarization allows calcium channels (called N and P/Q presynaptic channels) to undergo a conformational change, which opens a calcium channel and calcium ion influx further excites the neuron toward an actional potential and firing
- In cortical neurons, this excitation might initiate a seizure, and in peripheral pain or central thalamic neurons, may create sensitization whereby excessive pain signaling is created
- Theoretically, excitation elsewhere in the brain may create anxiety, insomnia, or the drive to drink alcohol
- Gabapentin (Neurontin), used in the current case, and its counterpart pregabalin (Lyrica), are both alpha-2-delta binding drugs
  - When either drug is introduced and binds to the alpha-2-delta subunit of voltage-sensitive calcium channels depicted in Figure 26.1, they close the channels because the protein structure of the channel changes, helping to narrow or close the channel passageway or central pore. Calcium ions cannot gain entry into the neuron
  - This pharmacodynamic activity diminishes excessive neuronal activity and theoretically lowers psychiatric symptoms as well as neurological symptoms
  - Although these drugs are structurally related to GABA, they are not true analogs and do not have direct actions on GABA-A receptors

Two-minute tutorial

pharmacologic strategies for alcohol cessation for use in a busy, office-based practice

- Psychopharmacologists seem to put off treating addiction symptoms while performing standard psychopharmacological outpatient practice
- Psychopharmacologists seem willing to become amateur neurologists when they treat EPS
- Psychopharmacologists seem willing to become amateur urologists when they treat sexual dysfunction caused by SSRIs
- Some psychopharmacologists seem willing to become amateur PCPs when they treat antipsychotic-induced weight gain, diabetes, or hyperlipidemia
- It is interesting in that psychopharmacologists are willing to go the distance, become educated about non-psychiatric medications and their application for use in off-label manners, but we often seem scared to use alcohol cessation medications that are clearly well studied and FDA approved and are de facto psychiatric in nature
- It is also interesting that, in a similar fashion, psychopharmacologists likely underutilize the smoking cessation medications of nicotine replacement therapy, bupropion-XL (Zyban) and varenicline (Chantix)
- Compared to other *DSM-5* disorders, nicotine use disorder and AUD likely have the largest impact on population health (morbidity, mortality, accidents), and we often minimally address these in the general adult psychiatric practice
- Consider learning about the following three approved AUD treatments *and* possibly employing them in day-to-day office-based psychiatric practice

Disulfiram (Antabuse)

- Is taken daily, 250 mg/d after initial loading with 500 mg/d
- Requires more informed consent and patient education, because if alcohol is ingested or absorbed, the patient may have violent nausea and vomiting
- It is an aldehyde dehydrogenase inhibitor
- It is aversive conditioning and a deterrent approach
- Patient must clearly be sober prior to starting
- This drug is harder to start in practice as it is time-consuming to educate the patient
- Often when patients refuse to go to a rehabilitation facility for 28 days, they can be offered daily disulfiram instead, where they are ideally observed taking it by a sober support person or in the office itself
- Both approaches theoretically can separate a person from ongoing alcohol use

- The rehabilitation facility has physical walls
- Disulfiram has mental walls due to the fear of vomiting

Naltrexone (ReVia)

- Is taken 50 mg/d after use of a titration protocol
- It is an opioid antagonist
- Theoretically, it dampens the positive reward feelings from binge alcohol drinking and decreases the likelihood of future use after being sober as it separates the stimulus–response nature of alcohol ingestion and feeling good afterward

Acamprosate (Campral)

- Is taken 666 mg three times a day
- It is a glutamate metabotropic receptor antagonist
- Theoretically, it dampens glutamate excitotoxicity when the influence of GABA-A PAM is withdrawn when alcohol sobriety occurs
  - GABA activity decreases and there is theoretically now unopposed glutamate hyperactivity
- This may reduce alcohol cravings and aid in sobriety maintenance
- For all agents, it is ideal if the patient achieves at least a few days of being sober prior to drug initiation

Posttest self-assessment question and answer

Which of the following are most accurate about gabapentin and its ability to treat psychiatric symptoms?

A. It alleviates mania
B. It alleviates panic attacks
C. It alleviates obsessive compulsive symptoms
D. It reduces alcohol consumption
E. A and C
F. B and D
G. All of the above

Answer: F

A review of off-label literature and review articles suggests a moderately stringent evidence base supporting the use of gabapentin to diminish panic, social anxiety, and alcohol consumption. There is much less evidence, and even negative outcomes, for treating mania. There is clear supportive evidence for its use in treating epilepsy and neuropathic pain disorders.

References

1. Myrick H, Anton R, Voronin K, Wang W, Henderson S. A double-blind evaluation of gabapentin on alcohol effects and drinking in a clinical laboratory paradigm. *Alcohol Clin Exp Res* 2007; 31:221–7.

2. Furieri FA, Nakamura-Palacios EM. Gabapentin reduces alcohol consumption and craving: a randomized, double-blind, placebo-controlled trial. *J Clin Psychiatry* 2007; 68:1691–700.

3. Bonnet U, Banger M, Leweke FM, et al. Treatment of acute alcohol withdrawal with gabapentin: results from a controlled two-center trial. *J Clin Psychopharmacol* 2003; 23:514–9.

4. Letterman L, Markowitz JS. Gabapentin: a review of published experience in the treatment of bipolar disorder and other psychiatric conditions. *Pharmacotherapy* 1999; 19:565–72.

5. Pande AC, Pollack MH, Crockatt J, et al. Placebo-controlled study of gabapentin treatment of panic disorder. *J Clin Psychopharmacol* 2000; 20:467–71.

6. Pande AC, Davidson JR, Jefferson JW, et al. Treatment of social phobia with gabapentin: a placebo-controlled study. *J Clin Psychopharmacol* 1999; 19:341–8.

7. Mula M, Pini S, Cassano GB. The role of anticonvulsant drugs in anxiety disorders: a critical review of the evidence. *J of Clin Psychopharmacol* 2007; 27:263–72.

8. Taylor CP, Gee NS, Su TZ, et al. A summary of mechanistic hypotheses of gabapentin pharmacology. *Epilepsy Res* 1998; 29:231–46.

9. American Psychiatric Association. *Diagnostic and Statistical Manual of Mental Disorders*, 5th edn. Washington, DC: American Psychiatric Association Press, 2013.

10. Stahl SM. *Stahl's Essential Psychopharmacology*, 4th edn. New York, NY: Cambridge University Press, 2013.

11. Stahl SM. *Stahl's Essential Psychopharmacology: The Prescriber's Guide*, 5th edn. New York, NY: Cambridge University Press, 2014.

The Case: Oops. . .he fell off the curve

The Question: What to do when patients lose too much weight

The Dilemma: In the era of weight-gain side-effect notoriety, the stimulants may cause equally problematic loss in weight and stature

Pretest self-assessment question (answer at the end of the case)

Which of the following do not appear to have marked weight-loss adverse effects when treating children with ADHD?

A. Guanfacine–ER (Intuniv)
B. Clonidine-ER (Kapvay)
C. Atomoxetine (Strattera)
D. Lisdexamfetamine (Vyvanse)
E. A and B
F. A, B, and C
G. All of the above

Patient evaluation on intake

- Nine-year-old presents with his parents who note that they are having a hard time managing him at home and at school
- He is "not like their other kids"

Psychiatric history

- At age six, they noticed increasing anxiety regarding things such as attending school, death, dying, and incurring illnesses
- He would often walk in circles and flap both arms intermittently throughout the day in response
  - This increases as his anxiety escalates
  - He is "thinking about things" and is restless
  - Thoughts may be positive, have a fantasy component, or be daydream-like while walking
  - Denies having negative, hostile thoughts
  - Does not feel controlled, like he is being forced or told to do this
  - Does not have hallucinations or delusions
  - Walking in circles does not seem to foster a reduction in anxiety and does not seem repetitive enough where he loses hours of productivity
  - He has no other stereotypic movement or functional fixedness issues
  - He does have tactile sensitivity with certain food textures and does not like to be hugged or touched, but is amicable and affable
  - He does not appear to be rigid or oppositional

- Around this age, he developed greater inattention, inability to focus, hyperactivity, and impulsivity, which have gradually escalated over the last two years
  - These symptoms now interfere with schooling and have caused him to be held back to repeat one grade
- He is a gregarious child who has friends and sustains reciprocal friendships and relationships
- There is no evidence of combativeness or violent behavior
- Walking in circles occurs at home only now as he is able to control this at school. However, his inattentive and hyperactive symptoms continue and are apparent at home, school, soccer, at the mall, etc., and are pervasive
- Recently, the patient is more aware that he is impaired and not moving through school at the same rate as other children
- He now finds things to be "difficult," "boring," problematic, and his self-esteem is suffering
  - At times he is sad, but there is no evidence of MDD, psychotic disorder, or bipolar disorder

Social and personal history

- Patient is a third grader
- Parents are married and he has three younger siblings
- He likes some sports, reads a lot, and plays video games
- He was born by normal delivery and reached usual developmental milestones

Medical history

- There are no acute medical problems
- Used to be roughly at the 50th percentile for height and weight, but since medications were issued by his pediatrician one year ago, he has dropped gradually toward the 10th percentile
- The pediatrician is not currently concerned as the family has shorter stature and feels the patient has not lost significant enough weight or "fallen off the growth curve"
- There is no personal, nor any family medical history of cardiac issues
- The patient does not have any tics or other abnormal involuntary movements

Family history

- Mother may suffer from GAD
- There is no clear family history of ADHD, intellectual or developmental disorders

Medication history

- Started an SSRI, fluoxetine (Prozac), 20 mg/d given by his pediatrician one year ago for the anxious symptoms
  - This has been moderately effective
  - Dose was lowered to 10mg/d two months ago as he developed enuresis, anorexia, and weight loss
- Started lisdexamfetamine (Vyvanse) 20mg/d three months ago in addition to the SSRI
  - Tolerating this well, but with minimal additional effectiveness
  - Previously, D-methylphenidate-XR (Focalin-XR) 10–20mg/d caused him to become sad and emotionally labile
  - Methylphenidate transdermal (Daytrana) patch caused heart palpitations and increasing anxiety at 20 mg/d, and was discontinued
  - The parents do not attribute his anorexia and gradual weight loss to these stimulant trials as this began earlier with the SSRI monotherapy

Psychotherapy history

- Sees a therapist every one to two weeks
- Parents have tried many positive reinforcement strategies with little effect

Patient evaluation on initial visit

- The patient presents with mild anxious symptoms, but reports his generalized worrying about multiple topics has greatly diminished, as has his walking in circles, since starting the SSRI
- The greater clinical problem is inattention, hyperactivity, and impulsivity, which have only minimally responded to an SSRI, low-dose stimulant, and behavioral modification attempts
- May now be underweight and short in stature

Current psychiatric medications

- Fluoxetine (Prozac) 10 mg/d (SSRI)
- Lisdexamfetamine (Vyvanse) 20 mg/d (stimulant)

Question

Is it possible that the SSRI is causing his weight loss instead of the more commonly accused and more often guilty stimulant?

- Yes, in depression and anxiety studies, the SSRIs have been associated with appetite suppression and weight-loss adverse effects. Anorexia is noted in 7% of adults treated acutely with fluoxetine and 4% with sertraline
- No, the SSRIs cause weight gain and appetite increase more often than weight-loss adverse effects

- No, the stimulants are well known for their approved use, and off-label use as appetite suppressants in obese patients
- No, the stimulants are well known for anorexia and weight-loss adverse effects while treating ADHD

Attending physician's mental notes: initial evaluation

- The patient's anxiety appears to predominantly contain multifocal worries consistent with GAD, but his repetitive walking behaviors seem to be more in line with OCD
- His repetitive movements and arm flapping could be related to mild ASD (formerly Asperger's disorder in *DSM-IVTR*), but he has no other ASP symptoms
- Regardless, his worries and repetitive behaviors seem controlled; but if history is accurate, his nearly curative SSRI is causing excessive weight loss and enuresis when used at higher therapeutic doses
- Does meet ADHD, combined-type diagnostic criteria, and these symptoms are the most problematic for now
- Case is complicated by current side effects and previous stimulant trials have been ineffective due to intolerability

Question

Which of the following would be your next step?

- Remove the SSRI as his weight loss is problematic
- Remove the stimulant as it is the most likely weight-loss agent
- Switch to another SSRI in hopes of better tolerability
- Switch to another stimulant in hopes of better tolerability
- Switch to a novel antidepressant class to continue anxiolysis
- Switch to a nonstimulant ADHD-approved medication
- Further maximize his current medication regimen

Attending physician's mental notes: initial evaluation (continued)

- Anxiety is so well controlled that removing the SSRI could make things worse
- ADHD is poorly controlled so the stimulant should be raised
- It is clear that his parents are concerned immensely about his weight and height but it is unclear if the patient is truly at risk or falling off his growth curve, as the pediatrician is non-committal about this finding currently

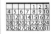

Case outcome: initial visit

- Parents are fully informed and educated about the risks and benefits of both his current medications

- After coming for consultation, they are ambivalent about *any* changes due to the fact:
  - That they have had negative effects from previous stimulants and increasing this one worries them
    ○ They refuse an increase in his dose, and state they will consider this and call back
  - That they have had good effects from the SSRI, and despite current side effects, would not want his anxiety to return
    ○ As the patient has been in remission from his anxiety symptoms now for several months, they do reluctantly agree to lower his fluoxetine (Prozac) down to 5 mg/d to lower his side-effect burden and hopefully continue its effectiveness

Further investigation

Is there anything else you would especially like to know about this patient?

- What about his collaborating pediatrician and his findings?
  - A release of information is obtained
  - The pediatrician states that starting the fluoxetine SSRI clearly promoted secondary enuresis at the higher 20 mg per dose
  - It is not clear if the weight loss and growth retardation is from the SSRI, the multiple stimulant trials, his genetics, or normal, as he has not fallen off his growth curve yet
  - His height and weight trajectories have diminished but are not an imminent problem
  - The pediatrician suggests that psychotropics continue to be prescribed as his psychiatric symptoms are the most disruptive and problematic now
  - He will consider endocrine and developmental geneticist consultations if these adverse effects worsen and become a clinical dilemma
  - He confirms there are no cardiac concerns for this patient and approves use of stimulants. An EKG is not warranted
- Is there any reason why he might be vulnerable to side effects from his low-dose psychotropics?
  - Fluoxetine (Prozac) is clearly known as a strong inhibitor of the CYP450 2D6 isoenzyme system in the liver
    ○ Psychopharmacologists often have to lower doses of other augmentation agents, such as aripiprazole, atomoxetine, desipramine, etc., when fluoxetine is part of the regimen
    ○ Amphetamine stimulants are a substrate for CYP450 2D6 and may need to be lowered when combined with fluoxetine in some patients, or they may experience stimulant intoxication or toxicity

    ○ Methylphenidate-based stimulants are unlikely to be subject to a drug–drug interaction involving his SSRI via CYP450 isoenzymes

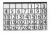

Case outcome: first interim follow-up visit two months later

- Between sessions, parents agree to increase lisdexamfetamine (Vyvanse) to 30mg/d and taper off fluoxetine (Prozac), as it is still thought to be the primary reason for weight loss
- ADHD symptoms improve markedly at school
- At home, there is still great difficulty in the mornings and late afternoons when the stimulant is not at peak plasma levels
- Enuresis resolves with tapering off of fluoxetine and he has no acute side effects from lisdexamfetamine increased dosing
- His pediatrician feels that annual monitoring is adequate for his height and weight
- He is 51 in and 56 lbs and has not lost weight recently
- All are happy with the patient's continued lack of anxiety recurrence and ongoing moderate ADHD improvements

Question

The patient has morning and late afternoon breakthrough ADHD symptoms; what might you suggest?

- Increase the stimulant in the morning
- Wake the patient up briefly an hour before his usual waking time and administer his stimulant then to improve morning symptom control
- Even though his stimulant is approved once daily, administer a smaller booster dose at lunch-time at school for better afternoon/evening symptom coverage
- As his stimulant is considered long acting, augment with a shorter-acting, amphetamine-based stimulant (d/l-amphetamine [Adderall]) in the morning and/or afternoon for better symptom control
- Augment his stimulant with a nonstimulant, longer-acting ADHD medication such as atomoxetine (Strattera), guanfacine-ER (Intuniv), or clonidine-ER (Kapvay)

Case outcome: interim follow-up visits three to six months later

- Lisdexamfetamine (Vyvanse) is increased to 40 mg/d to obtain better effectiveness and afternoon symptom control of ADHD
- Parents will attempt to awaken the patient earlier to dispense this medication for better symptom control at breakfast-time and on his bus ride to school
- There is no change in stature/height

- School reports good ADHD symptom control, but notice that patient seems to be worried about eating habits, bathroom habits, and appears to be more obsessive in general
- Sertraline (Zoloft) is started, fearing anxiety recurrence and in lieu of fluoxetine (Prozac)
  - It is started ideally to recapture an SSRI anxiolytic effect without the side effects of anorexia or enuresis
  - At 50 mg/d, anxiety symptoms normalize but secondary enuresis begins again
  - Sertraline (Zoloft) is lowered to 25 mg/d as a result; several weeks later, SSRI effectiveness was noted to return
- He continues with good effectiveness from both medications and enuresis is resolved

Attending physician's mental notes: follow-up visit, six months

- Two out of two SSRIs have caused enuresis, but the current low-dose SSRI seems to be fairly effective in lowering his anxiety without this adverse effect
- Increased stimulant dose has lowered his ADHD symptoms, improving his school performance, self-esteem, and lowered his parents' frustration at home
- Height and weight have not changed, so perhaps the previous weight loss was, in fact, due to SSRI fluoxetine (Prozac), which had been discontinued some time ago

Case outcome: interim follow-up visits eight to 12 months later

- Toward the end of this interval, the patient appears to have lost 5 lbs
- The parents ask for options outside the current medicine combination that might avoid weight-loss side effects
  - Pediatrician reports that he has now, in fact, fallen off the growth curve, is mildly concerned, and asks if medications can be switched or drug cessation offered over the summer
  - Drug cessation is not clinically warranted as the patient's esteem will suffer due to his ADHD symptoms, which would begin interfering with peer relationships and ability to go to summer camps
  - The patient refuses to drink protein-enrichment shakes, but is allowed to eat and snack *ad lib*, but he fails to gain weight this way
- Nonstimulant options are discussed and the patient is started on the ADHD-approved guanfacine-ER (Intuniv), an alpha-2 adrenergic receptor agonist, while the lisdexamfetamine (Vyvanse) is lowered to 30 mg/d in the hope of reversing the newest weight loss

- Guanfacine-ER (Intuniv) dose is titrated up and lisdexamfetamine (Vyvanse) dose is lowered in the hope of fully replacing the stimulant eventually
  - The patient becomes sedated and sleepy at school on 3 mg/d of guanfacine-ER and exhibits an increase in his ADHD symptoms on the remaining lisdexamfetamine 10 mg/d

Case debrief

- This patient may have a subsyndromal developmental disorder given his stereotypic behaviors, tactile sensitivity, and possibly genetic short stature
- He suffered a mixture of GAD and OCD symptoms that have been fully treated with low-dose SSRIs
  - This treatment clearly caused enuresis, and while on SSRIs, his normal weight gain seemed inhibited
- He suffered a moderate to severe number of ADHD symptoms, which were well treated once an adequate stimulant dose was achieved
  - This treatment in conjunction with SSRI use ultimately caused him to fall off his growth curve, instigating a change in medications away from the higher-dosed stimulant medication and SSRI combination
- The patient is currently taking
  - Sertraline (Zoloft) 25 mg/d
  - Lisdexamfetamine (Vyvanse) 20 mg/d
  - Guanfacine-ER (Intuniv) 2 mg/d
- He suffers no acute side effects and is functioning well at home and at school
- He appears to be maintaining his weight and height on this regimen and his loss of stature and weight has halted for the time being
  - There appears to be benefit now with minimum side effects on low doses of three complementary medications in a rational polypharmacy approach
- He functions better upon awakening and in the afternoons compared to using a stimulant alone to control his ADHD symptoms
- He is less anxious, and it appears that guanfacine-ER has also augmented his SSRI response in this area
- He has been sent for genetic testing to determine if he has a congenital stature disorder or a chromosomally based developmental disorder such as Williams' syndrome

Take-home points

- ADHD comorbidity in children is less prevalent than noted in adult patients
- Comorbidity does, however, occur sometimes and this case emphasized the overlap of ADHD, anxiety disorders, and ASD

- Like adults, adequate doses of psychotropics are generally needed to obtain good clinical responses
- Like adults, children develop side effects with the added complication that the medication may hinder normal growth potential
- These longer-term side effects must be monitored in collaboration with primary care clinicians

Performance in practice: confessions of a psychopharmacologist

- *What could have been done better here?*
  - The SSRI was effective for anxiety but problematic for inducing weight loss and enuresis; are there other options for anxiolysis in this patient?
    - ○ Atomoxetine (Strattera) is an ADHD-approved agent that is an NRI. Agents with this property sometimes act as anxiolytics
    - ○ BZ sedative–anxiolytics are frowned upon in children due to paradoxical agitation effects and addiction
    - ○ SNRIs have no approvals in this age group and possess SRI properties equivalent to those of SSRIs and are likely to have similar side effects, while the NRI properties might help the ADHD symptoms
    - ○ Buspirone (BuSpar) is a 5-HT1A receptor partial agonist that is approved for adults with GAD and it might be utilized off-label in children with anxiety
    - ○ The antihypertensive agents guanfacine (Tenex) and clonidine (Catapres) are sometimes used off-label to treat adults with agitation, anxiety, and insomnia as both are alpha-2a noradrenergic agonists
  - Slow-release preparations exist for both Intuniv and Kapvay, respectively, and are approved for treating childhood ADHD
  - In the future, it might be possible to discontinue this patient's SSRI to determine if guanfacine-ER (Intuniv) alone will treat his anxiety without enuresis or weight loss
- *Possible action items for improvement in practice*
  - Research the risks of stimulant use with regard to height and weight loss
  - Research the risks of stimulant use with regard to cardiac side effects and monitoring
  - Research nonstimulant options available for treating ADHD as they may carry less risk for short stature or weight loss

– Research strategies where polypharmacy may be rational and warranted to improve effectiveness while diminishing side effects

Tips and pearls

- When dosing stimulants in children and adolescents
  - Collaborate with primary care
  - Monitor height and weight
  - Monitor blood pressure
  - Monitor for abnormal movements such as tic disorders
  - Monitor for affective dyscontrol and acute onset of suicidal symptoms
  - Monitor for switches into mania if the patient has comorbid bipolar disorder
  - Monitor for substance abuse and drug diversion
    - Evidence suggests children and teenagers treated with stimulants often have better symptom control and less risk of addiction to drugs later in life
    - However, teenagers and young adults may divert and share their medications more often
  - Consider an EKG or further cardiac workup in patients with a severe family history of cardiac illness or early myocardial infarctions, or those with any current cardiorespiratory symptoms noted upon their own exertion
    - The American Heart Association issued a warning that all children should have EKGs prior to stimulant use
    - The American Association of Pediatricians has made similar comments but has since modified them, suggesting EKGs are needed only on a case-by-case basis
    - The FDA has issued warnings regarding the possibility of sudden cardiac death with stimulant use
    - The most current longitudinal studies suggest no added cardiac risk with stimulant use compared to that in children not taking stimulants

Two-minute tutorial

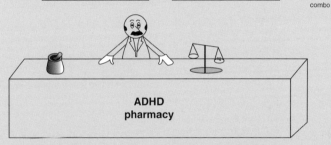

Figure 27.1. Attention deficit hyperactivity disorder pharmacy.

Medication management of ADHD in children versus adults

- First-line treatments for ADHD in children (Figure 27.1, left) include slow-release stimulants, while immediate-release stimulants, atomoxetine, and alpha-2a agonists (guanfacine-ER, clonidine-ER) are second-line options
- The classical stimulants have the largest effect sizes and greatest evidence base for ADHD efficacy
- The slow-release stimulants likely lower side-effect rates, given their lower and more consistent plasma levels, and improve compliance by once-daily dosing
- Third-line options include antidepressants with noradrenergic properties
- Adjunctive options include atypical antipsychotics or behavioral therapy
- For adults (Figure 27.1, right), first-line treatments include nonstimulants such as atomoxetine, guanfacine-ER, or perhaps off-label modafinil (Provigil), as well as slow-release stimulants

- Immediate-release stimulants and noradrenergic antidepressants are second-line options
- Adjunctive options may include atypical antipsychotics or drug-abuse treatments for patients with SUD
- In adults, there is greater risk of stimulant abuse or diversion, which warrants often starting with nonstimulant preparations despite their lower effectiveness at times

Posttest self-assessment question and answer

Which of the following do not appear to have marked weight loss adverse effects when treating children with ADHD?

A. Guanfacine-ER (Intuniv)
B. Clonidine-ER (Kapvay)
C. Atomoxetine (Strattera)
D. Lisdexamfetamine (Vyvanse)
E. A and B
F. A, B, and C
G. All of the above

Answer: F

A, B, and C are considered nonstimulant-approved treatments for child and adolescent ADHD. A plus B are alpha-2a receptor agonists and C is an NRI. Mechanistically and statistically, A, B, and C are associated with less apparent risk for abnormal weight and stature loss compared to the true stimulant medications such as lisdexamfetamine (D).

There does exist a controversy in that shorter-term studies of stimulants suggest weight and height loss, but prospective, longitudinal studies up to 10 years have most recently suggested no loss of weight or stature due to ADHD or stimulant use. Many initial studies followed biostatistics only for a few years or did not follow children into adulthood.

References

1. Stahl SM. *Stahl's Essential Psychopharmacology*, 4th edn. New York, NY: Cambridge University Press, 2013.
2. Stahl SM. *Stahl's Essential Psychopharmacology: The Prescriber's Guide*, 5th edn. New York, NY: Cambridge University Press, 2014.
3. Biederman J, Wilens T, Mick E, et al. Psychoactive substance use disorders in adults with attention deficit hyperactivity disorder (ADHD): effects of ADHD and psychiatric comorbidity. *Am J Psychiatry* 1995; 152:1652–8.
4. Wilens T, Faraone S, Biederman J, et al. Does stimulant therapy of attention-deficit/hyperactivity disorder beget later substance abuse? A meta-analytic review of the literature. *Pediatrics* 2003; 111:179–85.

5. American Psychiatric Association. *Diagnostic and Statistical Manual of Mental Disorders*, 5th edn. Washington, DC: American Psychiatric Association Press, 2013.

6. Biederman J, Spencer T, Monuteaux M, Faraone S. A naturalistic 10-year prospective study of height and weight in children with attention-deficit hyperactivity disorder grown up: sex and treatment effects. *J Pediatr* 2010; 157:635–40.

7. Faraone SV, Biederman J, Morley CP, Spencer TJ. Effect of stimulants on height and weight: a review of the literature. *J Am Acad Child Adolesc Psychiatry* 2008; 47:994–1009.

8. Swanson JM, Elliott GR, Greenhill LL, et al. Effects of stimulant medication on growth rates across 3 years in the MTA follow-up. *J Am Acad Child Adolesc Psychiatry* 2007; 46: 1015–27.

9. Poulton A, Cowell CT. Slowing of growth in height and weight on stimulants: a characteristic pattern. *J Paediatr Child Health* 2003; 39:180–5.

10. Fluoxetine. FDA Package Insert 2007, Eli Lilly Inc. http://pi.lilly.com/us/prozac.pdf. Accessed August 10, 2015.

11. Sertraline. FDA Package Insert 2014, Pfizer Inc. http://labeling.pfizer.com/ShowLabeling.aspx?id=517#page=1. Accessed August 10, 2015.

12. DeBattista DMH, Schatzberg AF, eds. *Black Book of Psychotropic Dosing and Monitoring*, 10th edn. New York, NY: MBL Communications, 2006.

13. Schwartz TL, Nihalani N, Jindal S, et al. Psychiatric medication induced obesity: an epidemiologic review. *Obes Rev* 2004; 5:115–21.

14. American Academy of Pediatrics, Committee on Quality Improvement, and Subcommittee on Attention-Deficit/Hyperactivity Disorder. Clinical practice guideline: treatment of the school-aged child with attention-deficit/hyperactivity disorder. *Pediatrics* 2001; 108:1033–44.

15. American Academy of Pediatrics. Diagnosis and evaluation of the child with attention-deficit/hyperactivity disorder. *Pediatrics* 2000; 105:1158–70.

16. Miller A, Lee S, Raina P, et al. *A Review of Therapies for Attention-Deficit/Hyperactivity Disorder*. Ottawa, ON: Canadian Coordinating Office for Health Technology Assessment (CCOHTA), 1998.

17. March JS, Swanson JM, Arnold LE, et al. Anxiety as a predictor and outcome variable in the multimodal treatment study of children with ADHD. *J Abnorm Child Psychol* 2000; 28:527–41.

18. Schelleman H, Bilker WB, Strom BL, et al. Cardiovascular events and death in children exposed and unexposed to ADHD agents. *Pediatrics* 2011; 127:1102–10.
19. Markowitz JS, Patrick AS. Pharmacokinetic and pharmacodynamic drug interactions in the treatment of attention-deficit hyperactivity disorder. *Clin Pharmacokinet* 2001; 40:753–72.

The **Case:** 54-year-old with recurrent depression and "psychiatric" parkinsonism

The **Question** (Pharmacogenetics, Part 1): How might psychopharmacology be delivered in the future?

The **Dilemma:** Can genotyping help predict successful treatment selection

Pretest self-assessment question (answer at the end of the case)

A 54-year-old patient has depression with prominent cognitive symptoms and also has the Val/Val genotype for catechol-O-methyltransferase (COMT). Based only on this genetic result, what treatment might be preferred for this patient?

A. SSRI

B. SNRI

C. NDRI

Patient evaluation on intake

- 54-year-old man was admitted to the hospital for an MDE
- Experienced his first MDE at age 30; since then has had periodic MDEs of two-to-three months duration almost every fall/winter

Psychiatric history

- At age 37 had first inpatient psychiatric admission
- Admitted again as an inpatient at ages 43 and 45
- However, received no psychopharmacologic treatment other than sporadic St. John's Wort for any of these episodes; he seemed to respond to this treatment plan
- At age 47 was again hospitalized with an MDE
  - Characterized by depressed mood, psychomotor retardation, cognitive impairment, reduced drive, sleep problems, delusions of guilt, and suicidal thoughts

Social and personal history

- Smokes cigarettes regularly, does not drink or use illicit drugs
- Is single and does not have any children

Medical history

- There are no current medical problems

Family history

- He does not have any significant family history of psychiatric disorder

Medication history

- At this admission to the inpatient unit, he was treated with prescription psychotropic medications for the first time
  - Mirtazapine (Remeron) 45 mg/d (NaSSA)
  - Risperidone (Risperdal) 3 mg/d (atypical antipsychotic)
  - Valproic acid (Depakene) 2000 mg/d (mood stabilizer)
  - Lorazepam (Ativan) 2.5 mg/d (BZ)
- Experienced slight improvement but continued to have reduced drive, concentration deficits, psychomotor retardation, and suicidal thoughts
- He developed EPS with risperidone treatment and was switched to another atypical antipsychotic, quetiapine (Seroquel) 400 mg/d, still with only partial MDD improvement
- Mirtazapine (Remeron) was then switched to the SSRI sertraline (Zoloft) 200 mg/d and experienced some additional improvement in his mood but not in his concentration or fatigue
- Next, received a series of 18 ECT sessions, while continuing only sertraline (Zoloft)
- He obtained full remission status post-ECT and was discharged, with maintenance ECT and continuation of his SSRI recommended
- Upon ECT service discharge, he was sent to outpatient psychiatry clinic for follow-up care

Patient evaluation on initial visit

- Presents now, at age 54, with depressed mood, severe lack of drive, concentration deficits, memory problems, slow thinking, extreme fatigue, rigid facial expressions and gestures, and suicidal thoughts
- His symptoms could be characterized in part as "psychiatric parkinsonism" with lack of drive and problems with concentration and memory, psychomotor retardation, slower thinking (bradyphrenia), and problems with facial expression and emotional gestures
  - These Parkinson's-like symptoms are caused by his MDD
- He is not currently taking any medications as he stopped sertraline (Zoloft) after inpatient care but before his visit to outpatient department

Question

Based on this patient's history and current symptom profile, testing of which of the following genes might be useful?

- SLC6A4 (SERT)
- SLC6A4 and COMT
- SLC6A4, COMT, and methylenetetrahydrafolate reductase (MTHFR)
- SLC6A4, COMT, MTHFR, and calcium channel voltage-dependent L-type, alpha-1c subunit (CACNA1C)
- SLC6A4, COMT, MTHFR, CACNA1C, and D2 receptor (DRD2)

Attending physician's mental notes: initial evaluation

- Testing of any of these genes may provide information that could be considered in the management of this patient
  - SLC6A4, 5HTTLPR Long(L)/Short(S) promoter insertion/deletion (rs63749047) and L(A)/L(G) (rs25531) polymorphism
    - This patient is homozygous (i.e., has two copies) for L(A)/L(A)
    - May indicate individuals who are more likely to exhibit response to SSRI treatment (compared to those with the S or L(G) allele)
    - They have more normal SERT function
    - They are hypothetically more resilient to stress-induced triggers for depression and suicide
    - L(A)/L(A) alleles are considered *good**
  - COMT, 158 Val>Met (472 G>A, rs4680)
    - This patient is homozygous for (158 Val/Val, 472 G/G)
    - May indicate individuals with depression who are more likely to experience associated cognitive symptoms such as slowness of information processing, difficulty with executive functioning, and problem solving
    - They have greater reductions in DA levels in prefrontal cortices
    - VAL/VAL alleles are considered *bad*
  - MTHFR, 677 C>T
    - This patient is homozygous for T/T
    - May indicate individuals with depression who are also more likely to experience associated cognitive symptoms, especially in those who also express the Val variant of the COMT gene
    - These patients utilize brain L-methylfolate inefficiently, thus lowering their ability to synthesis serotonin, NE, and DA
    - T/T alleles are considered *bad*
  - CACNA1C, G>A rs1006737
    - This patient is homozygous for (G/G)
    - The A allele (not carried by this patient) may indicate individuals with mood disorders who are more likely to experience frequent relapses and recurrences
    - They may lack neuronal membrane ion channel stability and allow excessive activity perhaps in limbic areas
    - G/G alleles are considered *good*
  - DRD2, -141C insertion/deletion (rs1799732)
    - This patient is homozygous for (Ins/Ins)
    - May indicate individuals who are more likely to benefit from augmentation with an atypical antipsychotic in the event that they do not respond to an antidepressant (compared to those who carry the Del allele)

- These patients hypothetically have more normalized function of the D2 receptors in associated neuronal pathways
- Ins/Ins alleles are considered *good*

*For simplicity and teaching purposes, the alleles in this case are labeled as *good* or *bad*. These are not basic science nor clinical terms. Instead, these terms are used to get the reader accustomed to alleles being protective against psychiatric symptoms and disorders or increasing one's risk of developing symptoms or disorders. *Good* means protective in general and *bad* means that risks increase. Additionally, the reader should be advised that it takes many alleles of many different genes interacting, and all of these interactions must work together with the environment (psychosocial stressors) in order for psychiatric symptoms to occur. For sake of simplicity, it is easier to start with *good* and *bad* to learn about the genetic underpinnings of psychiatric symptoms and how to bridge the gap between basic science and clinical application.

Case outcome: initial visit

- No psychotherapy is offered
- No prescription is issued
- In considering the potential future of psychopharmacology, the patient has his saliva or cheek swab analyzed and is tested for risk genes for MDD
- His results came back as listed in Table 28.1

Table 28.1. Risk genes for MDD

Pathway	Gene	Protein	Result
Serotonin	SLC6A4	SERT, also called serotonin reuptake pump, responsible for termination of serotonin action	**L(A)/L(A)**
Dopamine	DRD2	D2 receptor, target of antipsychotic drugs, theoretically overactive in psychosis and underactive in Parkinson's disease	**(Ins/Ins)**
	COMT	Enzyme responsible for degradation of DA and NE	**(158 Val/Val, 472 G/G)**
Glutamate	CACNA1C	Voltage-gated channel for calcium	**(G/G)**
Metabolism	MTHFR	Predominant enzyme that converts inactive folic acid to active folate	**(T/T)**

Question

Based on this patient's symptoms, history, and genetic testing results, which of the following would you prescribe?

- Serotonergic antidepressant
- Dopaminergic antidepressant
- Any antidepressant plus an atypical antipsychotic
- Any antidepressant plus a stimulant
- A prodopaminergic antidepressant plus L-methylfolate
- ECT

Attending physician's mental notes: initial evaluation (continued)

- Carrying both the COMT 158 Val/Val and the MTHFR 677 T/T genotype theoretically could result in increased degradation of DA in the prefrontal cortex, leading to decreased DA signaling there and associated cognitive dysfunction
- Theoretically, it is plausible that the effect of the COMT Val allele on DA neurotransmission, which is further enhanced by the epistatic genetic interaction with the MTHFR T allele, could be a central explanation for the severe cognitive impairments of this patient, particularly with regard to his executive functions ("prefrontal dopamine" hypothesis)
  - This patient cannot synthesize as much DA for later use (MTHFR T allele)
  - This patient breaks down DA at a higher rate (COMT 158 Val/Val allele)
  - The net effect is less globally available DA in the CNS
- In addition, these genotypes might also be a good theoretical explanation for the "psychiatric parkinsonism" symptoms: lack of drive and concentration, memory disorder, psychomotor retardation, slower thinking (bradyphrenia) and movement (bradykinesia)
  - The development of EPS in this patient on a rather low dose of risperidone (3 mg/d) is another sign of low DA function
  - The patient's genetic test results suggest that although he could respond to a serotonergic antidepressant (despite having failed monotherapy), a prodopaminergic drug might best address his symptoms as his "psychiatric parkinsonism" features might reflect poor dopaminergic clinical functioning
  - Prodopaminergic options include NDRI, MAOI, and possibly augmentation with a stimulant or wakefulness-promoting agent
- The patient's genetic test results might also suggest that he should not receive augmentation with an antipsychotic, as these agents are DA antagonists and he may not tolerate these very well, and thus potentially exhibit further EPS or cognitive decline
- To compensate the decreased capacity to convert folic acid to methylfolate (MTHFR: 677 T/T), L-methylfolate (Deplin) might be a beneficial augmentation strategy

– L-methylfolate (Deplin) is approved as a medical food capable of boosting antidepressant effectiveness

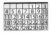

Case outcome: interim visit at six weeks

- Before the results of his genetic testing are known, sertraline 100 mg/d is reinitiated because of his previous response to it; lorazepam (Ativan) 2 mg/d is also prescribed during the first few weeks
  - As a carrier of the L(A)/L(A) alleles for SCL6A4, this patient may be more likely to respond to SSRI treatment than individuals with the S or L(G) alleles
  - Of the SSRIs, sertraline has the most dopaminergic activity (it has some ability to block the DAT, especially at higher doses)
  - However, the DAT is minimally present in the prefrontal cortex; thus, sertraline may benefit his "psychiatric parkinsonism" due to possible deficiencies of DA in the striatum, but may not address his cognitive symptoms from possible deficiency of DA in the prefrontal cortext
- Lithium was next chosen as an augmenting agent due to the frequency of recurrence of depressive episodes, but it was not tolerated (severe tremor) and was stopped after 10 days
  - Although this patient was not bipolar disordered, the cyclic nature of his MDEs suggested a rationale for mood stabilizer use
- He experienced sufficient improvement in his mood after four weeks on sertraline (Zoloft) to allow hospital discharge after six weeks
- If he continues to experience DA-related symptoms, and does not achieve remission, then the next step could be an augmentation with bupropion, a stimulant, or L-methylfolate

Case debrief

- This patient suffers from recurrent MDD, which is now considered to be TRD
- He had some previous treatment, but much was subtherapeutically delivered
- Genetic testing was ordered; suggested where his neurobiological vulnerabilities might lie and also indicated which antidepressants might be the most helpful first
- Instead of randomly choosing an antidepressant, or even choosing one based on clinical experience, preliminary genetic tests may allow the psychopharmacologist to choose the most likely agent for the patient to respond to first
- This may save weeks of non-response to agents unlikely to deliver good clinical effectiveness and also save weeks of depressive symptom suffering waiting for antidepressant effects to occur

- In this case, the clinician chose to optimize the SSRI and the results were reasonable
- If the goal is remission, or if this patient were to relapse, then use of an NDRI or L-methylfolate should be considered as these would also address the theoretically genetic vulnerabilities noticed in his testing

Take-home points

- Genetic testing as a clinical tool is still in its infancy, but has the potential to inform treatment decisions
- Genotyping may be especially useful for patients who do not respond to or tolerate drugs as expected
- Caution is essential when adopting genetic testing into the selection of treatments in clinical practice

Two-minute tutorial

A short tutorial on the scientific background of this case

- SLC6A4: the patient is homozygous for the Long(A) promoter alleles, L(A)/L(A)
  - Compared to patients with the L allele, the S allele results in decreased SERT expression, decreased presynaptic serotonin reuptake, and higher synaptic serotonin availability results
  - Patients who possess the L allele are also tested for the A>G polymorphism within the L allele itself; compared to the L(A) allele, the L(G) variant allele results in decreased expression of the SERT, and a phenotype similar to that of the S allele
  - Individuals with the S or L(G) alleles may be less likely to respond to SSRI-based antidepressant therapy, may be more likely to experience adverse effects from SSRIs, and may respond to SSRI therapy much more slowly
    - In summary, patients with the S or L(G) alleles have less SERT/reuptake pump availability, and therefore are less likely to respond to SSRI antidepressants
    - This patient does not have either of these genotypes, but conversely has the Long(A) allele and likely has adequate SERTs to respond positively to SSRI treatment, hence an SSRI was ultimately chosen, albeit at higher doses
- DRD2: the patient is homozygous for the -141C insertion allele (Ins/Ins)
  - Insertion/deletions of -141C in the DRD2 promoter may influence striatal DA binding and antipsychotic drug response
  - Individuals who carry the Del allele (Del/Ins or Del/Del) demonstrate less satisfactory antipsychotic drug response compared to patients with the homozygous Ins/Ins genotype

- Del allele carriers are also at higher risk of atypical neuroleptic-induced weight gain
  - In summary, this finding is likely not important in our current patient as he is not psychotic and an antipsychotic agent was not chosen as an augmentation
  - This patient was Ins/Ins and if he were to become psychotically depressed, then he more likely might respond to antipsychotic therapy
  - He would also be at less risk for AAWG
- CACNA1C: the patient is homozygous for the rs1006737 G allele (G/G)
  - CACNA1C gene alterations may lead to calcium channel disturbances, excess neuronal excitability, and excess glutamate
  - These alterations may lead to increased depolarization of selective limbic regions associated with mood and perception
  - Dysregulated calcium channels may lead to paroxysmal decompensations with increased risk of relapse in patients with mood disorders
  - The CACNA1C rs1006737 A allele has been associated with elevated rates of mood disorder recurrence
    - In summary, this finding might suggest vulnerability to recurrent mood episodes or cycling in affective disorders
    - This patient has the G allele and likely is not genetically vulnerable to mood cycling and decompensations on the basis of the genotype alone
      - However, his history suggests many unipolar depressive episodes hinting that the cause of his cycling is not related to this allele, or that despite the finding of his G allele, to diminished cycling; he has other vulnerabilities that overwhelm the positives of his G allele
- COMT: the patient is homozygous for the 158 Valine allele (158 Val/Val, 472 G/G)
  - The COMT 158 Val allele is a high-activity allele, leading to increased COMT activity
  - The COMT enzyme is responsible for degrading DA and NE, and the Val allele more aggressively decreases DA in the prefrontal cortex, which may lead to cognitive and working memory deficits where optimal DA levels and activity are needed
  - Patients with the homozygous Val/Val genotype may be less likely to respond to SSRI treatments
  - Individuals with cognitive symptoms who possess the COMT Val allele may theoretically benefit from agents that increase DA availability
    - In summary, Val alleles allow for increased COMT activity, decreased DA-availability, and resultant cognitive problems

- In this patient, he was exhibiting these symptoms, and choosing a DA facilitating psychotropic may have been warranted
- Interestingly, his SLC6A4 L(A) allele suggested this patient would be a good responder to an SSRI, but this COMT Val allele suggests the opposite
- Again, depending on the vulnerabilities a patient inherits, genetic testing can still only make suggestions on how to improve treatment. It will likely not tell the clinician which vulnerability is the most egregious as far as depressive etiology is concerned. Some findings are inevitably contradictory

- MTHFR: the patient is homozygous for the 677 T allele (677 T/T)
  - MTHFR is the predominant enzyme that converts inactive, peripheral folic acid to a CNS-available and active form of folate called L-methylfolate
  - The 677 T allele is associated with decreased MTHFR activity, causing there to be less L-methylfolate in the CNS
  - L-methylfolate is involved in the one-carbon cycle, which is required in the making of monoamine neurotransmitters, and theoretically may lower transmitter levels as a possible contributing etiology in MDD
  - The 677 T allele also may lead to increased homocysteine and decreased methylation capacity that can increase expression of COMT and lead to reduced DA
  - Elevated homocysteine and the MTHFR 677 T/T genotype have been associated with increased risk of schizophrenia, and particularly with negative and cognitive symptoms
    - In summary, the T allele allows for less L-methylfolate formation and less DA availability, which may contribute to depression
    - This patient possesses this vulnerability and treating with a dopaminergic agent or even L-methylfolate itself may be warranted

- MTHFR–COMT methylation interaction
  - Decreased methylation of COMT, caused by decreased function with the MTHFR 677 T variant as discussed previously, results in decreased DA signaling, and may ultimately lead to cognitive impairments
  - This effect is exacerbated in patients who carry both the MTHFR 677 T allele and the high-activity COMT 158 Val/Val genotype, with increased cognitive impairment
  - This effect has been demonstrated in schizophrenic patients but not in healthy controls
    - In summary, this patient carries both of these genetic vulnerabilities, but does not have schizophrenia
    - He does exhibit marked vegetative depressive symptoms, psychomotor impairment, and cognitive dysfunction

Patient's genetic summary

- In Table 28.2, findings in **red** suggest genetic vulnerabilities
- Genes (a person's genotype) code for proteins, i.e., receptors, enzymes, growth factors, and genetic regulators
- Proteins allow neurocircuits to be active at optimal performance levels
- Neurocircuits that are overactive or underactive likely lead to symptoms (a patient's phenotype or the symptoms we detect during interviews)
- Sometimes these inappropriately hyper- or hypofunctioning neurocircuits can be seen with functional neuroimaging techniques such as functional MRI (fMRI) or PET scans (called an endophenotype)
- If a patient inherits enough of these subtle molecular vulnerabilities (gene mutations), then s/he could theoretically collect numerous abnormal proteins, develop abnormally functioning neurocircuits, and show different psychiatric symptoms that may coalesce into a syndrome or categorical *DSM-5* diagnosis
- Findings in **black** suggest neutral or protective genetic vulnerabilities in this patient

Table 28.2. Genetic vulnerabilities in a patient with MDD

Pathway	Gene	Comments	Patient Result
Serotonin	SLC6A4	Carriers of the Short(S) or L(G) alleles may be less likely to respond to SSRIs, or may respond more slowly, and may be more likely to experience adverse effects from SSRIs	**L(A)/L(A)**
Dopamine	DRD2	Del allele carriers (Del/Ins or Del/Del) may demonstrate less satisfactory antipsychotic drug response compared to Ins/Ins individuals	**(Ins/Ins)**
	COMT	Patients with the homozygous Val/Val genotype may be less likely to respond to SSRI treatments	**(158 Val/Val, 472 G/G)**
Glutamate	CACNA1C	The A allele has been associated with elevated rates of mood disorder recurrence	**(G/G)**
Metabolism	MTHFR	Presence of the 677 T allele (C/T or T/T) is associated with decreased MTHFR activity, leading to increased homocysteine	**(T/T)**

Continued

Table 28.2. (cont.)

Pathway	Gene	Comments	Patient Result
		and decreased methylation capacity	
	MTHFR–COMT methylation interaction	Methylation pathways regulate the metabolism of neurotransmitters, particularly DA. In low methylation states, such as that caused by the MTHFR T allele, DA is degraded at a higher rate. This effect is exacerbated in patients who carry both the MTHFR 677 T allele and the high-activity COMT 158 Val/Val genotype	Patient has a gene–gene interaction noted

Posttest self-assessment question and answer

A 54-year-old patient has depression with prominent cognitive symptoms and also has the Val/Val genotype for catechol-O-methyltransferase (COMT). Based only on this genetic result, what treatment might be preferred for this patient?

A. SSRI

B. SNRI

C. NDRI

Answer: C

The Val allele, as in this case, codes for a protein (the enzyme COMT) that is now defective. COMT here is now overly active in degrading DA, thus depleting its availability in the synapse. This may lend to the possible etiology of MDD. Antidepressants that increase synaptic DA or dopaminergic neurotransmission may be the most likely to help. An NDRI is the most likely approved agent as it would be the most aggressive at DRI. Off-label stimulant use might be effective as well. Interestingly, the NETs in the frontal cortex also act as DATs. Therefore, the NRI half of the SNRI serves as DRI activity as well. The SSRIs, in general, have little impact on DRI except for minor effects associated with sertraline.

References

1. Arinami T, Gao M, Hamaguchi H, Toru M. A functional polymorphism in the promoter region of the dopamine D2 receptor gene is associated with schizophrenia. *Hum Mol Genet* 1997; 6:577–82.

2. Baune B, Hohoff C, Berger K, et al. Association of the COMT val158met variant with antidepressant treatment response in major depression. *Neuropsychopharmacology* 2008; 33:924–32.

3. Casamassima F, Huang J, Fava M, et al. Phenotypic effects of a bipolar liability gene among individuals with major depressive disorder. *Am J Med Genet B Neuropsychiatr Genet* 2010; 153B:303–9.

4. Ferreira MA, O'Donovan MC, Meng YA, et al. Wellcome Trust Case Control Consortium. Collaborative genome-wide association analysis supports a role for ANK3 and CACNA1C in bipolar disorder. *Nat Genet* 2008; 40:1056–8.

5. Gelernter J, Cubells JF, Kidd JR, Pakstis AJ, Kidd KK. Population studies of polymorphisms of the serotonin transporter protein gene. *Am J Med Genet* 1999; 88:61–6.

6. Heils A, Teufel A, Petri S, et al. Allelic variation of human serotonin transporter gene expression. *J Neurochemistry* 1996; 66:2621–4.

7. Jönsson EG, Nothen M, Grunhage F, et al. Polymorphisms in the dopamine D2 receptor gene and their relationships to striatal dopamine receptor density of healthy volunteers. *Mol Psychiatry* 1999; 4:290–6.

8. Kato M, Serretti A. Review and meta-analysis of antidepressant pharmacogenetic findings in major depressive disorder. *Mol Psychiatry* 2010; 15:473–500.

9. Kirchheiner J, Nickchen K, Bauer M, et al. Pharmacogenetics of antidepressants and antipsychotics: the contribution of allelic variations to the phenotype of drug response. *Mol Psychiatry* 2004; 9:442–73.

10. Kocabas NA, Faghel C, Barreto M, et al. The impact of catechol-O-methyltransferase SNPs and haplotypes on treatment response phenotypes in major depressive disorder: a case-control association study. *Int Clin Psychopharmacol* 2010; 25:218–27.

11. Popp J, Leucht S, Heres S, Steimer W. Serotonin transporter polymorphisms and side effects in antidepressant therapy – a pilot study. *Pharmacogenetics* 2006; 7:159–66.

12. Stahl SM. *Stahl's Essential Psychopharmacology: The Prescriber's Guide*, 5th edn. New York, NY: Cambridge University Press, 2014.

13. Tsai SJ, Gau YT, Hong CJ, et al. Sexually dimorphic effect of catechol-O-methyltransferase val158met polymorphism on clinical response to fluoxetine in major depressive patients. *J Affect Disord* 2009; 113:183–7.

14. Zhang J-P, Lencz T, Malhotra AK. Dopamine D2 receptor genetic variation and clinical response to antipsychotic drug treatment: a meta-analysis. *Am J Psychiatry* 2010; 167:763–72.

The Case: 55-year-old with depression not responsive to serotonergic treatment

The Question (Pharmacogenetics, Part 2): How might psychopharmacology be delivered in the future?

The Dilemma: Can genotyping help predict successful treatment selection

Pretest self-assessment question (answer at the end of the case)

A 55-year-old patient with depression has the S/S genotype for the SERT gene (SLC6A4). Based only on this genetic result, what treatment might be preferred for this patient?

A. SSRI

B. SNRI

C. Noradrenergic TCA

Patient evaluation on intake

- 55-year-old man is admitted to the psychiatric hospital because of MDD

Psychiatric history

- MDD symptoms present for approximately five months
- Admits to impaired concentration and a depressed mood with suicidal thoughts, insomnia, brooding, and feelings of guilt
- This is his first MDE
- He has had no psychotropic drug treatment prior to this hospitalization

Social and personal history

- Separated from spouse and has four sons
- Denies drug or alcohol misuse

Medical history

- Denies acute medical problems

Family history

- There is no family history of mental illness

Patient evaluation on initial visit

- He is diagnosed with single-episode MDD
- First is treated as an inpatient with the NaSSA mirtazapine 45 mg/d but exhibits no response

Question

Based on this patient's history and current symptom profile, testing of which of the following genes might be useful?

- SLC6A4 (SERT)
- SLC6A4 and COMT
- SLC6A4, COMT, and MTHFR
- SLC6A4, COMT, MTHFR, and voltage-dependent calcium channel L-type, alpha-1c subunit (CACNA1C)
- SLC6A4, COMT, MTHFR, CACNA1C, and D2 receptor (DRD2)

Attending physician's mental notes: initial evaluation

- Testing of any of these genes may provide information that could be considered in the management of this patient
  - SLC6A4, 5HTTLPR Long(L)/Short(S) promoter insertion/deletion (rs63749047) and L(A)/L(G) (rs25531) polymorphism
    - This patient is homozygous (i.e., has two copies) for S/S
    - May indicate individuals who are more likely to exhibit unsatisfactory or no response to previous SSRI treatment or who have developed treatment-emergent side effects on SSRIs
    - S/S signifies *bad* alleles
  - COMT, 158 Val>Met (472 G>A, rs4680)
    - This patient is homozygous for (158 Val/Val, 472 G/G)
    - May indicate individuals with depression who are more likely to experience associated cognitive symptoms such as slowness of information processing, difficulty with executive functioning, and problem solving
    - Val/Val equates to *bad* alleles
  - CACNA1C, G>A rs1006737
    - This patient is homozygous for (G/G)
    - The A allele (not carried by this patient) may indicate individuals with mood disorders who are more likely to experience frequent relapses and recurrences
    - G/G alleles are *good*
  - DRD2, -141C insertion/deletion (rs1799732)
    - This patient is homozygous for (Ins/Ins)
    - May indicate individuals who are more likely to benefit from augmentation with an atypical antipsychotic in the event that they do not respond to an antidepressant (compared to those who carry the Del allele)
    - Ins/Ins alleles are *good*
  - MTHFR, 677 C>T
    - This patient is heterozygous for T/C

○ The T allele may indicate individuals with depression who are more likely to experience associated cognitive symptoms, especially in those who also express the Val variant of the COMT gene

○ T/C equates to *fair* alleles (Remember T/T is the poorest allelic combination for risk for MDD)

Case outcome: initial visit

- No psychotherapy is offered
- No further prescription is issued
- In considering the potential future of psychopharmacology, the patient has his saliva sample or cheek swab analyzed for five genes, with the following results:

Table 29.1. Risk genes in another patient with MDD

Pathway	Gene	Protein	Result
Serotonin	SLC6A4	SERT, also called serotonin reuptake pump, responsible for termination of serotonin action	S/S
Dopamine	DRD2	D2 receptor, target of antipsychotic drugs, theoretically overactive in psychosis and underactive in Parkinson's disease	(Ins/Ins)
	COMT	Enzyme responsible for degradation of DA and NE	(158 Val/Val, 472 G/G)
Glutamate	CACNA1C	Voltage-gated channel for calcium	(G/G)
Metabolism	MTHFR	Predominant enzyme that converts inactive folic acid to active folate	(T/C)

Question

Based on this patient's symptoms, history, and genetic testing results, which of the following would you prescribe?

- Serotonergic antidepressant
- Noradrenergic and/or dopaminergic antidepressant
- Any antidepressant plus an atypical antipsychotic
- Any antidepressant plus a stimulant

Attending physician's mental notes: initial evaluation (continued)

- Carrying *both* the SLC6A4 S/S and the COMT Val/Val genotype theoretically would reduce this patient's likelihood of responding to an SSRI; thus, choosing an agent with predominantly noradrenergic and/or dopaminergic properties may be preferable
  - Consider an NDRI like bupropion-XL (Wellbutrin-XL)

- Consider a TCA with greater NRI potential like desipramine (Norpramin), nortriptyline (Pamelor), or protriptyline (Vivactil)
- Theoretically, it is plausible that the effect of the COMT Val allele on DA neurotransmission, possibly combined with the effect of the MTHFR T allele, could be a central explanation for the severe cognitive impairments of this patient, particularly with regard to his executive dysfunction ("prefrontal dopamine" hypothesis)
  - This finding might further support adding antidepressant agents or augmentation strategies with more robust dopaminergic mechanisms of action

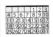

Case outcome: interim visit at four weeks

- He is switched to the TCA, nortriptyline (Pamelor), 200 mg/d
- This is considered a high dose, but his serum levels were previously lower while taking usual doses, so that this dose was required for his levels to reach the therapeutic range of 50–150 mcg/ml
  - Nortriptyline is chosen because, as a carrier of the S/S alleles for SLC6A4, this patient may be less likely to respond to SSRI treatment than individuals with the L(A) alleles
    - This way, a noradrenergic drug is used
  - Being a carrier of the Val/Val allele for COMT also theoretically suggests that he would be less likely to respond to an SSRI
- Quetiapine (Seroquel) is next chosen as an augmenting agent due to his delusions of guilt
  - 50mg/d titrating to 100mg/d given at bedtime
  - Being homozygous for the Ins allele for DRD2 could theoretically suggest that he may respond better to atypical antipsychotic augmentation in comparison to those individuals with the Del allele
- Lorazepam (Ativan) 2 mg/d is prescribed as needed for agitation or insomnia
- He experiences a good response to this regimen and is released from hospital
- If his symptoms relapse, augmentation with L-methylfolate could be considered as it would address his MTHFR solo T allele more directly

Case debrief

- This patient suffered from an index MDD episode with likely psychotic features
- He had no previous treatment, but his serious symptoms required inpatient hospitalization
- Genetic testing was ordered; suggested where his theoretical neurobiological vulnerabilities might lie and also indicated what antidepressant class (SSRI) might be the least helpful first and which class might be more helpful (TCA, antipsychotics)

- Instead of randomly choosing an antidepressant, or even choosing one based on clinical experience, preliminary genetic tests may allow the psychopharmacologist to choose more accurately the most promising agent for the patient to try first
- This may save weeks of non-response to unlikely agents
- This may deliver good clinical effectiveness and also save weeks of depressive symptom suffering waiting for antidepressant effects to occur

Take-home points

- Genetic testing as a clinical tool is still in its infancy, but has the potential to inform treatment decisions
- Genotyping may be especially useful for patients who do not respond to or tolerate a drug as expected
- Caution is essential when adopting genetic testing into the selection of treatments in clinical practice

Two-minute tutorial

A short tutorial on the scientific background of this case

- SLC6A4: the patient is homozygous for the Short promoter alleles, S/S
  - Compared to patients with the L allele, the S allele results in decreased SERT expression, decreased presynaptic serotonin reuptake, and higher synaptic serotonin
  - Individuals with the S or L(G) alleles may be less likely to respond to SSRI-based antidepressant therapy, may be more likely to experience adverse effects from SSRIs, and may respond to SSRI therapy more slowly
  - In individuals with unsatisfactory response to SSRI therapy and who possess the Short(S) (or the L(G)) alleles, treatment with alternative (non-SSRI) antidepressant mechanisms may be considered
  - Greater caution is recommended when initiating or discontinuing SSRI in individuals with the Short(S) (or L(G)) allele
    - In summary, patients with the S allele or L(G) alleles have less SERT/reuptake pump availability, and therefore are less likely to respond to SSRI antidepressants
    - This patient does have one of these genotypes and likely has inadequate SERTs, and will not respond clinically to SSRI treatment, hence SSRIs were not considered from the start!
- DRD2: the patient is homozygous for the -141C insertion allele (Ins/Ins)
  - Insertion/deletions of -141C in the DRD2 promoter may influence striatal DA binding and antipsychotic drug response
  - Individuals who carry the Del allele (Del/Ins or Del/Del) demonstrate less satisfactory antipsychotic drug response compared to patients with the homozygous Ins/Ins genotype

- Del allele carriers are also at higher risk of atypical antipsychotic-induced weight gain
    - In summary, this finding is important in our current patient as he is psychotic, he carries the Ins allele, and has a good chance of responding to antipsychotics
    - This might lead the clinician to use an atypical antipsychotic augmentation strategy earlier in care despite risks of movement or metabolic disorders
- CACNA1C: the patient is homozygous for the rs1006737 G allele (G/G)
    - CACNA1C gene alterations may lead to calcium channel disturbances, excess neuronal excitability, and excess glutamate
    - These alterations may lead to increased depolarization of selective limbic regions associated with mood and perception
    - These dysregulated calcium channels may lead to paroxysmal decompensations with increased risk of relapse in patients with mood disorders
    - The CACNA1C rs1006737 A allele has been associated with elevated rates of mood disorder recurrence
        - In summary, this finding might suggest less vulnerability to recurrent mood episodes
        - This patient has the G allele and likely is not genetically vulnerable to mood cycling and frequent decompensation, thus improving his long-term prognosis
- COMT: the patient is homozygous for the 158 Valine allele (158 Val/Val, 472 G/G)
    - The COMT 158 Val allele is a high-activity allele, leading to increased COMT activity
    - The COMT enzyme is responsible for degrading DA, and the Val allele has higher enzyme activity and thus decreases DA levels in the prefrontal cortex, which may lead to cognitive and working memory deficits where optimal DA levels and activity are needed
    - Patients with the homozygous Val/Val genotype may be less likely to respond to SSRI treatments
    - Individuals with cognitive symptoms who possess the COMT Val allele may theoretically benefit from agents that increase DA availability
        - In summary, Val alleles allow for increased COMT activity, decreased DA availability, and resultant cognitive problems
        - In this patient, he was exhibiting these symptoms, and choosing a DA-facilitating psychotropic may have been warranted
        - In this particular case, a noradrenergic TCA was chosen first, given the genetic findings, suggesting avoidance of the SSRI class
        - This TCA might increase NE in the CNS despite COMT aggressively degrading it

- MTHFR: the patient is heterozygous for the 677 T/C allele (677 T/C)
  - MTHFR is the predominant enzyme that converts inactive, peripheral folic acid to a CNS-available and -active form of folate called L-methylfolate
  - The 677 T allele is associated with decreased MTHFR activity, causing there to be less L-methylfolate in the CNS
  - L-methylfolate is involved in the one-carbon cycle, which is required in the making of monoamine neurotransmitters, and theoretically may lower transmitter levels as a possible etiology in MDD
  - The 677 T allele also may lead to increased homocysteine and decreased methylation capacity that can increase expression of COMT and lead to reduced DA
  - Elevated homocysteine and the MTHFR 677 TT genotype have been associated with increased risk of schizophrenia, and particularly with negative and cognitive symptoms
    - In summary, this patient is heterozygous where he has only one T allele. This situation allows for slightly less L-methylfolate production and DA availability than normal, which may contribute to depression symptomatology
    - This patient possesses this mild vulnerability and treating with a dopaminergic agent or even L-methylfolate (Deplin) itself may be warranted as an augmentation
- MTHFR–COMT methylation interaction
  - Decreased methylation of COMT, caused by decreased function with the MTHFR 677 T variant, results in decreased DA signaling, and may ultimately lead to cognitive impairments
  - This effect is exacerbated in patients who carry both the MTHFR 677 T allele and the high-activity COMT 158 Val/Val genotype, with increased cognitive impairment
  - This effect has been demonstrated in schizophrenic patients but not in healthy controls
    - In summary, this patient might be susceptible to this gene–gene interaction but he does not have schizophrenia
    - He is psychotic, depressed, and has cognitive dysfunction, which may be explained theoretically by this interaction

Patient's genetic summary

- In Table 29.2, findings in **red** suggest genetic vulnerabilities
- **Black** findings may be genetically protective
- Genes (a person's genotype) code for proteins, i.e., receptors, enzymes, growth factors, and regulatory factors
- Proteins allow neurocircuits to be active at optimal performance levels
- Neurocircuits that are over- or underactive likely lead to symptoms (a patient's phenotype)

- Sometimes these inappropriately hyper- or hypofunctioning neurocircuits can be seen with functional neuroimaging techniques such as fMRI or PET scans (called an endophenotype)
- If a patient inherits enough of these subtle molecular vulnerabilities (gene mutations), then s/he will collect abnormal proteins, develop abnormally functioning neurocircuits, and show different psychiatric symptoms that may coalesce into a syndrome or categorical *DSM-5* diagnosis

Table 29.2. Genetic vulnerabilities in another patient with MDD

Pathway	Gene	Comments	Patient result
Serotonin	SLC6A4	Carriers of the Short(S) or L(G) alleles may be less likely to respond to SSRIs, or may respond more slowly, and may be more likely to experience adverse effects from SSRIs	**S/S**
Dopamine	DRD2	Del allele carriers (Del/Ins or Del/Del) may demonstrate less satisfactory antipsychotic drug response compared to Ins/Ins individuals	**(Ins/Ins)**
	COMT	Patients with the homozygous Val/Val genotype may be less likely to respond to SSRI treatments	**(158 Val/Val, 472 G/G)**
Glutamate	CACNA1C	The A allele has been associated with elevated rates of mood disorder recurrence	**(G/G)**
Metabolism	MTHFR	Presence of the 677 T allele (C/T or T/T) is associated with decreased MTHFR activity, leading to increased homocysteine and decreased methylation capacity	**(T/C)**
	MTHFR–COMT methylation interaction	Methylation pathways regulate the metabolism of neurotransmitters, particularly DA. In low methylation states, such as that caused by the MTHFR T allele, DA is degraded at a higher rate. This effect is exacerbated in patients who carry both the MTHFR 677 T allele and the high-activity COMT 158 Val/Val genotype	This patient has a gene–gene interaction that may worsen symptoms

PATIENT FILE

Posttest self-assessment question and answer

A 55-year-old patient with depression has the S/S genotype for the SERT gene (SLC6A4). Based only on this genetic result, what treatment might be preferred for this patient?

A. SSRI

B. SNRI

C. Noradrenergic TCA

Answer: C

Carriers of the Short(S) alleles for the SLC6A4 gene may be less likely to respond to SSRIs, or may respond more slowly, and may be more likely to experience adverse effects from SSRIs. Therefore, choosing an SSRI first may be fraught with inefficacy or intolerability, thus wasting time clinically while trying to obtain a treatment response. Choosing an SNRI would carry similar problems in that SNRIs have full serotonin reuptake inhibition (SRI) function as part of their dual mechanism of action. Choosing a noradrenergic TCA, would avoid this SRI mechanism and be a logical first treatment choice.

References

1. Arinami T, Gao M, Hamaguchi H, Toru M. A functional polymorphism in the promoter region of the dopamine D2 receptor gene is associated with schizophrenia. *Hum Mol Genet* 1997; 6:577–82.

2. Baune B, Hohoff C, Berger K, et al. Association of the COMT val158met variant with antidepressant treatment response in major depression. *Neuropsychopharmacology* 2008; 33:924–32.

3. Casamassima F, Huang J, Fava M, et al. Phenotypic effects of a bipolar liability gene among individuals with major depressive disorder. *Am J Med Genet B Neuropsychiatr Genet* 2010; 153B:303–9.

4. Ferreira MA, O'Donovan MC, Meng YA, et al. Wellcome Trust Case Control Consortium. Collaborative genome-wide association analysis supports a role for ANK3 and CACNA1C in bipolar disorder. *Nat Genet* 2008; 40:1056–8.

5. Gelernter J, Cubells JF, Kidd JR, Pakstis AJ, Kidd KK. Population studies of polymorphisms of the serotonin transporter protein gene. *Am J Med Genet* 1999; 88:61–6.

6. Heils A, Teufel A, Petri S, et al. Allelic variation of human serotonin transporter gene expression. *J Neurochemistry* 1996; 66:2621–4.

7. Jönsson EG, Nothen M, Grunhage F, et al. Polymorphisms in the dopamine D2 receptor gene and their relationships to striatal dopamine receptor density of healthy volunteers. *Mol Psychiatry* 1999; 4:290–6.

8. Kato M, Serretti A. Review and meta-analysis of antidepressant pharmacogenetic findings in major depressive disorder. *Mol Psychiatry* 2010; 15:473–500.

9. Kirchheiner J, Nickchen K, Bauer M, et al. Pharmacogenetics of antidepressants and antipsychotics: the contribution of allelic variations to the phenotype of drug response. *Mol Psychiatry* 2004; 9:442–73.

10. Kocabas NA, Faghel C, Barreto M, et al. The impact of catechol-O-methyltransferase SNPs and haplotypes on treatment response phenotypes in major depressive disorder: a case-control association study. *Int Clin Psychopharmacol* 2010; 25:218–27.

11. Popp J, Leucht S, Heres S, Steimer W. Serotonin transporter polymorphisms and side effects in antidepressant therapy – a pilot study. *Pharmacogenetics* 2006; 7:159–66.

12. Stahl SM. *Stahl's Essential Psychopharmacology: The Prescriber's Guide*, 5th edn. New York, NY: Cambridge University Press, 2014.

13. Tsai SJ, Gau YT, Hong CJ, et al. Sexually dimorphic effect of catechol-O-methyltransferase val158met polymorphism on clinical response to fluoxetine in major depressive patients. *J Affect Disord* 2009; 113:183–7.

14. Zhang J-P, Lencz T, Malhotra AK. Dopamine D2 receptor genetic variation and clinical response to antipsychotic drug treatment: a meta-analysis. *Am J Psychiatry* 2010; 167:763–72.

The Case: 23-year-old with first depression...that's it!

The Question: How might psychopharmacology be delivered in the future: neuropharmacogenetic imaging?

The Dilemma: Can genotyping and functional neuroimaging help predict successful treatment selection

Pretest self-assessment question

A 23-year-old patient with her first depression has the S/S genotype for the SERT gene, the Del/Del alleles for the D2 receptor gene, the Val/Val alleles for the COMT gene, the T/T alleles for the MTHFR gene, and the A/A alleles for the CACNA1C gene. She also had a brain fMRI completed and it shows that her right insular cortex was hypoactive. Based only on these genetic results and neuroimaging findings, what treatment might be preferred for this patient?

A. SSRI
B. An atypical antipsychotic
C. Lithium
D. NDRI like bupropion
E. A noradrenergic TCA like desipramine
F. A mood stabilizer like lamotrigine
G. A folate-boosting product such as L-methylfolate
H. CBT

Patient evaluation on intake

*   23-year-old woman states that she feels "sad, down, and amotivated"
*   Admits to all MDD symptoms except for suicidality for the last two to three months
*   There was no psychosocial trigger and she reported that "life was going well"

Psychiatric history

*   There is no premorbid psychiatric history
*   This is her first MDE
*   There has been no prior psychotropic drug treatment before this hospitalization for suicidal thinking
*   There are no other comorbid psychiatric disorders present

Social and personal history

*   Graduated college with a business degree and has a good job as a manager in a local company
*   This job is going very well and with minimal stress
*   She is in a long-term relationship with a supportive boyfriend
*   There are no financial concerns

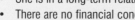

- Her upbringing was relatively stress free and her parents are supportive
- Denies any drug or alcohol misuse

Medical history

- Denies acute medical problems
- Takes no medications

Family history

- There is no family history of psychiatric disorder

Patient evaluation on initial visit

- She is diagnosed with single-episode MDD

Question

Based on this patient's history and current symptom profile, testing of which of the following might be useful?

- SLC6A4 (SERT) gene
- COMT gene
- MTHFR gene
- Calcium channel, voltage-dependent L-type alpha, 1c subunit (CACNA1C) gene
- D2 receptor gene (DRD2)
- fMRI of the insular cortex

Attending physician's mental notes: initial evaluation

- This patient is asking for a precise answer as to what type of treatment will "help her the most, the fastest, and harm her the least"
  - All antidepressants are equal per regulatory agencies
  - Her genetic testing is daunting in that she has the *bad* alleles for every gene (see Table 30.1)
    - She is less likely to respond to SSRI and may have more side effects
    - Her high-activity COMT will degrade DA more completely
    - She may be vulnerable to more cognitive depressive symptoms
    - She is less likely to respond to atypical antipsychotic augmentation
    - She may experience many recurring depressive episodes
- Testing of any of these genes may provide information that could be considered in the management of this patient
  - SLC6A4, 5HTTLPR
    - This patient is homozygous (i.e., has two copies) for S/S

- ° May indicate individuals who are more likely to exhibit unsatisfactory or no response to previous SSRI treatment, or who have developed treatment-emergent side effects on SSRIs
- – COMT
  - ° This patient is homozygous for (158 Val/Val, 472 G/G)
  - • May indicate individuals with depression who are more likely to experience associated cognitive symptoms such as slowness of information processing, difficulty with executive functioning, and problem solving
- – CACNA1C, G>A rs1006737
  - • This patient is homozygous for (A/A)
  - • The A allele may indicate individuals with mood disorders who are more likely to experience frequent relapses and recurrences
- – DRD2, -141C insertion/deletion (rs1799732)
  - • This patient is homozygous for (Del/Del)
  - • May indicate individuals who are less likely to benefit from augmentation with an atypical antipsychotic, in the event that they do not respond to an antidepressant (compared to those who carry the Ins allele)
- – MTHFR, 677 C>T
  - • This patient is heterozygous for T/T
  - • The T allele may indicate individuals with depression who are more likely to experience associated cognitive symptoms, especially in those who also express the Val variant of the COMT gene
- • As this is her index depressive episode, treating her to remission quickly and avoiding relapses and recurrences is the primary goal, similar to an index episode of schizophrenia or mania
- • It seems that no medication is an ideal choice and genetic testing really has failed to guide prescribing toward a clear, concise choice of antidepressant
- • Testing via fMRI suggests depression exists when the DLPFC is hypoactive and the limbic system is hyperactive
  - – This patient has this typical depression finding in her limbic area, which may help aid in diagnosis but does not help in treatment selection
  - – This patient also has a novel finding that her right insular cortex is hypoactive
    - • Initial studies suggest that this hypoactivity predicts a response to CBT but not SSRI
    - • Alternatively, if hyperactivity were detected, then response to SSRI is favored and CBT would likely be ineffective

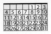

Case outcome: initial visit

- No psychotherapy is offered outside core therapeutic skills, support, and education
- No prescription is issued
- She is deemed to be a low suicide risk and should be amenable to outpatient therapy
- She is given advice about many medication and psychotherapy types to consider
- The patient states that she wants you to "pick the treatment with the greatest likelihood of helping her in the short term and with the least chance of harming her"
- In considering the potential future of psychopharmacology, the patient has a brain fMRI study completed. It is normal except that her right insula is noted to be hypoactive, the DLPFC is hypoactive, and the limbic system is hyperactive
- In considering the potential future of psychopharmacology, the patient has her saliva sample/cheek swab analyzed
- Like the previous two cases, **red** alleles in Table 30 are considered risky for depressive symptoms and drug responses
- The patient is tested for these five genes and her results are shown in the table

Table 30.1. Genetic vulnerabilities in a patient with single-episode MDD

Pathway	Gene	Protein	Result
Serotonin	SLC6A4	SERT, also called serotonin reuptake pump, responsible for termination of serotonin action	**S/S**
Dopamine	DRD2	D2 receptor, target of antipsychotic drugs, theoretically overactive in psychosis and underactive in Parkinson's disease	**(Del/Del)**
	COMT	Enzyme responsible for degradation of DA and NE	**(Val/Val)**
Glutamate	CACNA1C	Voltage-gated channel for calcium	**(A/A)**
Metabolism	MTHFR	Predominant enzyme that converts inactive folic acid to active folate	**(T/T)**

Question

Based on this patient's symptoms, history, genetic testing, and fMRI results, which of the following would you prescribe?

- SSRI
- An atypical antipsychotic
- Lithium

- NDRI like bupropion
- A noradrenergic TCA like desipramine
- A mood stabilizer like lamotrigine
- A folate-boosting product such as L-methylfolate
- An SSRI
- CBT

Attending physician's mental notes: initial evaluation (continued)

- Carrying potentially more risky alleles is problematic as it could diminish the usefulness of SSRI, SNRI, SSRI/5-HT receptor modulators, TCAs
  - Perhaps starting an MAOI as the first-line treatment will work
  - Perhaps sending the patient for ECT will work
  - Perhaps sending the patient for other neuromodulation will work, e.g., VNS, TMS
- Having a hypofrontal right insular cortex is a novel finding
  - This endophenotypic finding might suggest a preferential response to psychotherapy, specifically CBT, and a future riddled with non-response to antidepressants

Case outcome: interim visit through 16 weeks

- The patient is referred to an area CBT therapist and undergoes 12 weeks of manualized psychotherapy
- She reports that most of the MDD symptoms resolved and feels she is still gradually improving

Case debrief

- This patient suffered from an index MDD episode that was moderate to severe
- She had no previous treatment or family history to guide psychopharmacologic care
- Any first-tier antidepressant or psychotherapy could be selected in her case
- Genetic testing was ordered; suggested where her neurobiological vulnerabilities might lie and also indicated that many antidepressants could be ineffective
- Instead of going back to randomly choosing an antidepressant, or even choosing one that is more risky, second- or third-tier to start with, the fMRI allowed for a decision to opt out of psychopharmacology and advise the patient toward psychotherapy, specifically CBT in this case
- This could save weeks of non-response to unlikely psychopharmacologic agents

- This could save weeks of untoward side effects and medication intolerability

Take-home points

- Genetic testing as a clinical tool is still in its infancy, but has the potential to inform treatment decisions
- Genotyping may be especially useful for patients who do not respond to or tolerate a drug as expected
- Caution is essential when adopting genetic testing into the selection of treatments in clinical practice as the science is still in its infancy
- fMRI use is also in its infancy and its use clinically has not come to fruition in practice as there is less fMRI availability and it is expensive compared to genetic testing
- It is unlikely at this juncture that new patients with first-episode MDD will obtain genetic and functional neuroanatomic testing to delineate their genotype and endophenotype, but academically, the use of this science and technology could eventually guide the psychopharmacologist to more accurate and personalized treatment as is found in oncology practice
- Eventually, software could also be developed and used to calculate the percent chance of response, remission, side effects, etc. for each specific medication, psychotherapy, and device-based treatment. At initial or first follow-up encounters, the psychopharmacologist could have very clear guidance and direction as to which type of treatment to try first

Posttest self-assessment question and answer

A 23-year-old patient with her first depression has the S/S genotype for the SERT gene, the Del/Del alleles for the D2 receptor gene, the VAL/VAL alleles for the COMT gene, the T/T alleles for the MTHFR gene, and the A/A alleles for the CACNA1C gene. She also had a brain fMRI completed and it shows that her right insular cortex was hypoactive. Based only on these genetic results and neuroimaging findings, what treatment might be preferred for this patient?

A. SSRI

B. An atypical antipsychotic

C. Lithium

D. NDRI like bupropion

E. A noradrenergic TCA like desipramine

F. A mood stabilizer like lamotrigine

G. A folate-boosting product such as L-methylfolate

H. CBT

Answer: H

All of the medications listed may be fraught with greater side effects and greater ineffectiveness, given the alleles this patient has inherited from her parents. There is no easy or perfect choice for an antidepressant. The fMRI finding suggests similarly, at least, that SSRI will likely not help alleviate depression but CBT will.

For this final case of this psychopharmacology case-based textbook, the answer may not be to institute a psychotropic at all. This patient likely should be referred to a CBT specialist for psychotherapy.

References

1. Arinami T, Gao M, Hamaguchi H, Toru M. A functional polymorphism in the promoter region of the dopamine D2 receptor gene is associated with schizophrenia. *Hum Mol Genet* 1997; 6:577–82.

2. Baune B, Hohoff C, Berger K, et al. Association of the COMT val158met variant with antidepressant treatment response in major depression. *Neuropsychopharmacology* 2008; 33:924–32.

3. Casamassima F, Huang J, Fava M, et al. Phenotypic effects of a bipolar liability gene among individuals with major depressive disorder. *Am J Med Genet B Neuropsychiatr Genet* 2010; 153B:303–9.

4. Ferreira MA, O'Donovan MC, Meng YA, et al. Wellcome Trust Case Control Consortium. Collaborative genome-wide association analysis supports a role for ANK3 and CACNA1C in bipolar disorder. *Nat Genet* 2008; 40:1056–8.

5. Gelernter J, Cubells JF, Kidd JR, Pakstis AJ, Kidd KK. Population studies of polymorphisms of the serotonin transporter protein gene. *Am J Med Genet* 1999; 88:61–6.

6. Heils A, Teufel A, Petri S, et al. Allelic variation of human serotonin transporter gene expression. *J Neurochemistry* 1996; 66:2621–4.

7. Jönsson EG, Nothen M, Grunhage F, et al. Polymorphisms in the dopamine D2 receptor gene and their relationships to striatal dopamine receptor density of healthy volunteers. *Mol Psychiatry* 1999; 4:290–6.

8. Kato M, Serretti A. Review and meta-analysis of antidepressant pharmacogenetic findings in major depressive disorder. *Mol Psychiatry* 2010; 15:473–500.

9. Kirchheiner J, Nickchen K, Bauer M, et al. Pharmacogenetics of antidepressants and antipsychotics: the contribution of allelic variations to the phenotype of drug response. *Mol Psychiatry* 2004; 9:442–73.

10. Kocabas NA, Faghel C, Barreto M, et al. The impact of catechol-O-methyltransferase SNPs and haplotypes on treatment response phenotypes in major depressive disorder: a case-control association study. *Int Clin Psychopharmacol* 2010; 25:218–27.

11. Popp J, Leucht S, Heres S, Steimer W. Serotonin transporter polymorphisms and side effects in antidepressant therapy – a pilot study. *Pharmacogenetics* 2006; 7:159–66.

12. Stahl SM. *Stahl's Essential Psychopharmacology: The Prescriber's Guide*, 5th edn. New York, NY: Cambridge University Press, 2014.
13. Tsai SJ, Gau YT, Hong CJ, et al. Sexually dimorphic effect of catechol-O-methyltransferase val158met polymorphism on clinical response to fluoxetine in major depressive patients. *J Affect Disord* 2009; 113:183–7.
14. Zhang J-P, Lencz T, Malhotra AK. Dopamine D2 receptor genetic variation and clinical response to antipsychotic drug treatment: a meta-analysis. *Am J Psychiatry* 2010; 167:763–72.
15. McGrath CL, Kelley ME, Holtzheimer PE, et al. Toward a neuroimaging treatment selection biomarker for major depressive disorder. *JAMA Psychiatry (Chicago)* 2013; 70(8): 821–9.

Posttest and CME credit (optional)

CME online posttest and certificate instructions

The estimated time for completion of this activity is 55.0 hours. There is a fee for the optional posttest, waived for NEI members.

1. Read the book in sequence, evaluating the content presented
2. Complete the posttest and activity evaluation, available only online at www.neiglobal.com/CME (under "Book")
3. Print your certificate (if a score of 70% or more is achieved)
4. Questions? Call 888-535-5600, or email CustomerService@NEIglobal.com

Index of drug names

Index of case studies